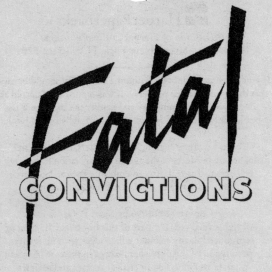

Fatal CONVICTIONS

A NOVEL BY

SHARI P. GELLER

ReganBooks

HarperPaperbacks
A Division of HarperCollinsPublishers

HarperPaperbacks
A Division of HarperCollins*Publishers*
10 East 53rd Street, New York, N.Y. 10022-5299

ISBN: 0-06-101223-8

A hardcover edition of this book was published in 1996
by Regan Books, an imprint of HarperCollins*Publishers*

Cover illustration © 1997 by Danilo Ducak

First HarperPaperbacks printing: January 1998

Printed in the United States of America

Visit HarperPaperbacks on the World Wide Web at
http://www.harpercollins.com

❖ 10 9 8 7 6 5 4 3 2 1

To the two brightest stars in the
galaxy of my life—
Joshua and Alexandra.
The book is for them—even if they
are years and years away
from being allowed to read it.

Acknowledgments

I have been given an extraordinary amount of support in writing this book and am grateful for the opportunity to be able to thank those who helped me along the way. First, my wonderful husband, Harvey. He has been my editor, my audience, and most importantly an unwavering cheerleader. Without his support and encouragement, I might still be saying, "Someday I'd like to write a novel." Next, my agent, Tina Bennett, who believed in this book from the first time we discussed it and never faltered in her efforts to guide it to a higher plane. She knew what could be done with the book, and did it. No writer could have a better champion in their corner. The terrific team at ReganBooks cannot be thanked enough, but I'll try. Judith Regan's clear and unwavering vision of what the book could be (and hopefully now is) was remarkable. Her instincts and insights were invaluable and her belief in the book was a constant source of inspiration. Judith's imprint can be found on every page and not just on the spine of the book. My editors, Jennifer Gates Hayes and Kristin Kiser, both deserve immeasurable recognition for all their efforts in putting this book together and keeping me relatively calm during the process. I also want to thank Elaine Brosnan, Shelly Peron, Nancy Peske, Todd Silverstein, and Sherri Weiss for doing their jobs so well. On a personal note, I owe an immeasurable debt of gratitude to my kids' surrogate grandmother, Mary Wittenberg, who entertained, babysat and, most importantly, loved my children and was always there for them. She will be missed. I also want to thank my mother-in-law, Gene Geller, who read two extremely unreadable early versions of the book and did not tell me to get a day job. And finally, I would like to thank Mark Wolf for making the catch of the year.

1

William Matheson resisted the lure of the air conditioner, deciding to stay on the balcony and nurse one last cigarette before having to deal with Kingsley. As blistering as it was outside, Matheson knew that it was going to be worse inside. At least for him. Even on the best of nights, two hours of contrived conversations, forced introspection, and feigned therapy were bad enough. But tonight, it was his turn on the hot seat.

"Hey, Bill, you got a smoke?"

"Huh?" he muttered in reply, oblivious to Larry's arrival, which was no mean feat given Larry's considerable size.

"A smoke? Can I bum one?"

"Yeah. Oh, sure," Matheson mumbled as he shook a cigarette from the pack.

Larry lit it and took a long drag, inhaling deeply before blowing the smoke out the corner of his mouth. "So where were you?" he asked finally.

"Just thinking about tonight," Matheson said with a hint of worry. He leaned back on the railing, watching the rest of the group slowly shuffle in.

"What do you care? You're almost a free man, you lucky bastard."

"Let's hope so," Matheson grumbled.

Larry perked up. "Why, did something happen?"

Matheson turned and flicked his ashes over the balcony. "You remember the meeting Kingsley set up with Ann and Laurie?"

"Yeah. What, it didn't go well?"

Matheson arched his eyebrows. "I suppose you could say that."

"Let me guess, they told you to fuck off?"

"Not exactly," said Matheson, grinning slightly.

Larry took the bait. "So what, then?"

Matheson paused to gaze off into the sunset, now afire in the lingering haze, and smiled broadly as he relived the moment. "I told them to fuck off."

"Oh, man, you didn't," Larry said with a schoolboy's snicker.

"I just lost it. I tried to be remorseful. I even practiced crying on cue. You know, I was ready to play along. But when I saw that little tramp and her butt-ugly mother, I just came unglued. I mean, that bitch practically hands me her daughter and says, 'Here, fuck her brains out,' and I'm the one who ends up almost going to jail? So I told them what I thought of them, and that it would be a cold day in hell before I'd apologize to them for the way they screwed me. Man, you should have seen their faces," Matheson crowed.

"Kingsley must have peed in her pants. Did she report you?"

"Not yet. She said she'd wait to see how tonight went."

Larry rested on the railing, which seemed to groan under the weight. "I'll bet she's gonna rake you over the coals."

"Look, there's no law against being an asshole, at least not last time I checked."

Larry snorted. "Lucky for you."

"Hey, screw you. Screw all of you. I've done my time. Five years showing up here and listening to their bullshit. Letting them try to 'rehabilitate' me," Matheson said sarcastically, "like I was some pervert. I didn't do anything wrong. She wanted it as much as I did."

"Well there's a line I've never heard before. Give me a break. She was, what, twelve?"

Matheson rolled his eyes. "Oh, please, save me the high-and-mighty crap. I'm a fucking saint compared to the rest of you. At least mine had pubic hair. You can't tell me Hillerman wouldn't have done the same thing in my shoes. They're just a bunch of hypocrites. I can't wait to blow this place for good."

"Well, you gotta admit, it sure beat going to jail."

"Not by much," Matheson said as he checked his watch. He looked back over at Larry and smiled. "Well, boys and girls, it's show time." Matheson took one last drag before twisting his cigarette into the ground. He turned and walked into the Oakwood Center with an oh-so-sincere look on his face and a well-timed apologetic bow of his head.

Inside, the air conditioner moaned noisily, straining to fend off the oppressive heat. Matheson took his usual seat and concentrated on maintaining his penitent posture, hoping that his performance would be up to its usual Oscar-winning caliber. When he saw Valerie Kingsley wearing an expression as dour as her severe navy business suit, he knew he'd have to be extra good tonight.

Matheson smiled at Kingsley, readying himself for tonight's challenge. She did not return the smile but walked briskly to her chair, clutching a manila folder tightly in her hands. She took her seat without her usual perfunctory greeting and opened the folder, taking roll as the room turned silent.

Matheson sat quietly, looking at Valerie and wondering why someone so attractive would work so hard to hide that fact. She tried all the little tricks, her long hair pulled back straight off her makeup-free face, oversized glasses working vainly to disguise crystal blue eyes, clothing selected for its ability to hide her slim figure. Little did she know she was fighting a losing battle. If she could have heard how the guys talked about her after group, it would have made her hair stand on end, he thought, amused.

"Bill, I'm really not sure where to begin," Valerie said finally as she snapped her file shut. "You sat here just last week and told us how you were looking forward to setting things straight with Ann and Laurie. You promised to finally take responsibility . . . to be accountable for your actions—for the pain that you caused. And then to go ahead and treat them like that?" Valerie's usual empathic demeanor gave way to a voice that was uncharacteristically hard, filled with anger and disgust. "How could you have done that?" Valerie stopped and stared straight at Matheson. He maintained the chagrined facade, looking apologetic and uncomfortable, yet saying nothing in answer to Valerie's pointed questions.

The awkward silence was broken by Frank LaPaca as he practically bounced out of his chair, waving his hand wildly, trying to get Valerie's attention. "Hello?" he sang out from Valerie's right. Frank was the resident busybody whose decidedly overly effeminate persona irritated his homophobic group members as much as his incessant interrupting irritated the therapist. Valerie looked over at him briefly and then looked back at Matheson, still waiting for his response. "Did I miss something?" Frank continued, ignoring Valerie's rebuff. "Was William a naughty boy?"

Valerie shot Frank an unamused glare. "Please, Frank. I want to hear from Bill right now." She turned

back to Matheson. "Why, Bill? Just help me understand how—after we all worked so hard with you, to
rehearse and prepare you for the session—how you
could have done that?" Matheson remained quiet,
confident that Frank would not and hoping the interruption would distract Valerie. He was not disappointed.

Frank leaned forward, unconcerned that it was not
his turn to speak. "What did he do, ask the girl to
blow him for old times' sake?"

Valerie's anger was sparked, but she kept her voice
level. She raised her hand to silence him. "Frank, I
think that's quite enough. Please let Bill speak."

"But, Valerie," Frank whined. "I think it would
really help the group if you tell us what happened."
He dropped into a low Joe Friday tone. "We need the
facts, ma'am, just the facts."

"Frank, in case you forgot, I lead the group here,"
Valerie snapped without looking his way, her eyes
fixed on Matheson.

Frank crossed his arms. "Jeez, have a hissy why
don't you? I just thought—"

Valerie spun around to face Frank. "You want to
know what happened? I'll tell you. It was a complete
and utter disaster. Bill walked in there and instead of
apologizing, he just sat there, letting them open up
their pain to him, and then when they were done he
literally laughed in their faces. He made a mockery
of the whole process. That's what happened."

Almost in unison the group members looked over
at Matheson. He took a deep breath, so that Valerie
would appreciate how hard this was for him, and
was about to begin his studied explanation. Instead,
Frank burst out laughing and slapped his legs excitedly. "I knew it. I just knew it. I told you all this
would happen, but who wants to listen to me? Didn't
I tell you that Bill's a class-A bullshitter? I know a big

ol' snowmobile when I see one," Frank said, smiling broadly.

Matheson's fellow group members couldn't believe that Frank was blowing such a great ass-kissing opportunity. They didn't come along very often, and the rest of the group certainly was not going to miss this one. "Bill, what were you thinking?" they chimed. "How could you have forgotten what we discussed?" "How could you let us down like that?" Each one in turn offering a heartfelt rebuke, infused with moral superiority.

As if any of you really gave a shit, Matheson thought. But that didn't stop him from shaking his head in mock disbelief at what he had done and muttering apologies brimming with feigned sincerity. He turned to his target, ignoring Frank and the rest of the group. "I don't know what got into me, Valerie. It's not like I enjoyed it." No more than winning the lottery, Matheson thought. "I really tried. I wanted the session to go well, for them, not for me." He fluttered his lashes, by now an instinctive move. Valerie seemed pleased by what she was hearing. She said nothing, just inclined her head slightly, encouraging Matheson to go on.

Matheson almost found this fun. On some strange level, he was going to miss yanking Kingsley's chain. She was so gullible, so full of love for her fellow man. She was just asking to be conned. How could he not oblige? He went in for the kill. "I just lost my head. I saw them there, accusing me, and I felt so"—he struggled for just the right word, then had to stifle a smile when he found it—"vulnerable. I just felt so vulnerable." He passed his fingers through his thick hair, the layers obediently falling back into place, and sighed deeply. "I'm so sorry that I let you all down," he continued as he looked around at his fellow group members, who sat in awed silence, mesmerized by the spectacle of such a sterling performance. Valerie nodded slowly, appearing to take in Matheson's words and trying to reconcile them with the rude utterances of last week. She sat silently, slowed down by his apparent contrition but not convinced of his sincerity.

Frank broke the silence. "Bravo, bravo," he shouted as he stood up, applauding. "That was wonderful. Best I've seen all year." His voice was choked with the same fake tears he dabbed from his eyes. "Now if you could've only done that last week, you wouldn't be in such hot water now," he taunted as he sat back down.

Any other time Matheson would have taken a shot at Frank, but Frank wasn't worth risking probation for. "I can't believe you, Frank. I mean, here I try to open up, to be honest about my feelings, and then you accuse me of . . . of acting. I'm hurt." Matheson put his hand up to his chest.

Frank leaned forward, pointing his finger at Matheson. "Listen, sweetheart, you've got nothing to be hurt about. Isn't that right, Valerie? Sounds like you're lucky they didn't carve you up like a pumpkin and stick a candle down your throat."

"Frank, I won't stand for you being so insensitive. I think Bill is really trying," Valerie scolded.

"Yeah, my patience."

"Frank!" Valerie's exasperation now focused on him.

"Fine, fine, do whatever you want." Frank waved his hand in the air, dismissively. "You're the boss. But if you ask me, I think you're letting him off way too easy."

"I'm not letting him off," Valerie protested. "I'm not going to defend what Bill did, but I think he knows he made a mistake and he seems genuinely upset about it. I'm happy to hear him express remorse for what he did. I think that's an important breakthrough for him. That's what's important here. Hopefully, we can all learn from this. Now, let's move on." Valerie looked around the room. "Does anyone have anything else to talk about?"

Matheson breathed a sigh of relief. He knew he had dodged a bullet. Kingsley was not about to report him now, and in one week he'd be done with his probation and the Oakwood. As soon as the session ended, he bolted out of his chair and headed to the door, elbowing Frank as he rushed by.

"Excuse me," Frank apologized with due sarcasm.

"Fuck you, butt boy," Matheson shot back. He stopped and poked his finger in Frank's chest, checking to make sure he was out of Kingsley's earshot. "And let me tell you something, you ever pull a stunt like that back there, and I'll—"

"You'll what? Are you threatening me? Oh, Valerie . . ."

"You just keep your fucking mouth shut or I'll make sure Hillerman gets what he needs to send your ass back to jail. I bet he'd like nothing more than to hear about your daily trips to the arcade. Just can't stay away from those young boys, eh, Frank?" Matheson turned and started walking away.

"Don't you threaten me," Frank shouted after him, but Matheson just kept on walking. "Two can play that game."

Matheson figured that he had just enough time to grab dinner and rush home to catch the last few innings of the seventh game of the World Series. He drove quickly down a relatively deserted Roscoe Boulevard, passing more strip malls and 99-cent stores than any city would want, let alone need, before finally arriving at the only true landmark in the San Fernando Valley—Tommy's Burgers. The drive-thru was quick tonight.

With the aroma of a double chili cheese filling his car, Matheson wound his way back to the dilapidated two-story apartment complex in North Hollywood he called home. His cramped one-room apartment looked to be decorated, if one could use that word, with the remnants of a failed garage sale. It pissed Matheson off that he had to live in a place where the only real piece of furniture he had, a soiled and foul-smelling green convertible sofa, doubled as his bed and his dining room table. His kitchen consisted of a small countertop burner and a refrigerator that, at best, could keep beer European warm. Dishes collected in a filthy, rusted sink that backed up more than it went down, and his bathroom had more leaks than a congressional committee. Still, it was cheap, and it was all that he could afford.

Matheson flipped on the game and plopped himself down on the sofa. It took him a minute to realize that the banging he heard was not the guy downstairs beating his wife again but was at his front door. He was startled and looked at the door. He wasn't expecting company. Someone had a lot of nerve to interrupt both the game and his dinner. "Who is it?" Matheson shouted with a mouthful of cheeseburger. He didn't hear a response. "Damn it, can't I just watch the goddamn game?" Matheson grumbled as he walked to the door.

"I said, who is it?" He looked through the peephole. Matheson saw only black just before the bullet punctured his eye. He fell back several feet, landing heavily on the worn brown carpet, now stained with his blood.

Two more shots helped open the door. "So nice of you to see me this late. You *can* still see me, can't you?" The killer bent down for a closer look. "Whoa, maybe not. That's some nasty hole you've got in your head. You ought to have someone take a look at that."

The killer stood up and walked over to the sofa, looking at the opened wrappers and half-eaten food. "Where's mine? That's no way to treat your company." The killer picked up the cheeseburger, examined it more closely, then threw it back down on the sofa. "On second thought, forget it. This stuff can kill you. Although, I guess you can afford to splurge tonight. It's not like you have to worry about your health anymore."

Matheson watched as the killer surveyed the apartment, his good eye straining to make out the figure. "You know, you really should get someone to come in and clean this dump. It's a disgrace. And your blood certainly isn't helping matters. No offense, Bill, but this place gives me the creeps. So forgive me for not staying too long. I hope you understand."

The banter didn't register with Matheson. While he heard the sounds, the burning in his head prevented them from becoming words. Matheson's anguished wail filled the room, his warm blood streaming off his face.

"I'm sorry, are you trying to say something? You should probably save your breath. I'm really not that interested in hearing anything you might have to say. You've said quite enough for one lifetime."

Matheson groaned indecipherably—feral, nonhuman sounds his only reply.

In a moment, Matheson felt a warm whispering voice in his ear. "You know, I'm sorry about having to do this. Really I am. It pains me greatly." The killer stood back up and laughed. "Although, maybe not as much as it's paining you." The killer thought for a moment, then spoke again, this time adopting a more melancholy tone. "Oh, who am I kidding? This doesn't pain me at all. It's just something that must be done—a job's a job, you know. So, why don't we see if we can get this over with quickly and still enjoy ourselves while we're at it? Okay?"

The killer circled Matheson, the gun fixed on him. "Now, I have three more bullets. Tell me, where should I shoot next?" When Matheson didn't respond, the killer's voice became more demanding. "Surely you must have some suggestions. Oh, c'mon, play along with me. Don't die without giving me some fun. How boring would that be?"

A low mewling sound emanated from somewhere deep within Matheson's shuddering body.

"What did you say? Speak up. The bullet's in your eye, not your mouth. You haven't lost your ability to talk, have you?" the killer asked with a voice filled with exaggerated shock. "I guess the bullet didn't penetrate as far as it should have. Why do you think that is? You know quite a lot about penetration, don't you?"

Matheson's breathing became more rapid, his panic spreading. He heaved himself up on all fours, instinctively trying to crawl away.

"Now where do you think you're going?" A shot blasted through his body, shattering Matheson's left leg. The killer blew the smoke that drifted out from the barrel of the gun. "Nice shot, cowboy."

Matheson collapsed into a fetal position, a feeble whimper his only response.

Another shot rang out, this time exploding Matheson's right knee. "Now you don't have a leg to stand on. Get it?" The killer laughed uncontrollably. "Oh, c'mon, lighten up. Don't worry, be happy."

Matheson lay motionless, each remaining breath growing more plaintive. His one good eye fixed on the shoes pacing back and forth in front of him. Waiting. He struggled to look up, to face his attacker. When he opened his bloody mouth in an attempt to speak, a faint, high-pitched cry was all that came out.

"Well, it's getting late, I guess I should be going. You may not have to get up tomorrow, but I do." Matheson saw one last flash of light just before the other side of his head disappeared into the floor. The killer stopped and looked back. "Please, don't get up. I'll let myself out."

2

Saul Glassman had long since retired and had little else to do with his time other than check on his rentals each day. With the crime in the neighborhood, he was accustomed to finding new graffiti in the morning, maybe a stripped car, or a jimmied lock. But Matheson was his first dead body. The sight of Matheson's faceless body caused Glassman to retch, bringing up his morning cup of coffee in a distasteful acid wash. His nausea followed him into the hallway as he sought to find a phone, the walls continuing to move ever so slightly out of his reach. By the time he called 911, he had regained enough of his composure to relay the relevant where and what of his emergency call.

Officers Sam Johnson and Ron Halloran arrived in under fifteen minutes and were met in front of the apartment building by a man waving his arms excitedly, as if a simple gesture would have been ignored.

"You must be the one who called the police?" asked Halloran. The shorter, pudgier of the two young officers, he had a hint of powdered sugar on the front of his rumpled uniform. His partner by contrast was an LAPD poster boy—fit, trim, and mustachioed, in his neat and stiffly pressed blues.

"Yeah. Saul Glassman." He held out his hand. "I'm really glad you're here." Halloran clasped Saul's clammy palm.

"Look at me, I'm soaked," Glassman said, wiping his hands on his shirt, next to the still damp coffee splatters. "I've never seen anything like this before. I mean, there's nothing left to him."

"Nothing left to who?" Officer Johnson asked as they walked down the hall.

"Well, I assume it's the guy who rents the apartment, but I didn't look too closely."

"What's his name?"

"Matheson, I—I don't remember his first name. He's been living here for about a year. Follow me," Glassman motioned. He led the officers up the front staircase. "It's the one at the end." Glassman pointed down the hall.

"Did he live alone?"

"Yeah, far as I know. He better have—he only paid for a single."

The officers walked down the quiet, musty hallway—courtesy of the rotting AstroTurf that passed for carpeting—and were struck by the near desolation of the apartment building. "Did you happen to notice anyone else around the apartment?" Halloran asked.

Saul shook his head. "No. I was just walking through the building, you know, checking it out, when I saw his door was open a little. When no one answered, I peeked inside. Just to make sure there was no problem. When I saw him on the floor, I just ran out of there and called you guys."

Officer Johnson took note of the blown-out doorknob. "Hey," he called to his partner, "whaddya think, forced entry?"

Halloran laughed. In the last hour of a ten-hour shift even marginal jokes seemed funny. "Maybe he forgot his keys and didn't want to pay for a locksmith."

With his club, Johnson carefully pushed open the door. The sight of a freshly rotting murder victim was never pleasant, but Johnson and Halloran were getting used to it. Glassman, however, was not so numb to society's ills. He stayed outside. He had seen enough.

"Would you look at this?" Halloran pointed to the ring of blood around where the peephole used to be. He bent down to examine Matheson more closely. "Oh man, he must have been shot while looking through the peephole!" Halloran winced at the thought.

"That must have been a surprise. 'Who is it?' Boom." Johnson shuddered slightly.

Johnson walked over to check out Matheson for himself. "Nice." Johnson noticed the blood smears on the carpet. "It looks like he was trying to crawl away. Not very far to get in this little dump, though. No offense, Saul," he said toward the door.

"None taken," Saul muttered as he retreated a few steps further down the hall.

Halloran looked around the cramped apartment. "Well, I doubt robbery was the motive. Not much to take. Although some guys'll kill you for a quarter these days. What's your guess?"

"Probably some personal dispute—family or business. Or maybe a drug deal gone bad, something like that." Johnson looked forward to the time when it would be his turn to solve the murders, not just to find the bodies. "Tell you one thing. He definitely pissed somebody off good."

"You got that right."

"Why don't you talk to Saul and see what he knows and I'll tape off the area and call Homicide."

"Hey, Saul," Halloran shouted out the door, "did you touch or move anything?"

"What, are you kidding me?" Saul poked his head around the corner and forced his eyes to stay fixed on Officer Halloran rather than looking at his former tenant. "When I looked inside and saw him, I just ran out."

"So what do you know about this guy?" asked Halloran as he walked up to Glassman.

"Not very much. I think he once told me that he was divorced. I don't really remember though. I know he's got a stepdaughter who he's not on real good terms with. I think he got in trouble for"—Saul looked around uncomfortably—"you know, shtupping her or something like that."

"Where'd you hear that?"

"I'm walking around here one day and I see this girl snooping around here. Pretty blonde, long legs. Real nice-looking. Anyway, she has her ear up to his door and I ask her what she's doing and she says she's his probation officer and was making a surprise home visit."

"And she told you about Matheson's background?"

"No, she wouldn't tell me anything. She left right after that. I told her I'd let her in, but she said no, she wanted to see him. Anyway, she didn't tell me what he was on probation for, so I asked him about it. I don't like criminals in my buildings. They always stiff me on the rent. When I asked him, he told me about it. Said it was no big thing, so they let him off with just probation. It didn't sound like anything I should worry about. And like I said, he always paid on time. He was no trouble."

"Did you ever see anyone else go into Matheson's apartment?" Halloran asked.

"How would I know who goes in and out?"

Glassman shrugged. "If a tenant pays his rent, I stay away."

"Does anybody live in the apartment next to Matheson's?"

"No, it's been vacant for six months. But you're welcome to talk to the other people in the building. Maybe they heard something. But don't count on it. You know, in this neighborhood, people keep pretty much to themselves. A moving van can back up to one of my apartments, clean out all the furniture, and nobody would see anything. You know how it is."

"Sure do," Halloran said. He took Saul's statement—scribbling what little Glassman knew into his notebook—and thanked him for his help, promising to contact him if he learned anything about the killing and asking Saul to do the same.

Halloran and Johnson left after briefing Homicide and headed back to the station to make their report. Not surprisingly, their sweep of the apartment complex produced no witnesses. Nobody heard or saw anything. Typical Valley homicide.

The local midafternoon newscasts initially ignored Matheson's murder. With so many killings in Los Angeles and its surrounding areas, another dead body just wasn't all that interesting. But when the police revealed Matheson's criminal record, an otherwise routine release of information, the TV news departments now found an angle that made the murder newsworthy. This was the second murder in less than two months of a convicted child molester. Although the police had officially classified the first as a failed car jacking—a man shot to death in the garage of his apartment building—they were never able to confirm their suspicions by finding a suspect.

Now, with a second murdered child molester turning up only a few miles from the first, it didn't take long for the media to circulate the idea that there might be a vigilante on the loose—a theory that the police had not yet embraced, but one that made the local news directors salivate.

By Tuesday night, Matheson's murder was all over the news. Handsome, professionally coiffed anchors were chirping about his killing, barely masking their appreciation for the juicy tidbit *de jour*. Channel 6 interspersed their evening fare with blaring promos about "second child molester found brutally murdered—details at eleven." Channel 10 promised their special extended coverage of this "late breaking" story, with the obligatory body bag visual accompanying the clip. Channel 3, already branding the murder a revenge killing, went so far as to set up a phone-in poll on whether vigilantes were saints or sinners, the Charles Bronson position prevailing handily with the callers.

Tom Baldwin, a deputy district attorney for the City of Los Angeles for longer than he'd care to remember, fifteen years next month, watched the TV accounts of Matheson's murder with a vague feeling that he'd heard of Matheson before, but he couldn't quite place the name. The next morning, as he read the *Los Angeles Times'* account of the murder, he remembered why Matheson's name had seemed familiar. Tom wondered if Rebecca had heard. He called, but there was no answer, so he showered and dressed without disturbing Claire. He left his house to fight the morning traffic, hoping that he would get to deliver the news.

Like so many of his co-workers, Tom was just putting in time as a prosecutor, hoping that a judicial appointment would be in the offing. If it weren't for the lure of the black robe, Tom might have gone the way of most D.A.s, leaving his low-paying job for a more lucrative, if less honorable, practice as a criminal defense attorney. But the D.A.'s office also offered the job security of civil service, and Tom liked knowing where his next paycheck was coming from, even if he also knew it wasn't getting any larger.

Tom arrived at the office at half past eight, dropped off his briefcase, and headed for the kitchen. Rebecca was standing by the coffeemaker, looking exhausted and careworn, trying for the caffeine jolt to get her through the day. By tonight, she would be sitting on the back deck of her sister's house in San Francisco, watching the thick fog slowly envelop the sparkling bay below, sipping a double mocha and listening to the new CDs she'd picked up for the trip. A few days off would do her good. She had just finished the Robertson case, a three-week trial involving a twice-convicted child molester who, two weeks after being released, raped a seven-year-old boy and cut off his penis because the boy had the audacity to cry the entire time that he was being raped. In all her years as a district attorney, the last eight of which she had spent prosecuting child molesters, Rebecca could not remember a more heinous crime or a more despicable criminal, and was both emotionally and physically drained from the trial.

Even before the Robertson case, Rebecca had grown to hate a job she had once loved so dearly. Having to listen to the endless stories of abuse, each more wrenching and pathetic than the one before, watching the endless parade of blank-eyed little survivors struggling to stay strong for their trip through the misnamed justice system, tore her apart. But she knew it was her calling. Someone had to be there for these children. In her mind, child molesters committed crimes far worse than murder. They killed not the body but the spirit of their victims. They betrayed the faith of the most trusting, and they stole innocence from the most guileless. As the courts looked the other way, the child molesters preyed upon the one sector of society least able to defend itself. They were consummate manipulators, always ready with an excuse, some bullshit rationalization. It was never their fault or their problem. "She wanted it; she enjoyed it; I thought I was helping her; it was only once; it was therapeutic; she was asleep; she was too young to remember." Rebecca had heard it all, and the weight of all this suffering was pulling her down with it. It had made her hard and cynical, and she didn't like the change.

"So, did you hear about William Matheson?" Tom asked. He leaned back casually on the counter, looking relaxed if monochromatic, from his wavy brown hair and brown wire-rimmed glasses, down to his brown wool Pierre Cardin suit and matching brown Nunn Bush.

Rebecca broke into a broad smile. "And they say there's no good news anymore. I almost broke a nail changing channels on my remote so fast. I don't know why all I found was a picture of the outside of his apartment building, though. Where was the body bag shot? I couldn't get enough of it, it was so . . . perfect." Rebecca laughed as her eyes narrowed to cool gray slits. "That makes two now. First Penhall, now Matheson. Things are really looking up, don't you think?" She lifted her coffee cup in a toast. "Here's to justice."

Tom now regretted wanting to be the messenger. While he knew Rebecca wouldn't exactly be grieving over Matheson's death, the intensity of her enjoyment still startled him. "Rebecca, I know how you feel about these guys, but you can't celebrate the killing of anyone, even a child molester."

"I can't?"

Tom sighed. He grabbed the coffee pot and poured himself a cup, taking two long sips. How swiftly and effortlessly Rebecca had put him on the defensive. She was good at that. "Listen, I don't want to be in the position of having to defend child molesters. This is all I'm going to say on the subject. There's a reason we have a criminal justice system." His voice sounded like a frustrated preschool teacher trying to convince a toddler that you don't hit someone back for hitting you. "Besides, child molestation isn't a capital offense."

Rebecca saw no reason to let Tom off easily. After all, *she* hadn't promised not to say anything more. "Well, it should be. Unfortunately, our male lawmakers don't share my view. Hey, if it were up to me, it would be one strike and you're gone, literally. These creeps should never get another chance to hurt a child." She shook her head, trying to release years of pent-up anger. It didn't help. She put her mug down on the linoleum counter. "Look, the guy got a slap on the wrist—probation, for God's sake! So excuse me if I think maybe someone handed him a more fitting punishment."

"I gather you won't be attending his wake?" Tom cracked.

"Hardly." Rebecca was not in the mood to laugh at herself.

Tom held back on any more retorts. He knew they would never have a rational, unemotional discussion on the topic. Yet he couldn't quite shake his frustration with her intransigent position. "You're something else."

"I'm something else?" Rebecca bristled. "Because I'm happy that Matheson's dead? I'm not going to pretend that I'm not happy about this because it looks unseemly to you."

He knew he should concede the point and move on, but he couldn't drop it. "I didn't say it was unseemly. I just think that you are a little too happy."

"Look," she said, exasperated. "Don't get me wrong. I just think that maybe the killings will focus the attention where it should be—on changing the law to mandate stiffer sentences. Sometimes drastic times call for drastic measures."

"Okay, okay," he said. "Truce. Look, I didn't mean to get you going." He decided to change the subject before they went any further down this well-worn path. "I heard you were out sick yesterday."

Rebecca nodded. "Migraine." She took a deep breath and held it, letting it out slowly, afraid that by saying the word she would somehow bring it back. Superstitions die hard. She was relieved to feel no pounding coming on. "I got lucky this time. It only lasted a day."

"So, you working on anything this morning? I could use some help on the Fleischer case."

Rebecca gave him an I-don't-think-so look. "Sorry, but I'm not really here today."

"You're not?"

"Nope. I just came in for a few minutes to check my messages, make sure there are no emergencies, and then I'm heading up to Elizabeth's for a few days."

"Well, good for you. From the sound of it, you could use some distance from this place. Have a good time. And be sure to say hi to Little Mary Sunshine for me," Tom said brightly, his sarcasm coming through the false smile as he walked out of the kitchen. He was not fond of Elizabeth and the feeling was more than mutual. Elizabeth blamed him for breaking Rebecca's heart and Tom blamed her for blaming him. So all Rebecca could do was roll her eyes at Tom's mild slur and say nothing, staking out her neutral position.

Rebecca went into her office, which was small and cluttered with files, books, and mounds of paperwork. As with most government offices, it consisted of a pale green metal desk and four overflowing beige file cabinets. At times, it more closely resembled an army recruiting center rather than a lawyer's domain. Rebecca had done little to decorate the place except to bring in a treasured picture of her and Elizabeth from her law school graduation and one ficus tree, which seemed to be in a perpetual state of autumn brown, with more leaves on the worn-out carpet than on the tree itself.

Rebecca opened the file cabinet behind her desk and pulled out Matheson's file. She hoped that with his death, maybe now the sting of one of her defeats would begin to dull. While she silently scanned the trial transcript—a transcript she could probably recite verbatim—her co-counsel in the Matheson case, Ralph Simpson, poked his head into her office. "Hey, Becky, did you hear about Matheson? Horrible."

Rebecca did not know what she hated more, Ralph or being called Becky. He always seemed to sympathize with the molesters, repeatedly telling Rebecca that she just did not understand the man's viewpoint. "What do you want?" Rebecca said, clearly irritated. So much for her plan on getting out of the office without running into Ralph.

He sauntered over to her desk, looking for goodies. "Boy, are we a little testy today?"

Rebecca quickly pulled the jar of M&M's away and put it in her desk drawer. He could buy his own candies, she wasn't about to treat him. "Ralph, get lost. I'm trying to get out of here."

"Well, show a little sympathy. The poor bastard

got killed in the middle of his Tommy's burger. How unfair is that?"

Rebecca eyed Ralph as she rested her chin on her hand. "How'd you know it was Tommy's?"

He stuck out his chest. "I have friends in high places."

"I'm shocked. I didn't even think you had friends in low places." Rebecca smiled broadly at her joke, then as quickly dropped the smile. "And, no, I don't feel sorry for him." She looked out her door, shaking her head. "I just had this discussion with Tom. What is it with you guys? Matheson was a despicable vermin who we're all well rid of. Look," Rebecca said, annoyed, "just leave me alone so I can get out of this place." She turned back to her desk.

"You know, Becky, you're much too young to be such a tired old bore." Ralph, satisfied at having the last word, turned and walked out leaving Rebecca to contemplate how true his words might be.

3

I see you made the paper," Jack Larson said as he walked past his partner waving this morning's *Times*. He sat down at his desk across from hers and donned his new reading glasses—a necessary but troubling reminder that the still boyishly handsome detective had just hit the big four-oh—and in his best Cronkite read: "Asked whether there is a connection between the Matheson murder and that of Eric Penhall, Detective Jennifer Randazzo stated, 'We have not yet reached any conclusions about a possible connection between the two killings. At this point in the investigation we are following all possible leads.'" The glasses came off, revealing soulful green eyes, and he pretended to pout. "You could have mentioned your partner, the senior detective on the case."

"I said 'we,' didn't I?" Randazzo stressed with due sincerity. She walked over and sat on the edge of his desk and bounced her low-heeled beige pumps under her partner's wounded face, excited, as usual, about the new murder investigation. Petite and cute, with large chocolate brown eyes and an expressive, upturned mouth, Jennifer Randazzo, formerly Josephina Maria Louisa Randazzo until she read *Love Story* and, as her only adolescent rebellion, decided to change her name, seemed in perpetual motion even when seated.

"And here I thought you'd snubbed me. My apologies. So how many copies did you send back to Mom and Pops?" Larson asked, tossing the paper on his desk.

"None yet, but I better soon. Dad wanted to show everyone back at his old precinct. He said that three generations of Randazzos walking the beat in Brooklyn never got their names in the paper, and here I do it in my first year as a detective."

"So Papa Randazzo is proud," he added, with a smile. "His little girl's done good."

"Yeah, I suppose," she mumbled, a little embarrassed. "Mom said to say hi," she added, quickly deflecting the compliment.

"And how is she?"

"Fine." It came out "foin," eight years on the left coast not completely obliterating her Brooklyn accent. "A little bursitis and my dad driving her crazy. She wishes he'd never retired. Now he's decided to take up cooking to help her out. She said he took eight pots to make one lasagna and guess who got to clean them all? Some help. Oh, and Mom wanted to know if you were seeing anyone nice." Randazzo smiled, her eyes crinkling around the edges.

"I guess she won't rest until I settle down with the next Mrs. Larson," he kidded. A two-time loser in marriage and a multitime loser in love, he wasn't so eager to try matrimony again.

"Don't feel bad. She doesn't leave me alone either." Randazzo switched into her mother's New York by-way-of-Naples accent. "'When you gonna give me a grandchild? You and Ben gonna make such beautiful children, when you gonna get working on it? You not getting any younger, sweetie.' I mean, what's gotten into her? My whole life I'm the baby of the family, now all of a sudden I'm ready to collect Social Security? Do you see any gray?" she asked, moving her hands through her shoulder-length coal black curls.

"Don't listen to her. You're still a baby. Look, you haven't even reached your full height," the six-foot-four Larson kidded his foot-shorter partner. "There's still time. I don't wanna lose you so soon."

"I'm not going anywhere."

"Good." He'd had as much luck with partners as he'd had with wives and wasn't about to lose the first partner he'd clicked with in years. "So what time are we heading out?"

"I need to return a few calls first."

Larson nodded and sat back to read his junk mail—two credit card applications and three magazine solicitations—before closing his eyes for a little nap. The soft morning hum slowly turned into a loud roar with the arrival of the rest of the A.M. crew. A few of the other detectives in the station stopped by Larson's desk to kid him about Randazzo's quote in the paper, asking him if he was going to take early retirement now that the torch had been passed. For the most part, he ignored the ribbing, his ego intact, but his nap interrupted.

Randazzo hung up from Toxicology and called over to him. "Well, no help there. Matheson was clean." She smiled, a proud, borderline smug smile. "You know, my dad said that's what we'd find. He didn't think this was about drugs." Her father had long since retired from the force, but he always told his daughter that his instincts were still as sharp as ever. Larson tended to agree.

"What else did Pops have to say?" he asked as he rolled his chair over to her.

"He thinks it's the ex. But then, he always suspects the spouse. He likes to say that murder's usually a family affair. Plus, living in New York, he's big on revenge killings. And Matheson's ex had plenty of reasons to want revenge."

"That's an understatement. The daughter too. She's old enough now—she could've done it."

Randazzo nodded, wondering if she should voice her theory. She checked herself—when did she suddenly become shy about speaking up? "You know, I'm not so sure we're looking at the usual case here. I mean, it sure is strange that another two eighty-eight was killed so recently."

"So? A lot of guys who've got records get killed." Larson rolled back to his desk.

"Yeah, but this seems different. And the reporters sure think the two cases are related. They're really playing up the connection."

"Now, Jennifer," he began paternally, "you can't let a bunch of news reporters direct the investigation for you. You're the detective, you don't have the luxury of jumping to conclusions, they do. Now there may be a connection there, but you let the investigation lead you to the answer. Don't let yourself get sidetracked by amateur speculation."

"Yes, sir," she said, bowing her head. After a moment, Randazzo's face grew serious. "But, what if it's true? What if someone is out there targeting child molesters?"

"Well, just my guess, you and I wouldn't win any medals apprehending someone who kills perverts. I'm not even sure why we'd want to."

"What are you saying?" She lifted her eyebrows in disbelief.

"Oh, c'mon. Think about it. Why should we bust

our butts to find someone who kills child molesters? Seems like the killer would be doing us all a favor." Larson wadded up a piece of paper and lobbed it toward the trash can next to Randazzo's desk, a mindless pastime he had picked up in his early days on the force.

"You're kidding, right? In case you forgot, we get paid to catch killers. It's in the job description, remember? Pretty well near the top, in fact."

Larson tried a hook shot that bounced on the rim then fell out, proving once again that height did not always equate with athletic ability. "Maybe so. But it seems to me that it'll strike a lot of people that these guys are simply getting their just deserts."

Randazzo crossed her arms defiantly. "Is that how it strikes you?" she asked.

"Well, how does it strike you?"

She did not respond.

"Come on, you've got to admit, on some level it makes sense. If it saves some kid from being molested, isn't it worth it?" he prodded. Randazzo continued to look unfazed. "Okay, what if some creep molested your kid? Wouldn't you be happy if somebody killed him?" This time, Jack thought he saw a reaction.

"That's an unfair question and you know it."

"See? It's not that easy when the shoe's on the other foot, is it, Miss Smarty Pants?" Larson flashed his signature smile that even his partner couldn't resist. "So now tell me, is killing a child molester a good thing or a bad thing?"

Too stubborn to give in, Randazzo decided to drop the subject with no points to either side. "We'll talk about this later. Right now I've got to go over to the lab. I'll meet you back here in half an hour. We've got a lot of work to do."

Larson settled back into his chair as he lobbed

another shot her way. "Well, wake me up when you get back."

Randazzo grabbed the high arching shot in midair. "Nah-uh. Why don't you try doing something useful."

"Like what?"

"Like talking to the D.A. who prosecuted Matheson. She wasn't in when I called."

"Boy, you sure give me all the fun jobs. I hate talking to attorneys," he said, unavoidably reminded of his two divorces. "Who is it, anyhow?"

She flipped through her notes. "Uh . . . Rebecca Fielding."

"Really!" He sounded just a little too excited.

"Let me guess, you know her?" she asked warily, fully expecting to hear another chapter of Larson's greatest sexual conquests.

"Yeah, she used to date a good friend of mine. A definite nine. You know, she would have gotten a ten, but she's a lawyer, so there's an automatic deduction. But, she was drop-dead gorgeous, golden hair, long legs. . . ." Larson's mind was momentarily diverted until he remembered he was supposed to be talking about work. "Sure, give me the number, I'll call her."

Randazzo put her hands on her hips. "You are such a pig."

"Is that pig as in cop or pig as in chauvinist?"

"The latter. And I suppose that the best way to find out what she knows is over dinner, right?" Randazzo teased.

"No, breakfast would be okay too, if she lets me wake her."

She shook her head, her dark curls bobbing around her oval face. "Why do I even talk to you? See what you can do about charming her into an interview today. Okay, lover boy?" Randazzo turned and left, knowing the phone call was in good hands. What Larson lacked in drive, he more than made up for in his ability to charm women.

Larson looked down at Rebecca's name on the slip of paper Randazzo had given him and wondered whether the statute of limitations had run out on her relationship with Tom. Under normal circumstances, Larson knew he'd never get Tom's blessing to ask her out, but now he had a perfectly acceptable excuse for meeting with her. He grabbed the phone and punched up the D.A.'s office, only to learn from the receptionist that Rebecca was on vacation. Jack didn't want to end up on the bottom of a stack of unreturned message slips. "Well, then, why don't you give me her secretary?" he said.

After a couple minutes, Rebecca's secretary answered the phone curtly. "This is Joan." Apparently the receptionist had clued her in to his persistence.

Larson figured he might need his best sugary sweet voice for this one. "Hello, my name is Jack Larson. I'm a detective from East Valley Homicide. I'm trying to reach Ms. Fielding, but I was told she's on vacation."

"That's correct. Until Monday. Would you like to leave her a message?"

"Well, I really wanted to talk to her today about a murder I'm investigating. The Matheson murder." How could she not help now, he wondered. It was on TV for heaven's sake.

"She'll be back in the office Monday. If you leave your number, I'll have her call you when she returns," Joan said deliberately, like a teacher repeating an instruction to her slower students.

"I'd prefer not waiting until Monday. Can't you just tell me where to reach her?"

His insistence was starting to irritate her, but Joan stood her ground. "Is there some urgency, Detective?

She's just gotten over a difficult trial and she needs a few days off."

Larson hated loyal secretaries, so he did what any self-respecting man would do—he gave up. "I'll tell you what, why don't you leave a message that I called—555-0804—and then just transfer me to Tom Baldwin?" Joan was only too happy to oblige.

Larson whistled softly out of tune as he sat on hold, thinking. It seemed wrong, somehow, using Tom to get to Rebecca. But then what were friends for? Besides, Randazzo would kick his butt if he didn't accomplish something before she got back. And he remembered just as Tom picked up that there was the matter of a small bet to settle as well.

"Tom Baldwin."

"Tommy, my boy. Wasn't that a great game? Who woulda believed the Mariners could've pulled it out? If Griffey's not a Hall of Famer, I don't know who is," Jack gloated.

"You schmuck." Tom laughed. "If Justice hadn't whiffed four times, it wouldn't have been a contest."

"Since when do lawyers put their faith in justice?"

"Wait, is that a joke? You've got to warn me before you come up with zingers like that." Tom enjoyed the repartee. He certainly didn't get much levity at home. "Listen, did you call for a reason or just to harass me? You'll get your money . . . eventually. By the way, did you know that gambling is illegal in this town?"

"You know, I was thinking. Why let a little thing like money get in the way of a wonderful friendship? I'd be happy to forget the whole thing if you just do me one small favor."

Tom shifted the receiver from one ear to the other, using the split second to think. He had never known Jack to let him out of a bet yet and was quite suspicious. "Forget it. Whatever it is, forget it. I've long since retired from the favor business. I'll messenger you the money."

"Oh, come on. I'm working on the Matheson case and I'd just like to chat with Rebecca Fielding. She prosecuted Matheson, right? I need to talk to her, but she's not in the office and not at home and her secretary's guarding her whereabouts like it's a state secret. Do you know where she is?"

"Yes, but she's on vacation for the rest of the week. You know, rest and relaxation. Can't it wait?"

"Not you too. What are you, her mother? You're as bad as her secretary. C'mon, it won't take long, I just have a few questions for her."

Tom sighed. It was a pretty easy way to get out of the bet, and a hundred bucks is a hundred bucks, after all. "Listen, if I tell you where she is, you forget where you got the number from. You understand?"

"I understand."

"She's at her sister's house."

Larson paused. "I think I'm going to need a little more than that."

Tom reluctantly gave him the number, hoping that Rebecca wouldn't ask where he got it. Larson saw the 415 area code—the Bay area. Nice choice for a vacation, he thought approvingly. Too bad he couldn't convince the brass to send him up there to interview her personally. He thanked Tom and hung up, then dialed the number only to reach a recording. As he started to leave a message for her, Rebecca thought about ignoring the call and honoring her vacation, but her curiosity got the best of her. She reached across the bed and grabbed the phone off the nightstand.

"Hello, I'm here."

"Ms. Fielding, thank you for picking up the phone. I'm sorry about calling you on your vacation. My name is Jack Larson and I'm investigating the

Matheson murder. I was hoping I could talk to you about the case." It felt odd being so formal, but Jack was unsure how to approach his best friend's ex, even though he had wanted to for years.

With a rueful smile she pushed aside the paper she'd been lazily reading. Even when she tried to leave work behind, it followed her, intruding right in the middle of Herb Caen. "I'm not sure what help I can be, Detective," she said.

"Well maybe none or maybe a lot. Do you have a few minutes to talk?"

She leaned back on one of the pillows, getting comfortable. "Sure, shoot. Oh, I guess I'm probably not supposed to say that," Rebecca said with a laugh.

"That's okay. Unless it was a Freudian slip."

"Am I a suspect, Detective?" Rebecca asked in mock seriousness.

"No, I was just kidding." Larson could have kicked himself. Less than a minute into the conversation and already he was sounding like an idiot.

"No apologies necessary. So, what can I help you with?"

"Well, I suppose the best place to start might be with Matheson's case. I don't know much about his history."

She sat up on the bed. "Have you talked to Ann and Laurie?"

"Not yet," Larson responded. "My partner's setting that up."

Rebecca held the portable in her hand, got up, and walked from her guest room into the family room. "I suppose in some ways it was a rather routine case." One that made me vomit after agreeing to the plea bargain, Rebecca thought to herself. "Matheson was twenty-eight when he started forcing Laurie to have sex with him. I think, if I remember correctly, she was twelve. Her mother was older than Matheson, midthirties, and not half as attractive as Laurie. It went on for two years before Laurie had the courage to tell a friend what was going on. Matheson was arrested after the friend told her mother what she had learned."

"What happened after he was arrested?"

"Well, to begin with, it wasn't at all certain that charges would even be brought against him," Rebecca said with disgust.

"Huh?"

"I don't know how much you know about incest cases . . ."

"Not much," Jack offered.

"Well, it's hard to get these cases filed and then even if you get that far, very few actually go to trial. Most are plea-bargained."

"Why is that?"

Rebecca looked down at her hand, tightly gripping the railing separating the family room from the breakfast nook, released her grip and started pacing. "Sometimes there's little physical evidence, sometimes the victims are too young to testify or too reluctant, and sometimes the mothers don't want their children to testify. In Matheson's case, we had a little bit of all of those. Although the biggest problem was Ann's—the mother's—reluctance," Rebecca said, trying to sound unaffected. "She was the one who bailed him out, if you can believe it. She didn't want him prosecuted at all."

"You're kidding?"

"Nope. In the beginning, she didn't believe Laurie. Even though all the signs were there—she and her husband hadn't had sex in over a year; he was showing an inordinate amount of interest in Laurie, taking her shopping, running her baths, combing her hair. Ann just ignored it. So when it came out what had been going on, she went straight into denial. Laurie had absolutely no support from her mother." A deep sigh betrayed her attempts to appear detached from the story.

Jack noticed the sadness in her voice. "That must have been difficult," he said softly.

Rebecca closed her eyes and felt the pang of just how difficult it was. "Well, I had hoped in time Ann would come around, but it never happened. Even after she heard the evidence we had, she still wouldn't believe Laurie. You know, it's hard enough trying to convince the victim to testify in incest cases without having to deal with mothers who can't see where their allegiances should be."

"The mother actually came out and took Matheson's side?" Larson asked, stunned by the idea.

"I've seen it many times before. The father is the breadwinner, after all, and the mothers don't want their world turned upside down. Having him thrown in jail can financially devastate a family. The mothers also don't want to deal with knowing that their husband preferred the daughter to them. There's this insane jealousy, as if they were competing with a sorority sister. Laurie's mother fell into the same trap—if you blame the daughter, both you and your husband come out unscathed. Without Ann's support, Laurie didn't want any part of a trial."

"What did you do?"

"I tried to act as a surrogate mother, telling her how I believed her, how I wanted to help her. I tried to explain how confused her mother was. She trusted me and agreed to go to court."

Jack paused to jot down a few notes. "So what happened?"

Rebecca stopped, realizing that her nervous pacing during this conversation was wearing down Elizabeth's new carpet. She sat down at the counter in the kitchen, took a sip of lukewarm tea, and plunged into the hardest part of the story. "I started to put on my case. I put the friend on the stand and then those who had investigated the charges. I probably screwed up. I should have put Laurie on first, when she still had her nerve. But sitting in court, looking at Matheson, she started losing it. He kept leering over at us, smirking at us, taunting us. He was intimidating her. When I tried to bring it to the court's attention, the judge said if he saw anything, he would put a stop to it, but men never see these things." Rebecca winced as she heard her blanket anti-men stereotyping. "Sorry, that didn't come out right."

"That's okay. No offense taken."

"Anyway," she continued, "when it was Laurie's turn to testify, she just panicked. I had worked with her for weeks, I thought she was going to be able to handle it. But instead, when I called her name, she grabbed my wrist and practically pulled me back down. She started crying, I could barely understand what she was saying, but the message was clear. 'Don't make me go up there.' I asked for a recess and tried to calm her down, but she was hysterical. Matheson's public defender came over to me as we were leaving the courtroom." She dropped her voice slightly to mimic the lawyer. "'I can see you have a bit of a problem,' he said. 'Maybe a good time to talk about a deal.' He'd been trying to get me to agree to a plea all along, but I wanted the guy to do time. He didn't deserve to walk."

"But now he had the advantage?" Larson asked.

"Yep. He had me over the barrel. So we agreed to a plea of guilty on only one charge of lewd and lascivious, with a recommendation of straight probation. I figured this way at least he'd still have a record and he'd have to register as a sex offender wherever he moved." Rebecca sighed deeply, and a long pause followed. "But it really wasn't enough, you know."

"You did what you had to do," Larson offered.

"I know I didn't really have much choice. But you should have seen the guy's face. He could barely control himself. He had repeatedly raped a twelve-year-old girl in her home and now he was going to rape us in court. He shot me one of the most smug, self-satisfied looks I'd ever seen. I've never seen eyes like that. That man was evil." Rebecca closed her eyes and Matheson's face came quickly in focus, bringing with it the memory of the moment, every thought, every sensation she felt then as clear as if it were happening again. Anger, hurt, frustration, and powerlessness overwhelmed her.

"Well, you'll be happy to know that the last time I saw his face, it didn't look too smug."

Larson's words helped bring Rebecca back to the present. She opened her eyes and nodded appreciatively. "That's the way it should be," Rebecca said, "but it's still little consolation for what he put us through. He may be dead, but he still got to live almost five years thinking he'd really pulled a fast one on us. He should have been rotting in jail the whole time instead of free and happy that he'd outfoxed us and pretty much gotten away with murder himself."

Jack registered her continued use of the word *us*. Perhaps she was overidentifying with the victims? But don't we all break the world down into us and them, he thought to himself. He quickly wrote down a few of Rebecca's key phrases on his notes. "Do you think Ann or Laurie were capable of killing him? From what you know about them," he asked.

"Oh, no. I'm sure they couldn't have killed him," she said quickly. "Laurie was more hurt than angry, Ann more confused than anything else. But I haven't kept in contact with the family. It's been almost five years." She paused and thought about his question some more. "No, I'm sure that they didn't do it. Anyway, if they wanted revenge, why wait so long?"

"Good question. While you were preparing for trial, did you turn up anything on Matheson that might help us in this investigation? Any prior victims, for example, or anyone else that would like to see him dead? Any dirt, so to speak?"

Rebecca hesitated, running the file through in her head. "No, sorry. The last person he had lived with before he married was in her early twenties, no children. She dumped him when she found someone with a better job. His ex-employer reported he was a fair worker, no hassles on the job, no drinking or fighting. Just not very hardworking."

Larson sat back, watching as two detectives dragged an unwilling suspect into one of the conference rooms for a little chat—an overly endowed prostitute he recognized as a regular around the station. He always marveled at her luck in having a butt large enough to give her counterbalance, but now he found her vast physical attributes distracting. He thought about any other questions he had for Rebecca, hoping for something that would help focus him in the right direction, but all he could think of was why anyone would pay for a piece of that.

"Well, I probably shouldn't keep you any longer. Especially since you're on vacation. How is it up there, anyway?"

Rebecca had forgotten where she was, being so caught up in replaying the Matheson trial. She took the phone through the French doors in the brightly lit family room and out to the panoramic balcony, looking out at the tranquil waters surrounded by crescent hills, the city a medley of blues and greens with a majestic orange bridge hanging above it all. Her voice softened along with her mood. "Just gorgeous, as always. I swear, even when the weather is bad—which is just about every time I manage to make it up here—San Francisco is always beautiful."

"You're lucky. The Santa Anas are blowing strong. Kinda feels like the proverbial blast furnace in Hades down here." Larson couldn't think of anything else to talk to her about, although he was enjoying the conversation. Then he remembered Randazzo's concern that Matheson's murder might not be an isolated one. "Oh, I almost forgot. You didn't also happen to prosecute . . . oh, what's his first name . . . Eric, Eric Penhall?"

"Yes, I did. It was a few years back. Oral 'cop' on a minor, his seven-year-old daughter. Another prince," she said, her voice hardened and sarcastic. She took a couple steps back into the family room and sat down on the couch. "I'd heard he was killed recently too, but nobody ever talked to me about him. Why are you asking? Do you think there's some connection between the cases?"

Larson hedged his answer. "It's something we're exploring. Two murder victims who both happen to be convicted child molesters. Seems more than a coincidence, don't you think?"

"I try not to think at all when I'm on vacation. It only gets me into trouble."

"Well, let me get you off the phone, then. Again, thanks for your time. If you think of anything that might be helpful, please give me a call."

"I will."

Rebecca put the phone down and walked back out to lean on the railing. She stared out at the glistening sapphire water and the flotilla of tourist-filled bay cruisers. Nearby, sailboats displayed their bright colors like peacocks in search of a mate. Rebecca imagined vacationing families huddled together against the brisk sea breeze and felt a little lonely. Elizabeth was her only family, and while there was a deep bond between them, they were never as close as she wanted to be. Aside from Elizabeth, Rebecca had no one else in her life, having done too good a job of keeping most everyone else at arm's length. She went back inside and grabbed some files she had brought with her and did what she always did to maintain a safe distance from everyone and everything—bury herself in work.

"You ready to go?" Randazzo asked Larson.

"Sure am."

"Did you talk to the D.A.?"

"Sure did. Got some background from her." He stared down at his notes, a confusing mess of seemingly random words and phrases taken from the conversation. He tossed the useless notes aside. "How 'bout if I just explain it to you?"

"Great. You can update me on the way. I'll drive."

In their government-issue, I'm-an-unmarked-police-car dark brown Cutlass, complete with the obligatory DARE bumper sticker, Larson recalled his conversation for Randazzo. "Fielding remembered the case quite clearly. The daughter, Laurie, she freaked at the thought of testifying and Fielding had to scramble to get something to stick. She had Matheson plead to one charge, a two eighty-eight, in exchange for not seeking any jail time. She thought Matheson was pretty smug about the whole thing, and that seemed to rattle her. She didn't paint a picture of an angry, vindictive victim or family. They seemed pretty pathetic, actually."

"How so?"

"Ann, the mother, had sided with Matheson, hadn't come to Laurie's defense. At trial, Laurie didn't have it in her to go forward and testify against him. It was sad."

"Did Fielding think Matheson had threatened Laurie?"

"She didn't say. She seemed to think it was more intimidation than explicit threats. He would glare at Laurie in court, that sort of thing. She never mentioned any physical threats, though."

Randazzo looked at Larson as they sat at a red light. She noticed he was uncustomarily quiet, almost pensive, a trait she ordinarily wouldn't associate with him.

"You look puzzled."

"No, not really. It was just odd. Fielding seemed to take it kinda personally. I just wonder how she can keep her sanity if she let all of her cases affect her like that."

4

Ann Jenkins, the former Mrs. Matheson, wasn't surprised when the call came from the police. She was, after all, the angry and bitter ex-wife, and her daughter the wounded victim—both ample fodder for vengeance theorists everywhere. She assumed they'd be questioned, especially after their recent encounter with Matheson. She had tried to talk to Laurie about what lay ahead, more dredging up of the painful past and more reminders of scenes better left buried along with Matheson, but Laurie understandably had trouble listening to her mother when it came to Matheson.

Ann greeted Larson and Randazzo at the door with an uneasy smile. Her drab pageboy, the puffy, sallow face, and dull gray, heavily lidded eyes revealed a woman well beyond her best years, who stood in stark contrast to her captivating daughter. Laurie must get it from Dad's side of the family, Larson mused. She had a heart-shaped freckled face with sparkling hazel eyes and loose golden curls that tumbled down her back. But Larson noticed a certain somberness, unusual for a teenage girl.

Ann looked about nervously, unsure of the protocol for such a visit. After leading the detectives into
the living room, she offered them coffee, needing to
do something to calm herself. She retreated briefly
into the kitchen as the detectives struggled to make
themselves comfortable on the overstuffed sofa. She
returned with a large tray, as if she were serving tea
for the ladies' club. Larson took the requisite appreciative first sip, then began. "I can imagine this is
very difficult for you to talk about, Ms. Jenkins.
Thank you for agreeing to see us so quickly."

"I'm still pretty much in shock . . . I'm not really
sure what to say."

"Well, let me ask you a few questions," said
Larson. "Maybe we can start with the last time you
saw Mr. Matheson?"

"Okay," she began, a deep breath providing the
needed emotional kick start. "It was about a week
ago at the center where he was in treatment. We,
Laurie and I, were invited there by his therapist,
Valerie . . . Kingsley, I think that's her name, for a
joint session with Bill. The way she explained it, Bill
was supposed to tell us what he had learned in therapy and offer an apology. She thought it might be a
good healing experience for Laurie and me."

"Mom, I think it was meant more for my benefit,"
Laurie said coolly.

"Yes, of course, that's what I meant." Ann stopped
to catch her breath. She took a long sip of coffee and
looked out the living room window at the small garden, her uneasiness with the past plain for all to see.

"So you agreed to go to the center?" asked
Randazzo quickly, trying to avoid the tension that
now filled the room.

"Well, not right away. I'm not that dumb, Detectives." Ann laughed nervously, her self-consciousness
painfully clear. "Laurie and I talked about it. I called

everyone. Laurie's old therapist, Bill's probation officer, the district attorney, just to help make the decision. I really was at a loss. I didn't know what to do."

"What did they say?" Randazzo asked.

"Well, I realize now that Laurie's therapist was trying to advise us against it, but it's not her style to just come out and say, 'No, don't do it.' She just laid out the options and had us discuss our feelings. I wish she'd just said it was a stupid idea," Ann said with a hint of resentment. "I thought I was doing the right thing." Her voice faltered and she looked lost.

"After what you went through, Ms. Jenkins, I'm not sure I could ever go to a meeting like that," Larson interjected, immediately aware by seeing her reaction that he had apparently just said the wrong thing.

"Well, Detective, be glad that you never had to face a decision like that," Ann said defensively. In her mind, she was being blamed for everything that Bill ever did, from the molestation to his arrogant insolence at the last meeting, and she was tired of it.

Laurie knew well her mother's touchiness on the subject—much deserved, she thought—and she wanted to avoid the unnecessary distraction of her mother's hurt feelings. "Look," she said quickly, "for whatever reason, we trusted Ms. Kingsley. She laid it on so thick about how great the clinic was, what wonderful work it did, what great results they were having with the men who went there. She told us that my step . . . that he was eager to 'set things right'—those were her exact words—and that he was ready to apologize. She made him sound like a whole different person. I thought if we went, he'd drop to his knees and beg me for forgiveness. And I wanted to see him do that, just once. I guess I should have listened to Ms. Fielding instead. She told us she thought it would be a mistake to trust him. She said, 'Once a manipulator, always a manipulator.'"

"That's the second time we didn't follow her advice, and both times she turned out to be right," Ann added, staring into her coffee cup. She took a sip and looked back up at the detectives. "You know, I called her after the meeting and told her what had happened. I expected her to say 'I told you so.' I guess I figured I deserved it. But she was really nice about it. She just said how sorry she was that we had to go through that again. She told me it was Bill and Ms. Kingsley who both should be ashamed of themselves, not me."

"You mentioned before that was the second time you didn't follow her advice. When was the first?" asked Randazzo.

"At the trial. She really wanted to see Bill punished, so did we, of course, but we just didn't have the strength to prosecute." Larson took note of Ann's use of the word *we*. Apparently revisionist history had Ann at Laurie's side during the trial. "I know she was greatly disappointed in us, that we didn't go all the way with the case. But it was taking too much of a toll on Laurie. She just wasn't up for a battle."

"I was too weak back then," Laurie interrupted. "I was afraid of him, afraid of how I would look to a jury. I thought they'd blame me for everything. If I'd told what happened and they hadn't believed me, well. . . . I knew Ms. Fielding believed in me, she really wanted me to testify against him and put him away. But I was too embarrassed to get up there in front of all those people and tell them what I did, I mean, what he did to me. Ms. Fielding promised to take care of me, promised to make it as comfortable as possible, but I guess I didn't really believe she could protect me. Nobody had before," she said softly. Randazzo noticed Ann visibly wince at Laurie's comment and felt a little uncomfortable witnessing this private moment.

Larson missed it, distracted by what Laurie had said. "So you both spoke with Ms. Fielding recently? About Matheson?" he asked, surprised that Rebecca hadn't mentioned this to him.

"Yes, as I said, we talked, I'd say, a week or so before the meeting," Ann replied, nodding in Laurie's direction for confirmation.

"So what specifically happened at the session?" Larson asked.

Ann took another deep breath. "We went into the session and instead of apologizing the— the— I know he's dead, but . . ." Her voice filled with rage. "The bastard! He turned the whole thing around, said he'd been pressured into the session, that he had no intention of apologizing, that in three weeks we could all kiss his ass. I was stunned, I couldn't speak. It was just horrible."

"I'm sorry we have to talk about this, I can see how upsetting it is for you," said Randazzo. Larson was glad to have Randazzo as a partner. At times like this he was usually at a loss for comforting words.

"I was so angry. Ms. Kingsley realized the session was a disaster. She tried to talk us into coming back to 'work on our feelings.'" Contempt replaced Ann's anger now. "Can you believe the nerve? She begged me not to make a big deal about this, but you know, I've already talked to an attorney. She thinks I could sue the center for what they put us through."

"Laurie, can you add anything to what your mother described about the last session with Mr. Matheson?" Larson asked.

Laurie stared off, her eyes sad and distant. "You know, what made it all worse was how Ms. Kingsley had built my hopes up. She told us how sorry he was. I really wanted to believe her because the last time I heard anything from him he was still saying it was all my fault. I know that's what she thought, too," Laurie added, looking over at her mother. There was no sound in the room until Laurie suddenly burst into tears, her shoulders heaving with the force of each sob.

Ann sat staring at Laurie, embarrassed and immobile. Larson did not handle displays of emotion well, especially ones that went uncomforted. He tried not to look at the women and instead studied the cover of an old magazine on their coffee table a bit too intently. It was Randazzo who tried to console her. She reached over to touch Laurie gently on the shoulder. "That's silly. Of course it wasn't your fault."

"It's not silly," Laurie cried. "It's something I live with every second of every day. That something *I* did made him do it. How can you not blame yourself when your own mother doesn't believe you? I was so scared and so embarrassed and I didn't know what to do to make him stop." Her words came rushing together, her voice choked by sobs. She dropped her head and closed her eyes and she was alone, speaking to no one, and everyone, wanting finally to rid herself of the pain. "It's like a virus that I can't get out of my head. I still get that sick feeling in my stomach every night before I fall asleep, sometimes so bad my whole body shakes. Even when I wake up I can't stop feeling that fear. I can't make it go away." Laurie buried her head in her hands.

Her daughter's accusation rang in Ann's head and she felt the cold, reproachful stare of the detectives and quickly issued a protective denial. "I wish I had known what was going on."

Laurie snapped around to look at her mother, the pain contorting her face. "How could you not know what was going on, when he snuck out of your room night after night and then moments later you'd hear me crying. What the hell did you think was going on?"

Ann seemed to fold up on herself and looked away, her face pulled down by the weight of Laurie's words. Larson and Randazzo realized they had walked into more than they had expected. Randazzo reached for Laurie's hand and held it gently. "I'm so sorry. I didn't mean to minimize your pain."

"It's okay. I know." Laurie angrily brushed the tears off her cheeks. "Dammit, I'm not going to cry about this anymore. Crying's not going to change anything that happened. I just have to move on. It probably sounds weird, but now that he's dead, I feel like I can really do that now—get on with my life."

It didn't sound that strange to Randazzo. Yet she couldn't help wondering whether either of these women had a role in his death. No one spoke for an excruciatingly long time until Randazzo turned to Ann and asked the inevitable question. "Ms. Jenkins, where were you on Monday night?"

"I was at home," Ann replied.

"By yourself?"

"Why . . . yes, Detective. I was home, by myself, reading. I don't have an alibi, if that's what you're asking. I'm not sure I need one. Did I hate Bill? You bet. But I didn't kill him."

She sounded convincing, even to Larson who'd heard more than his share of false alibis. No attempt to take herself out of consideration as a suspect, just a simple direct denial.

"Laurie, on Monday night . . . ?" Randazzo began.

"Monday? I was at a friend's house. We were watching the game. If you want, you can talk with some of my friends."

"Laurie, if you would make us a list, with their

numbers, that would be a great help." Randazzo tried to sound friendly, but it was hard when she knew that Laurie realized she and her mother were suspects.

As Larson and Randazzo returned to their car, they looked at each other in disbelief at the strained scene they had just witnessed. "I can't believe Laurie still has anything to do with her mother. Can you believe Ann stood by that creep after what he did to her daughter?" Randazzo stood by the trunk, emotionally drained and still in shock over what she'd observed.

"Not really, but then I don't have a great track record for figuring out women," Larson said as he instinctively walked around to the passenger side. He hated driving. Plus, he liked the idea of being chauffeured around. It was one of the perks of being the senior officer—that and not having to be the first one over the wall when chasing a suspect.

Randazzo slid into the driver's seat and slammed her door a little harder than usual, underscoring her aggravation with what she'd just witnessed. She pulled away from the curb and headed down the narrow, overgrown Santa Monica street. Fifty years ago the street shone with brand-new bungalow houses built for the returning GIs. Each house was handsomely landscaped with young trees and flower beds filled with impatiens—a staple for any beach community. Today, though, the street bore little resemblance to its earlier days, or even to the wealthier sections of town north of Montana.

Randazzo drummed her hand on the steering wheel. "Well, take it from me. There is no excuse for a woman letting something like that happen to her own daughter. I can just imagine what my mother would have done if any guy tried to molest me—he'd be pissing out his ear by the time she was done with him."

Larson had seen the pictures of Randazzo's mother—a slight, weathered woman who looked as if she would be lifted off the ground by the faintest gust of wind—and smiled at the idea of her beating up some guy. But he didn't question Randazzo's estimation of her mother's abilities. "Not everyone is as tough as your mom. Look at Ann. She probably figured Matheson was her last chance. So maybe she felt trapped."

Randazzo turned onto Pico Boulevard, one of the many streets in Santa Monica that showcased the city's burgeoning homeless population. "Oh, please. Save me the Phil Donahue garbage. Women like Ann who put up with crap from guys get what they deserve. You can't just blame the guy. If you stay there, you're just as much at fault," Randazzo stated with absolute resoluteness.

Jack looked up the street in search of a drive-thru, his rumbling stomach demanding to be filled. "I guess maybe for some it's not that easy to leave." Jack figured that this was a safe, politically correct statement to make, which he wouldn't have to defend, since he was saying it to a woman. He guessed wrong.

"That's just a cop-out. Weakness. I'm tired of hearing that." Randazzo was silent for a moment. "I once had a boyfriend who hit me," she said suddenly. Larson looked over at her, as much surprised by what she was saying as the fact that she was saying it. She usually kept her feelings on personal matters to herself. "You can bet he never got a chance to do it again."

"You never mentioned that before."

Randazzo shrugged it off, glancing out her window,

waiting for the light to change. "The guy tried to be a big shot. He shoved me against the wall to show me how tough he was, then he slapped me in the face. So I kneed him with everything I had and I got the hell out of there. Then I had Pops make a little visit to him to make sure he knew not to do that to anyone ever again." She nodded to herself. "That's how you deal with men who give you trouble."

Larson turned a doubting face toward her. "I think you're simplifying something pretty complex. Not every girl can drop-kick a guy two city blocks like you can."

"They should learn to."

He wouldn't give in. "And not every girl has a dad who'll always come to her defense like yours."

"So they should do it for themselves."

Larson just smiled. He knew he was outgunned and outmanned. To Randazzo everything had an easy answer, there were no conundrums, no hard calls. So he dropped it. He looked back down the street and saw a drive-thru just up ahead. Larson pointed to it like a bird dog to a dead pheasant. His partner instantly understood and signaled to turn in.

"So what else did you think of Ann and Laurie?" he asked.

"They may as well have had 'suspect' tattooed on their foreheads. 'We hated him, he deserved to die, we're glad he's dead, and, by the way, two weeks ago he spit in our face.' Well this is a new tactic—look as obvious as possible and no one will suspect you," she said as she pulled up to the window.

"You suspect them?"

Randazzo shook her head. "No, not really."

"So, see? It works."

✛   ✛   ✛

The intercom buzzed. "Valerie, your favorite person is on line one."

"Oh, not again. That's the third time today." Valerie sighed.

"What do you want me to tell her?"

"Tell her . . . oh, forget it. Just put her through." Valerie rubbed her face with her hands, trying to get ready for another round. "Yes?"

"Ms. Kingsley, hello. This is Rebecca Fielding. I'm sorry for calling again, but I have a few more questions I forgot to ask you." Rebecca sat at Elizabeth's kitchen table, which she had turned into a makeshift office with her papers spread all around and by the phone a long list of calls to make.

"About Mr. Matheson?"

"No, I don't think there's any need to talk about him anymore. Do you?"

"No, I guess not. So why are you calling then?"

"I'm updating my files and need some information on Bradley Knight."

"Brad's not being treated here anymore."

"Since when?" Rebecca demanded, her anger apparent. "He's not off probation yet. What do you mean he's not being treated there anymore? Where is he?"

"Ms. Fielding, I can only answer one question at a time." Valerie deflected Rebecca's harsh tone. "He wanted to finish up at Elmhurst, so that's where he is," she said flatly. She left off the "get over it."

"Why wasn't I notified about this?"

"I'm sure we sent a report about it, I guess it never made it to you. But his probation officer, Velma Martinez, knew. He left a few months ago." Bored, Valerie began doodling little cubes on a piece of notepaper, first the shape of a square, then the lines out to the imaginary horizon, connected on two sides. Dozens of little, perfect boxes. She wondered how she'd get through these calls if phones with picture monitors were ever installed.

"That's great for Velma, but I haven't seen any reports on him for over a year," Rebecca fumed. "Why did he switch centers?"

"He was having trouble getting along with some of the people here, so he just decided to leave," she said while squelching an "it's none of your damn business" retort. "You know, it is his decision, along with the probation department, where he goes for treatment. Not the district attorney's office."

"I don't understand how he could leave so close to the end of his probation. How can the court get a reasonable assessment on his progress if there's no continuity in his treatment?" Rebecca asked, exasperated. She had promised herself not to let work irritate her on vacation. But then, weren't most promises made to be broken? "I just don't understand how this could happen!" she blurted out.

"Well, it's really not such a big deal. He was here for almost the whole time, so he got the benefit of our treatment."

"Oh, well there's a comforting thought," Rebecca grumbled under her breath.

"Excuse me?"

"Nothing," she said quickly. "Never mind."

"Why are you so concerned, anyhow? You're not his probation officer. I think it's really up to Velma, don't you?" Valerie stifled the suggestion that Fielding should get a life rather than pester her nonstop about her patients.

Rebecca gave the receiver an extra squeeze as she closed her eyes. "I guess I don't view my role as limited as you do," she said finally.

Valerie couldn't contain her annoyance anymore. "I guess not. You call here every week to see if anyone has blown their nose without your permission," she fumed. "I don't need you breathing down my neck all the time. Neither do the other therapists for that matter. We're doing what we're supposed to do and that's all you need to know." Valerie stopped before she said anything else. A hostile relationship would serve neither of them well, so Valerie softened her tone in spite of her exasperation. "Look, you don't believe in treatment and there's nothing we can say to change your mind. You'll just have to accept that we're taking care of what needs to be done."

"Well, I suppose if I knew that were true, I wouldn't be so concerned," said Rebecca. "But I can't trust that any of you are doing the right thing. All that treatment seems to do is keep the jails from getting overcrowded. I'm sorry, but when I hear that someone is allowed to bounce around to whatever treatment facility suits his fancy, well, that doesn't fill me with confidence. In fact, it makes me wonder just how well you are doing your job."

Valerie clenched her teeth, fighting to remain calm. She started on a new piece of paper, switching from cubes to little arrows, starting from the outside of the page and moving inward, one connecting to the next, over and over. Her pen pushed hard into the paper, leaving deep crevices. "Last time I checked, it wasn't up to you to decide how we do our job," she blurted. Valerie paused, inhaling deeply, forcing herself to think and choose her words carefully. "Look, we're not a prison and we're not an arm of the police department. We are a treatment and counseling facility. And we provide a valuable service to troubled men who need our help."

"I honestly do not understand you people—"

"You people?" Valerie jumped on the perceived slight.

Rebecca sighed deeply. "Look, you and I, we

obviously come from different directions. We just see things differently."

Valerie took Rebecca's comment as a sign of conciliation and she calmed herself. "Ms. Fielding, it's your job to prosecute these men. But after they're sent here, then it becomes my job. And I'm doing the best I can."

Rebecca bristled at her words. "But if your best is not enough, then someday you're going to have to hear about your client abusing some other child. That's what's at stake here. If you fail with one of these guys, somebody will be hurt."

"I understand that. But I don't think you understand that your involvement after their cases are over may contribute to their inability to get better. You're a constant reminder of their offense and you're impeding their recovery."

"I see. So it's all my fault that your patients leave therapy no better than when they started?"

Valerie threw her pen down. "This conversation is not getting us anywhere."

"Of course not," Rebecca said acerbically. "Why should it? It never does."

5

D r. Robert Hillerman had run the Oakwood Center blissfully undisturbed for over a decade, treating a broad range of sex offenders mandated into therapy by judges who hoped that there was a cure for what was euphemistically referred to as "inappropriate sexual urges." For a treatment center whose very existence depended upon no one questioning the effectiveness of its approach, obscurity was its most important commodity. Now, however, the Oakwood's thin veneer of anonymity was giving way to the publicity surrounding the Penhall and Matheson murders. Dealing with this unwanted attention was foremost on Dr. Hillerman's mind—and not the fact that two of his patients had turned up dead—when he was startled by the buzzer on his intercom.

"Dr. Hillerman, Detectives Larson and Randazzo from the LAPD are here to see you regarding Mr. Matheson," a pleasant voice chirped.

Either he had suddenly developed Alzheimer's or this had not been scheduled. "Why didn't they call first?" Hillerman demanded of his receptionist. Hillerman hated surprises, particularly when they came from someone making minimum wage.

"They did, Dr. Hillerman, I—uh—I'm sure I left you a message slip," she stammered apologetically.

"How many times have I told you that you can't just leave me a note? You must tell me!" he barked into the speaker. He looked around his desk, trying to find the missing note. Right on top—in red. He crumpled the paper and threw it angrily in the wastebasket. "We'll talk about this later. Just send Valerie in here and tell the detectives I'll be with them in a minute." Hillerman stood up, hesitated, and then sat back down, not sure what he wanted to do first. He worked to prioritize his thoughts, rubbing his temples furiously. He grabbed the receiver and quickly dialed Stan Berman, his attorney for the last twenty years, but instead of getting the live version all Hillerman got was Stan's annoying voice mail. He angrily left a message for him to call back immediately and slammed the phone down, irritated that he had to do this alone.

"You wanted to see me, Dr. Hillerman?" Valerie asked, entering Hillerman's office, unaware of the reason for the meeting. As always, she looked professional, dressed today in a tan suit with a scoop-necked cream-colored silk blouse. Her hair was pulled back in a loose ponytail, leaving a few strands to softly surround her delicate face. She exuded a gentleness that was as intriguing as it was befitting.

Hillerman ordinarily would have stopped to appreciate her attractiveness, his eyes lingering appreciatively on every curve of her body while he pretended to engage her in some dialogue, but this morning his attention was directed elsewhere. "There are two detectives here to see me about Matheson. I suspect they will also want to speak with you, since you were his treating therapist. Now I want you to listen to me very carefully." Hillerman paused, waiting to continue until their eyes locked. "You may answer their questions with short, succinct answers only. I do not want you volunteering any information. Whatever you say can have profound repercussions for the clinic, and you must keep that in mind at all times. Keep on your guard when you speak." Hillerman swiveled his chair abruptly and pushed the receptionist's button, convinced he'd been waiting hours for Stan's return call. "Has Stan called back yet?" he shouted into the intercom.

"No, Dr. Hillerman, but I'll put him through the minute he does," she said earnestly.

"Fine. And bring another chair in here."

Valerie watched the veins pop out along Dr. Hillerman's forehead, making crisscrosses with the creases in his deeply tanned skin. Valerie tried to remain calm and not let his urgent demeanor and brusque manner rattle her, but she could feel her heart move to her throat.

Hillerman turned toward Valerie, the furrows in his brow deepening as he scowled. "Now, I doubt we will be able to avoid discussing Matheson's last session with his ex-wife and stepdaughter, but we have to keep the center from looking bad. Matheson caused us enough trouble while he was alive. Now that he's dead, we can spin things in our favor." As usual, Valerie thought silently. "Just remember, do not allow yourself to become intimidated just because they are the police. It was your call—your professional judgment as the therapist—whether Matheson was ready for such a session."

Hillerman hoped Valerie understood that he was preparing her speech. He intoned deliberately to stress the importance of his words. "You believed, based on his statements in group, that he was going to participate in the session in good faith. He surprised you by saying what he did. It could not have been predicted based on your prior sessions with him. We need not discuss the testing that had been done and the results, do you understand?"

Valerie nodded.

"Good. The family seemed upset and you offered your services to them, but they declined, correct?"

"Yes, Dr. Hillerman," Valerie said.

"And even though the meeting went poorly, there was nothing that you could have done differently. It was a totally unexpected, unfortunate episode."

"I understand." She removed her jacket and positioned herself under the air vent, trying in vain to cool her body.

Hillerman leaned forward, his hands crossed in front of him on his uncluttered cherrywood desk. Valerie always marveled at his desk—the wood was so shiny and unblemished, not a scratch in sight, as if the wood dared not show a flaw. She stood straight waiting for him to continue, fully aware of the only noise in the room—the soft hum from the computer on the corner of his desk, its large off-white monitor a looming presence in an otherwise traditional office decorated in rich, dark hues.

"Now, we will not be discussing what an utter failure Mr. Matheson turned out to be as a clinical patient. Thank God that's not important anymore. Let's focus on our successes. Do you understand?" Hillerman demanded.

Valerie managed to force a yes through her tightening throat.

"Good." The pretty dark-haired receptionist carried in a chair almost as big as she was and set it next to the other guest chairs across from Hillerman. "Thank you, Elena," Hillerman said, forming the longest pleasant exchange in the four years she worked there. "I believe we're ready. You may send them in."

Elena returned to her desk and slid back the glass window. "Dr. Hillerman is ready to see you," she said brightly.

Larson stopped his pacing and waited for Randazzo to put down the magazine she had been thumbing through as they waited. Randazzo had tried to get Larson to join her on the green plaid sofa—offering him a copy of the latest *Psychology Today* magazine—but Larson, who viewed the psychological profession as barely a step up from voodoo, declined, unamused. Randazzo tossed her magazine down and stood up, allowing Larson to go first as they were escorted out of the waiting room and down the long, narrow hallway. As they headed to Hillerman's office, passing a number of people along the way, Larson wished that he had a VISITOR badge so no one would mistake him for one of the center's patients.

Dr. Hillerman welcomed Larson and Randazzo from behind his desk, getting up only briefly to shake their hands, a saccharine smile replacing his usual disdainful frown. He lingered more with Randazzo, clasping her hand between both of his and adding a dulcet "Charmed" in greeting. After he sat back down, he introduced Valerie to the detectives dismissively, as if she were some clerk typist and not Matheson's primary counselor. Randazzo thought Hillerman looked like an aging pampered East Coast aristocrat—tall, tan, and trim with a shock of prematurely gray hair, a small pouty mouth, and long thin nose. She thought Valerie was attractive, if a little prim, with her conservative suit and large tortoise-shell glasses.

Larson had been more intrigued by the wall

behind Hillerman, which seemed to be a shrine to his own self-importance covered with diplomas, credentials, certificates, and awards, some with more Latin in them than a pre–Vatican II mass. Larson was not impressed with the display of academic excess, because it had long ago occurred to him that those who were truly brilliant didn't need to hang the proof on their walls.

Hillerman held his head high and back straight so that he could literally look down his nose as he spoke. "Detectives, my secretary failed to notify me of this appointment, so we're going to have to make this quick."

"This won't take very long, Dr. Hillerman," Randazzo replied as she flipped open her notebook. "We'd like to see the clinic's records on Mr. Matheson."

Hillerman looked pained and a little off guard. He hadn't thought to cleanse Matheson's file of unwanted matter. He rubbed his chin and sat quietly, to appear as if he were considering their request. "I'll, of course, need to speak with our attorney to see if we can do that. There are issues of confidentiality, as you know. I'll have to get back to you on that." Hillerman stood up. "Now, if that's all you need—"

"Uh, no, we also need to talk to Ms. Kingsley. Of course, if you'd like, we can get out of your way here." Randazzo smiled at Valerie, including her among the "we."

"What is it you'd like to know?" asked Hillerman, settling back into his chair to make it quite clear that he had no intention of going anywhere.

Randazzo turned to Valerie and noticed a certain tenseness in the way she sat with her back stiff, her hands clasped on her lap, her legs tucked under her chair. She smiled to ease Valerie into the interview.

"How long were you Matheson's therapist?" Randazzo asked, offering up a slow pitch.

"For almost two years. I took over the group from someone else." She spoke quickly, her words running together.

"So you weren't his first therapist?"

"No," Hillerman interjected, as if the question had been directed toward him. "The Oakwood is a training facility as well as a treatment center. We bring therapists like Ms. Kingsley into existing groups the same way that new members join as old members graduate. You see, while the actual group participants may change from time to time, there is always continuity in the groups themselves. This continuity is essential for developing group cohesiveness, for establishing and maintaining group norms, for facilitating self-disclosure, and for increasing participation."

Larson and Randazzo exchanged a fleeting "Oh, brother" look. Randazzo forced her eyes to stay fixed on Dr. Hillerman and not roll up in their sockets in involuntary reaction to his speech. "Dr. Hillerman, since I'm not familiar with your clinic, why don't you tell me about the groups, how they're formed, what the therapist is supposed to do with them? That sort of thing," Randazzo asked. She figured if he was that eager to do the talking, she'd get the background information out of him first. Then maybe she'd get the chance to have Valerie answer her specific questions about Matheson.

Hillerman was only too happy to oblige. He had started the center—and a small cottage industry treating sex offenders—and reveled in sharing his "baby" with others. He took Randazzo's opening as an opportunity to give the unabbreviated speech. "The clinic has a number of different groups comprised exclusively of sex offenders. We also see some of the men on an individual basis, if they are in crisis or need additional therapeutic support as an adjunct to the group. We treat men suffering from the whole gamut of paraphilias, from the voyeur to the predatory child molester. But our approach is the same regardless of the patient's particular predilection. We utilize a cognitive-behavioral approach to therapy, not focusing on the underlying psychological issues but instead addressing the thoughts and behaviors that lead to sexual offense."

"Uh-huh," Randazzo said slowly, not out of a lack of understanding of what he was saying—she'd majored in psychology in college and had a good appreciation for various treatment approaches—but as a simple "go on."

Dr. Hillerman misread Randazzo, taking her interjection as a sign of ignorance and decided to elucidate. Had he guessed that Larson was lost, though, he would have been right. "Let me illustrate. One school of thought is to focus psychodynamically on why the offender acts out—what occurred in his history that may explain the offense. This approach seeks to help the men understand where their deviant behavior comes from as a way to help them overcome their impulses. We, by contrast, do not believe that understanding one's history is the answer. Instead, we look to what thoughts he uses to convince himself that it is all right for him to act inappropriately and teach him how to stop those thoughts and replace them with rational, healthy thoughts."

By now Larson had almost counted all the holes in one of the ceiling tiles, and made his boredom obvious for all to see. Randazzo did not have the luxury of being able to kick him under the table, so she did the next best thing. "Dr. Hillerman, maybe you could give my partner an example. I think it might help him understand what you are saying."

Randazzo was quite pleased with herself. Larson, on the other hand, was not as amused.

"Of course." Hillerman turned his attention to Larson. "Here's a hypothetical. A man has an adolescent daughter. He and his wife are having marital difficulties. Maybe he's having problems at work. He takes to drinking a little more than usual. His daughter is young, vivacious, carefree. With his wife or with his boss he may feel insecure or inadequate, but with his daughter he still feels powerful. He still feels like a man. At this point, normal prohibitions would warn the man to keep the relationship on a father-daughter plane, not to sexualize the relationship or make it more than it is. It is what helps us all to control negative impulses. I like to explain it as the Jiminy Cricket we carry with us on our shoulder that tells us right from wrong. But these men lack normal mental prohibitions. Instead, they use mental gymnastics called rationalizations, denials, or minimizations to give themselves permission to do that which they know on some level is improper."

Hillerman took the time to fill and light his pipe, allowing the information to soak in. He preferred talking about the center to discussing the unpleasantness surrounding Matheson. After a few successful puffs of smoke, he resumed. "Thus, in our scenario, the man would tell himself that his daughter is flirting with him, that she finds him sexy. He tells himself that she's more of a wife to him than his own wife. He tells himself that she appreciates him like his boss fails to. He tells himself they have a special relationship, and that it's okay to act out how he feels. He tells himself it's mutual. Basically, he tells himself whatever he has to in order to make it all right.

"As therapists, we teach him to go back to the very beginning, to identify all the points along the way where he failed to think and behave rationally—when he failed to heed the small voice that told him what he was doing was wrong. What we do is plot out a line, a continuum from the beginning of an irrational thought to the end where the man acts out. We train the men to recognize when they make the first lapse, as we call it—the first errant step along the continuum—the first irrational thought that he uses to justify behavior that any rational person would consider unjustifiable. Because if he can stop himself there, he won't get to the end point where he acts out. That's why I believe this approach is the most successful." He turned and tossed a patronizing smile at Randazzo.

Randazzo sat quietly, contemplating what she'd heard. She thought back to all she'd learned in school, and it all seemed inconsistent with what Hillerman was saying. Then again, it had been several years since her last class, and she would be the first to admit that she knew enough about psychology to get into trouble, but not enough to get out. "I don't know," she said finally, shaking her head. "I know a lot of people try behavior modification to stop smoking or overeating, but they go right back afterward. If you can't get people to stop these habits how are you going to get them to stop being pedophiles? I mean, if someone is turned on by a child, how are you ever going to change that?"

Hillerman scowled at Randazzo, who refused to flinch in return. He certainly didn't feel the need to be lectured by a cop on his therapeutic techniques. "With all due respect, Detective, as therapists we obviously do not ascribe to the theory that people do not change. None of us is a perfect person, with no ugly impulses or inappropriate thoughts. What separates the majority of people from the men in here is that the rest of us can control our negative impulses and not act upon our negative thoughts. By mastering our techniques, the men leave here knowing how to do just that. Our statistics show us to be very successful."

"I suppose that depends on how you measure success," Randazzo said, still unconvinced. "If success means they're cured, then I'd agree. But if all it means is they know what to do, but still can't control themselves, then I'd say that's not very successful." Larson was finding the whole thing rather funny. Here they came to talk about Matheson and instead Randazzo was debating treatment theories. He smiled to himself, knowing that Hillerman was about to learn what he already knew—Randazzo was a lot like a pit bull who after latching onto something just couldn't let go. "Do you know that the guys leaving here will absolutely never offend again?"

Hillerman's eyes narrowed at the not-too-veiled reproof. "Since there are no absolutes, it would be a waste of time to speak in those terms. We believe progress is success. That's how we measure success."

"And what if they haven't shown progress?" Randazzo pressed on. "What do you do then?"

"That's not a situation we face very often, I'm pleased to say. The proof of our success is in our high referral rates from the courts and the probation officers. And we are very near national accreditation from the Association for the Treatment of Sex Offenders. We do good work here, Detective. It's a simple fact. If we weren't successful, we wouldn't be in business."

And you'd have to get a real job, Randazzo thought to herself. She wanted to continue the debate but decided that she didn't have the academic credentials to convince Hillerman that he was wrong. Although she figured common sense alone should have told him that. Randazzo switched the focus to Valerie. "How was Matheson in group? Did he get along with the other group members?"

Valerie thought about the question, wondering whether the answer might be a reflection of her leadership skills. Hillerman was watching, after all. "Yes and no. When he first came here, he was in a different group, but he left because of some personality conflicts."

Yes and no. Gee, thanks for the definitive answer, Randazzo thought. "Did he get along better with the men in the second group?"

"I think so. There were still some personality clashes." Valerie looked over at Hillerman, trying to make eye contact, to see if she was on safe territory. He gave her a slightly raised eyebrow in response, then cast a quick glance over at Randazzo, who noted the cue and frowned her displeasure at Hillerman. "It's difficult to get a dozen people to sit around and discuss their personal lives and not have some friction develop," she continued. "Not everyone sees the world the same way. Different backgrounds, different personalities make for potential disagreements. But that's what group is all about—learning to handle each other's differences, how to resolve conflict." She smiled to herself, knowing she had covered herself well.

"So, does that mean that you believe that whatever clashes Matheson had with the other group members were nothing out of the ordinary?"

"Exactly. At times, he would push someone's buttons, and at other times someone would push one of his. But no different from anyone else in group." She seemed anxious to paint her group sessions as ordinary.

"What was your opinion of Matheson as a group member?" Randazzo asked.

"I thought he was doing fine. He wouldn't usually

bring up anything to talk about, but if I pulled him into a discussion, his participation was fine. He'd share his experiences. He'd give his opinions. I found him fairly supportive of the other men in group," Valerie said, looking at Hillerman for an approving nod, but his face betrayed no opinion about what she was saying.

"How did he explain his offense?"

"He didn't talk about it much. When he first would try to give his view of what happened, it was always watered down. He would say that the D.A. blew it out of proportion by filing so many charges against him when all he had done was 'cop a feel.'" Valerie put the phrase in quotes for the detectives. "But more recently he said he understood how his drinking and loneliness led him to turn to Laurie for comfort."

"That sounds like he was still making excuses," Randazzo said, her smooth brow furrowed.

"Well, you're right, of course," Valerie replied defensively. "Technically, they're excuses. But for him, it was an improvement, and we were pleased with that. Detectives, you must remember, therapy is a process. With Matheson, I tried to have him recognize how his relationship with his wife and stepdaughter had all the earmarks of trouble early on, so that in later relationships he could stop before problems develop."

"Did you feel that he was getting it?" asked Randazzo.

Valerie paused and looked out the window to the dreary industrial center across the street. Trying to think of the right answer, Randazzo wondered. So much of what she had said up to this point seemed so automatic, almost canned. "Oh, definitely," she said unconvincingly. "He clearly had made progress within the confines of the group. But he had difficulty reaching the final step. So many of the men here seem to reach an epiphany during their last year. As if all the years preceding had laid the foundation for the realization of what we were trying to teach them. It takes a long time to break down the wall of resistance, but eventually they get it. But I wasn't sure we were there with Matheson yet. I thought he was close, but—" Valerie saw Hillerman blanch and stopped midsentence.

"Yes?" Randazzo prodded.

"Well, I had set up a meeting with Matheson and his ex-wife and the stepdaughter." Valerie felt Hillerman's eyes burning her skin. Tread carefully.

"And how did the session go?" Randazzo asked, curious to see if everyone's spin on the meeting was the same.

Valerie paused, looking down quickly. "Not well," she said with a slight shake of her head. Valerie recrossed her legs and leaned in toward the detectives, looking over at Hillerman for support. Hillerman avoided her eyes, instead staring intently at the ever changing screen saver on his computer. His sudden distance worried Valerie, but she pushed on with the story. "Ann and Laurie told him how they felt about what he had done, what they had done to heal themselves, and where they were today. It was not confrontational, just an honest expression of their feelings. They really opened up their hurt and pain to him. I don't know what I expected him to feel about what they were saying, I couldn't read him, but he seemed to be really listening, taking it all in."

Valerie flashed on the memory of Matheson, the smirk that started slowly after Laurie had finished talking, which erupted into a loud belly laugh dripping with disdain. How do you describe that, she wondered, without angering Hillerman? "Well, when it was finally his turn to speak, he leaned back in his seat and just spewed out about five minutes of meanness—not what we'd rehearsed, not what he was supposed to say, but just about all the wrong things you could imagine saying under those circumstances. I didn't know what to do. It all happened so fast. He went from what I thought was silent contrition to outright contempt in nothing flat. I just don't know what happened."

"What did you do?" Randazzo asked.

"What could I do? At that point, it was too late— Ann and Laurie just about ran out of there—so I told Bill we'd discuss it in group. And we did. The whole group wanted to talk about it. They were as shocked as I was. He said he was sorry. He was just taken by surprise by the whole meeting. It really stirred up a lot of feelings in him that he just didn't know how to handle. But I think he really felt bad about what he had done. Unfortunately the family wasn't there to hear it—to know he was sorry."

"Did you report the incident to the court?"

"That wasn't necessary," Hillerman quickly blurted out. "He really couldn't be punished for what he did."

"Maybe he was," Randazzo suggested.

"What do you mean, Detective?" Hillerman asked.

"Well, I'm sure the thought that his killing was for revenge must have crossed your mind. Just a week after he tells his stepdaughter and his ex to go screw themselves, he gets whacked." Hillerman looked at Randazzo blankly. "It never crossed your mind that they might have killed him to get back at him for that?"

"Actually, no," Hillerman equivocated. "I don't think in terms of getting even. I think in terms of getting better. My efforts, my life's work, is to rehabilitate these men. So maybe I do have difficulty fathoming someone who would repudiate my work at the barrel of a gun."

Randazzo raised her eyebrows in a "you've got to be kidding me" expression. "You mean to tell me that no one here has ever received hate mail or death threats or anything like that?"

"No, of course not. Why would we?"

"I would imagine that not everyone is fond of your patients," Randazzo suggested.

Larson didn't want his two cents to go unspent. "You see, Doctor, as a layman, it seems to me that many people might think castration would be more appropriate treatment for your clients than weekly rap sessions, don't you think?"

"Detective, I don't find comments like that to be the least bit humorous."

"I didn't intend it to be funny," Larson said.

Hillerman relit his extinguished pipe, puffing furiously and sending a cloud up in front of him. "No, I don't think the public really wants revenge. I think there is a lot of misunderstanding about what we do here, but if the public understood and appreciated what we do, they would support it wholeheartedly. Perhaps that might be a side benefit of this unfortunate situation. Maybe the attention cast on the clinic will rally support for our efforts to treat and rehabilitate rather than punish. One must always look for the silver lining, Detec-tive."

Larson was ready to throw up, but he was afraid Hillerman would take it as an offer to discuss his feelings. So he looked over at his partner to see what else she wanted to ask. As she sat there thinking about her next question, Randazzo was suddenly struck by the fact that in all the time they'd been there, Hillerman never asked any questions about the murders or whether they had anything to do with the Oakwood. "Dr. Hillerman, do you have any explanation for the fact that two of your patients have been killed?"

Hillerman stiffened. "I thought *you* were the detectives."

Larson saw Randazzo's dark eyes flash and stepped in before she could give Hillerman reason to regret his sarcasm. "Two of your patients have been shot to death in the last two months. Now there are only two possibilities—they are either unrelated murders or someone is targeting your clients. What Detective Randazzo is asking is from where you sit, what's your take? Do you think your clients are at risk? What are you going to tell them when they ask if someone is targeting them?"

"I'll tell them to call you," Hillerman said, a phony smile splashed across his face.

Larson decided he'd heard enough from Hillerman for one day. He directed his next question toward Valerie. "Let's put Matheson aside for now. While we're here, is there anything you can tell us about Eric Penhall?"

"I wasn't his regular therapist, Detective." Valerie looked over at Hillerman, who was suddenly nervous about not having had the opportunity to prepare Penhall's therapist, Janet Chapin.

"Uh, Valerie, why don't you go grab Janet and fill her in on what the detectives want to discuss?" Hillerman hoped Valerie understood.

The intercom buzzed and Hillerman snatched the phone. "Yes," he demanded.

"Mr. Berman on line one."

Hillerman looked over at the detectives, sitting too quietly for his comfort. "Good. Tell him I'll be done with my meeting shortly and that our meeting will go on as scheduled."

Valerie felt more relaxed, a spring returning to her step as she headed down the hall to Janet's office.

"Jan, your turn," she said gaily, happy to be passing the baton.

Janet was busy typing, finalizing one of her many monthly reports to the probation department, this one on an exhibitionist who used to park along the street, call women over asking for directions, and when they naively approached his car, whip out his manhood for them to see and ask them if they wanted to pet Sparky. "My turn for what?" she asked as she kept banging away at her keyboard.

"Hillerman's with some cops. They want to talk to you about Penhall."

Janet stopped typing and turned around. "Why do they want to talk to me?"

"Because I told them you killed him," Valerie kidded. "Hey, if I have to be grilled about Matheson, you get the heat on Penhall—he was yours. And by the way, Hillerman wants you to make sure that you extol the virtues of this place."

"Great," she said in all insincerity. She hit save and went over to grab her file on Penhall, then headed to Hillerman's office. She greeted the detectives, shaking their hands, lingering a bit longer with Larson. Being grilled by him wouldn't be that bad, she thought.

Randazzo snapped Janet out of her momentary hypnosis. "Ms. Chapin, we're investigating whether the murder of Eric Penhall may be related to the murder of William Matheson and we were wondering what you could tell us about Mr. Penhall. Any reason why anyone would have wanted to kill him?"

"No, none that I could see," Janet said. "He never said anything in group about having any enemies— he got along okay with his ex, all things considered. I don't think I'll be able to help you much. Eric was pretty quiet in group. He'd figured us out. You know, we can't put a man in jail for not talking. Although I drew the line at him trying to bring in reading material—that was a bit much," she joked, flashing a coquettish smile to Larson. With makeup she might have caught Jack's eye, but Janet never bothered with makeup at the office. Too much work for no payoff, she figured. Today, though, she thought she might have figured wrong. Hillerman cleared his throat deliberately and glared at her, hoping she would get the hint to temper her overly forthright answers.

"Did Mr. Penhall participate in a face-to-face meeting with his victim like Matheson did?" Randazzo asked.

She paused and considered her answer. "No, I didn't think he would make a good candidate for a meeting like that."

"So you hadn't had any problems with Mr. Penhall before he was killed? Nothing out of the ordinary?"

Janet shrugged. "No. He was getting close to the end of his probation and I tried to get him to talk about what he'd learned. He said, 'Don't have your daughter give you a blow job.'" Janet just sighed, her eyes downcast as she felt the disappointment again. "It was too bad. He knew what he'd done was wrong, but beyond that he never wanted to discuss it. So I had some concerns about how he'd handle life after probation. You know, we provide a safety net for these guys. Once they're gone, it's too easy to fall into old bad habits. I talked to the D.A. about it, but she said she needed some proof he was violating probation or her hands were tied. I told her I didn't have any. So that was the end of it. He was killed before we had to worry about his release."

Having checked and rechecked his watch repeatedly without anyone taking the hint, Hillerman decided for a more straightforward method of ending the discussion. "We are more than happy to help the investigation in any way we can, Detectives. But for now, I hate to call this to an end, but I really must be getting on to my meeting." Hillerman spoke as he rose from his chair, arm extended to signify it was time for them to leave. "If you need any more from us, just give us a call and we can set up another time."

Larson and Randazzo were ushered out with only a thick color brochure on the Oakwood Center. They took the stairs down from the second-floor office to the street level and walked along a narrow path, stepping over a homeless man asleep under a pile of blankets despite the heat, to the parking lot in the back. "Maybe they should rename the center the Tower of Psychobabble," Jack said finally.

Randazzo laughed in agreement. She unlocked the doors and took her usual seat behind the wheel, pulling out of the lot and onto the dreary street. In the last dozen years this part of the Valley had changed from middle class to poor, where the only new paint on houses was graffiti. Larson no longer noticed the change, and Randazzo, a transplant from the East, had no knowledge that things had ever been different. They drove past houses where families seemed to live outside on the front steps, sidewalks, and street as much as they lived inside, which was in stark contrast to the more affluent communities, where no one was ever seen on the streets. Here, on front lawns children and women gathered next to stacks of clothes and random household items, laundry hung limply on clotheslines, and peddlers pushed small food carts up and down the narrow streets.

"So what were they talking about?" Larson asked. "They can't possibly believe all that mumbo jumbo they were spouting, can they?"

"'Fraid so." Randazzo turned onto Sepulveda, a boulevard that in most towns was wide enough to be considered a freeway, lined with shops, food joints, and gas stations, with nary a tree in sight. "You hungry?"

"You have to ask?"

She thought about Tommy's, but the memory of the flies buzzing around the remainder of Matheson's last meal still lingered. She figured she might never be able to eat there again and resented Matheson for that. "How 'bout Pink's?" Pink's was their favorite hot dog stand, where on a particularly hot day like today the server's dripping sweat added a nice salty bite to the chili dogs. To some it was gross, but to true aficionados, it was a little bit of heaven on a bun. "It's on the way to the probation department."

Jack laughed. Pink's was over the hill in Hollywood, which was about ten miles out of the way, a half-hour by freeway. "No it isn't."

"I'll make you a deal. If you say yes, I'll buy you a chocolate chip sweet roll at Canter's." Canter's—the deli of the gods. How could Jack resist?

"You're the one driving," he said.

Randazzo turned onto the freeway and settled back in quiet anticipation of a meal that would have no nutritional value whatsoever. Even before she had merged into traffic, Jack had dozed off. Her mind drifted as she thought back to the interview with Hillerman. "You know," she mused, "if they really believe they're doing any good, they may be as dangerous as their patients."

6

As Stan took his seat, Hillerman made a notation of their start time. At $350 an hour, he wasn't going to pay for a minute more than he had to. Stan was still unpacking his briefcase when Hillerman began. "Well, I just had an absolutely delightful conversation with two of L.A.'s finest regarding our dearly departed," he said.

"Did they give you any trouble?" Stan asked as he searched for his pen.

Hillerman scoffed at the notion, leaning back in his chair comfortably. "No, not really. They're obviously clueless and just came by to poke around."

"Did you tell them anything I should know about?"

"No. You would have been proud of me. They left here knowing little more than when they came in."

Stan dropped three sugar cubes into the black coffee that Elena had brought him and swirled them around until they melted. "Well, that's good. The last thing we need is snooping cops."

"Not to worry. I gave them the fifty-dollar speech

about our noble endeavor, and that seemed to leave them satisfied, if not a little confused."

"I'm sure they left here quite impressed with you. Even if they didn't understand what you were saying." Stan laughed. "Heck, I don't even know what you are saying most of the time." Hillerman did not return the laugh. Stan shifted in his seat and cleared his throat. "So if the meeting with the police went fine, why do you seem so upset?"

Hillerman reached over and grabbed his pipe from its holder, tapping it upside down against the trash can to empty it out. He spoke as he cleaned out the last few stubborn remnants of tobacco. "It's not just the police. It's all the attention on the clinic. The phones have been ringing off the hook. People are hanging around outside. We can't have this level of scrutiny."

Stan shifted in his chair again, trying to get comfortable. A large, heavyset man, he disguised his weight problem with oversized Hugo Boss suits. He was less successful in trying to hide his receding hairline by parting his hair at his ear and plastering the thin strands across his head. "Well, as far as the publicity you're getting goes, there's not a lot we can do, unless it's false or paints the clinic in a bad light. You know, like claiming it's a dangerous place. Really what you need is some good publicity to counteract the bad. I've got a friend at the *Reporter* who owes me. Maybe I can get him to write a favorable piece about you and the clinic."

"Good, good. I'd be happy to give an interview, anytime." Hillerman eyed the clock. "Now, what do we do about Ms. Fielding's latest missive to the board?"

"Well, we could pay off the mailroom clerk to burn the letter," Stan said with a little laugh. Hillerman's sour expression denoted no trace of humor. Stan cleared his throat again and resumed a more serious posture. "I think our only choice is to ignore it and continue our efforts to paint her as a crackpot who's out to close the center for her own personal reasons. We need to work on satisfying the board so that they feel their concerns have been addressed. But I don't think we have to respond directly to the points in her letter."

"I don't see how you can ignore a shark that's nibbling at your toes. It's only a matter of time before you're swallowed whole." Hillerman had spent most of his energy over the past few months having to fend off attacks from Rebecca on a number of fronts and was not interested in hearing that he should ignore her. He wanted something concrete, a way to silence her for good.

Stan took a quick sip of his coffee, thinking of what he could say that would possibly satisfy Hillerman. "I understand your concern, Bob. There's no question that she'd like nothing more than to put you out of business. I guess she thinks that since you're the biggest clinic out there, if she can get to you, getting the rest shut down will be easy. And she knows that you're on probation, so this is the time to strike. But what you have on your side is your expertise. If you can present data that satisfies the board, that will carry more weight than her shouting."

Hillerman continued fiddling with his pipe, filling and refilling it, tapping it down each time to get the right concentration, before lighting it. A large cloud of vanilla-scented smoke drifted toward Stan. "I'm not sure I can get that together as quickly as we need it. You know, I've been working on a plan to get the Oakwood off probation, but I need more time. After all these years in business, now suddenly everyone wants proof. Proof! As if we were working with something that was easy to quantify. This is not accounting."

Hillerman sucked on the pipe but nothing happened, the fire had extinguished. "Dammit! The last thing I need is that bitch—"

"Look, we've been lucky so far. I don't think the board finds her terribly credible," Stan said, trying to reassure Hillerman.

"Credible? She's a loon, for god's sake. She seems to think that if she shuts us down, suddenly all sex offenders will get life sentences. It's ludicrous."

Stan tapped his notepad with his pen absentmindedly. "Unfortunately, Bob, she does have a right to her opinion."

"Not when her opinion is taking direct aim at me. Isn't there anything you can do? What the fuck am I paying you for?"

Stan ignored the attack, maintaining a calm demeanor. He knew that the answer was that he was paid as much for putting up with Hillerman as for his actual legal advice. "Why don't we try a different tack with her? We already have all the dirt on her that we need, so let's save it for now. Why don't you try meeting with her? Maybe extend her an olive branch."

"And what if that doesn't work?" Hillerman snapped.

"Well, let's try it and see what happens." Stan paused, carefully watching as Hillerman considered his options.

"Fine. But if it doesn't work, we'll continue with my approach."

Stan bowed his head slightly. "Of course," he said. He knew that, ultimately, it always came down to doing things Hillerman's way—save the clinic at all costs.

So much paint had peeled off the glass door that Larson and Randazzo appeared to be visiting the

Van Nuys office for the L S ANG L S C NTY PR B T N D P RT. Inside the rambling one-story office building, it was clear that none of the county's funds were going toward upkeep. Half the ceiling tiles were missing, exposing pipes, vents, and insulation. The vast waiting area consisted of dozens of cracked, plastic chairs in putrid greens and yellows, all lined up on one side leaving a large expanse suitable for nervous pacing. At least the industrial-grade linoleum flooring was holding up nicely.

As Larson checked in, Randazzo stood observing the odd assortment of folks waiting for their five-minute probation checkups: a cowboy, a guy with a three-foot-long braid, baggy-clothed homeboys and girls, some with their kids in tow, laborers with work-worn hands, and a businessman with a folded hand-kerchief popping out of his breast pocket. She was particularly intrigued by one man who looked like Fu Manchu and was offering a bag of Cheez-Its to a well-behaved toddler who beamed with appreciation at the unexpected gift. She couldn't help but wonder what offense the kind stranger had committed to get himself sent here.

Velma greeted the officers graciously, her wide smile and warm brown eyes creating an instant bond. She was a short woman with dyed orange-red hair styled in a shoulder-length bob, oversized matching red glasses and full makeup. The orange spandex pantsuit she wore colorfully enveloped her two-hundred-pound frame, and she maintained the color scheme down to her inch-high sandals and painted toes.

"Thanks for seeing us on such short notice. We really appreciate your help," Randazzo said as she shook Martinez's hand.

"Oh, please. Call me Velma."

Velma walked the detectives to her office, past dozens of other small cubicles where probation officers sat leaning forward, speaking earnestly to their apparently indifferent probationers. The noise level in the large room was a constant loud murmur punctuated by the occasional raised voice, slammed file cabinet, or tearful outburst. Velma apologized for the mess in her office, which seemed pretty well organized to Larson. The cold, partitioned cubicle was decorated with pages from a 1989 Ansel Adams calendar and a decade's worth of postcards from her probationers in an effort to make her four-by-six working space more livable.

"I'm sorry I don't have anything to offer you. I usually bake something, but last night I just was too tired." Velma's lilting Mexican accent rose and fell in undulating rhythms as she spoke. "I like to make things for my guys, it helps break the ice, you know, and keep things friendly. I mean, as long as they're not getting into any trouble, we don't need to be fighting. Don't you agree?" She was so sweet, so sincere, how could they not? Randazzo and Larson nodded their assent. They sat down in small metal framed chairs, Larson's knees bumping up against the front of Velma's desk. She shrugged apologetically as Larson struggled to move his chair into a comfortable position. He finally settled on sitting with his chair facing Randazzo. Randazzo noticed Larson's predicament, and after fighting off the temptation of doing a long interview, she decided to do the abbreviated version.

"Ms. Martinez . . . I mean, Velma. Was Mr. Matheson in any kind of trouble recently?"

Velma thought for a moment then shook her head. "No, no, nothing. That's why I was surprised by what happened. He never got in any trouble." Velma paused and looked over at the picture on her desk, a posed family portrait with her sitting among three smiling teenagers. She lowered her eyes for a moment, then looked up at Randazzo, her easy smile replaced by a somber expression. "It's just so terrible what's going on in the streets, so much violence. No one's safe anymore."

Randazzo nodded, even though she wasn't sure that was the answer to what happened to Matheson. "So he never got in trouble while on probation?" Randazzo asked. She cast a quick glance over at her still uncomfortable partner. Larson's neck was hurting from his contorted position trying to face Velma, so he gave up and turned back toward Randazzo. Over her shoulder he watched a heated conversation between a large male probation officer in a wrinkled gray polyester suit and a skinny, young gangbanger wearing pants that were eight sizes too big and a red bandanna around his head. The contrast, with each wearing their unofficial uniform, was striking.

"The last couple of years, no, he never gave me any problem. Now when he was first assigned to me, he did. He skipped a lot of therapy sessions and missed his makeups. So I wrote him up and he had to go back to court. The judge told him that not going to therapy and missing his meetings with me could land him in jail." Velma paused for the punch line. "He cleaned up his act real fast. That boy did *not* want to go to jail."

"So I take it after that the two of you got along well," Randazzo said. She turned to look outside of Velma's cubicle and noticed the argument that was keeping Larson amused.

"Yeah. The only problems we ever had after that was when he'd start up with how he wasn't a criminal. He'd say things like he really didn't do anything the girl didn't want him to do. That kinda garbage. So I had to keep telling him, 'William, we're stuck with each other for a long time and it's going to be even longer if you gonna spend your time lying to me.' So he just sits there, pouting like a baby. 'No one wants to hear my side of the story,' he says to me. 'I'm telling you the truth. She was blackmailing me.'"

Velma rolled her eyes and the corners of her mouth turned up. "Like I never heard that one before. So, I stop him right there and tell him he pled guilty and that's the end of it. And then he says to me women shouldn't be allowed to judge him because we don't understand the temptations men have to deal with. He asks me how'd I'd like it if someone came into my house and paraded a plate of brownies in front of me every day—how long would it be before I just had to eat one? I tried telling him that the difference was my brownie didn't care if I ate it."

"Jeez. Did you talk with his therapist about this? That therapy wasn't working for him?" Larson asked.

"Velma!" It was the young kid with the bandanna, pleading with Velma for help. "Will you talk to this guy? He don't listen to me! He says he don't let no one come in here in colors. These ain't colors," he said, pulling on his clothes. "Velma, tell him, I ain't got no other clothes. You know." He had a heavy Mexican accent, which he seemed to exaggerate when talking to Velma about her Caucasian co-worker.

Velma got up, walked over, shaking her head. "Mario. What I tell you about staying out of trouble? Now you go down to the thrift shop"—Velma grabbed her purse and put a twenty-dollar bill in the boy's hand—"and pick up something nice. You get something that fits. I ain't gonna let you walk around in that either. What you doing comin' in here like that?" Velma threw her hands up in the air, frustrated, then came back with a two-minute barrage of Spanish that Randazzo and Larson did not understand—except for the tone. Velma's tirade made Mario noticeably shrink, and he nodded weakly as he slinked away, his pants dragging on the ground.

Velma sat back down and smiled at the detectives. "Just 'cause I'm off the gang detail doesn't mean I still can't kick 'em in the butt when they need it."

Larson and Randazzo laughed, intrigued by the different Velmas. They liked her. For a government employee she really seemed to care about what she was doing, and they weren't used to seeing this. "Looks like you're doing a good job," Randazzo said.

Velma visibly puffed up at the compliment. "I try. These kids need a mom."

"So going back to Matheson, did you think he was doing well in therapy?" Randazzo asked. Based on his views about women, it didn't seem so to Randazzo.

"No. He was just doing his time. You know, as my mama used to say, 'you can lead a horse to water, but you can't make him drink.' Just 'cause we make 'em go to therapy, doesn't mean they're gonna change," Velma said matter-of-factly. "It didn't help that they have a revolving door at Oakwood. You know, Matheson had three different counselors in five years. I didn't get the feeling any of them were making any progress with him. But you couldn't tell from the reports they'd write about him. Especially the last one. She made him sound like he was doing great. You can read it, I have it here." Velma got up and dug into the file cabinet behind her desk, pulling out a thick file. She opened the file, pulled out a one-page report, and handed it to Randazzo.

Randazzo looked it over, focusing on the glowing summary of Matheson's "great progress" at the end, then looked back up shaking her head. "Doesn't sound like they were talking about the same guy."

Velma gave Randazzo a knowing look, letting her know she just hit on an important point. "That's the problem with these guys—they're always trying to con you. I'm used to it, but I guess the counselors don't know they're getting snowed."

"But shouldn't they know?" Randazzo asked, stating what to her seemed to be obvious.

Velma shrugged. "It's really frustrating. I get these reports from them, just like that one on Matheson, and they go on about how great these guys are doing and how they've made such great progress. But I don't see this big change. They all sound the same at the end of probation as when they started. Seems to me that therapy's just a big waste of time." Velma shut the drawer on the file cabinet and turned around with a smile. "But no one ever asks my opinion."

Randazzo and Larson exchanged glances—apparently Velma shared their opinion of Oakwood. Randazzo checked her notes one last time, but it looked as if all her questions had been answered for now. "So is there anything else you can think of that might be helpful?" she asked.

Velma thought for a moment, looking off in the distance, slowly shaking her head as nothing more came to mind. "I can think of a lot of my guys that I would have expected to turn up dead before this one. I still can't believe it."

Randazzo stood up to leave. Larson was much slower as he tried to unravel his body. "Okay. Well, thank you for your time. If you think of something that might help us later, please give a call. Here's my number." Randazzo offered her a business card as she said to Larson, "Let's go, old man."

"So?" asked Larson as they walked out of Velma's building and onto the street. The wind the night before had left the sidewalk covered with newspapers and fast-food wrappers. Hearing the trash crunch under their feet as they walked to their car reminded Larson that this was as close as anyone ever got to autumn in Van Nuys.

"So what?"

"So we didn't learn anything we didn't already know," Larson complained. "What do you think?"

"I think that Matheson was an asshole."

"You didn't like Matheson's brownie analogy?" asked Larson.

"Not after having met the brownie." Randazzo shuddered.

When they reached the car, Randazzo started walking over to the passenger side. "I don't want to drive."

"Let's flip for it. Call it," Larson said as he threw a quarter in the air.

Randazzo seemed distracted. "No, you drive, I need to think."

While Larson readjusted the seat and then started to drive off, Randazzo kept staring at her notebook. She threw her head back when she realized what had been bothering her in the meeting. "Did you notice something?"

"No, what?"

"Well, unless I need glasses, that was not the woman who Saul Glassman saw at Matheson's apartment. Remember? He described the P.O. as leggy, blonde, and pretty and, no disrespect to Velma, but if you were gonna describe her, those are not words that immediately pop into your mind."

"So what does that mean? He must have misunderstood who the lady was, or maybe Matheson had more than one P.O."

"No, she said she had him from the beginning. So who would be snooping around there posing as his P.O.?"

Larson broke into a broad smile. "Good question. Nice catch, partner."

"All in a day's work," Randazzo said as she jotted a memo to herself to find the mystery P.O.

7

For the second time in as many nights, Elizabeth was greeted at the door by exotic aromas wafting out of her kitchen, a room not accustomed to such delicious excess. This time, it was garlic wallowing in lemon, olive oil competing with dill, and mint simmering over a moistened lamb. Another of Rebecca's great meals awaited. "Bec, you're spoiling me. I may never let you leave," she called toward the kitchen.

Rebecca came out to meet Elizabeth, looking tired but happy. She blew a few strands of hair off a flushed face. "Hey, I may never go. I'll tell you what, why don't you hire me to cook for you? That'll kill two birds with one stone—I won't have to deal with the office and you won't have to feel guilty about letting such a beautiful kitchen go to waste."

"Waste? Hey, if it weren't for the kitchen, I'd have no place to plug in my coffeemaker," Elizabeth said with a laugh. She walked into the living room, tossed her purse on the couch, then took off her overcoat and draped it across a chair. She picked up the stack of mail and quickly thumbed through it before tossing it all on the coffee table. "Just junk and bills."

"So how was work?" Rebecca asked, leaning up against the wall leading to the living room.

Elizabeth stood, stretching her back, trying to loosen the effects of a too-long drive home. She was a couple inches taller than her sister, about five ten, and a little thicker around the waist—courtesy of too many meals at places where fat and sugar were considered major food groups, but the Fielding genes came out in the fair coloring and good bones. "Fine, no emergencies," Elizabeth said. "How 'bout you? Did you spend the day on the phone with the office?"

"No, just a quick call for messages," Rebecca said proudly. She avoided mention of the dozen other work-related calls she did place. After all, Elizabeth had asked only about calls to the office.

Elizabeth's eyes narrowed suspiciously. "I'm not sure I believe you."

"You don't trust your own sister?" Rebecca said, her hand to her chest.

"Not really, but I guess it's good that you're at least paying lip service to taking it easy." Elizabeth headed upstairs to her bedroom to change her clothes, with Rebecca following behind. "Now if only I could convince you not to spend the rest of your vacation slaving away in my kitchen. You know, San Francisco has some of the best restaurants in the world. At least let me take you out tomorrow night for your farewell dinner."

Rebecca smiled and nodded. "It's a date."

"Don't get me wrong. It's not like I don't appreciate all your hard work. But I thought you came up for a rest. You look more ragged than when you got here." Elizabeth kicked off her shoes and peeled off layers of work clothes, leaving a trail of laundry in her path.

"Thanks a lot!" Rebecca exclaimed with a laugh. "I thought I looked pretty good. Besides, I'm having a great time. It's nice, quiet. I love having someone to cook for. And the best thing is, the phone doesn't ring with some idiotic defense attorney trying to sell me some deal. I like playing housewife. I could get used to it."

"Oh, you'd go crazy if you stayed home all day."

Rebecca lay down on Elizabeth's bed, sinking deep into the white down comforter. "I'm afraid I'm gonna go crazy if I stay at work much longer," she said finally.

"Boy, what happened to the days when—"

"When I loved my job? That was a long time ago," Rebecca said wearily. "When I still thought I could change the world."

"Yeah, those days. Why the change?" Elizabeth pulled on a pair of sweatpants, then fumbled in her drawer for a top.

Rebecca stared absentmindedly at the slowly swirling ceiling fan. "It's not any one thing. It's a lot of things over time. I don't really want to get into it, I wouldn't know where to start."

Elizabeth walked over and sat down at the edge of the bed. "C'mon, talk to me. I'm a doctor, remember?" Elizabeth looked over at Rebecca, hoping her professional credentials would do what their sibling relationship never quite accomplished—break down the communication barrier between them. Yesterday she could see Rebecca was troubled, and yet the whole night had been spent in superficial conversation. Now she sensed Rebecca was looking to open up, so Elizabeth gave her the chance. "So what's got you so down?"

Rebecca thought for a moment, searching for the right words. "It's just that place," she began at last, sighing heavily. "I've got to get out of there. I am so far beyond being burned out, it's incredible. I just don't know what to do." She grabbed a pillow and tucked it under her head then pulled it out, fluffed it up, then replaced it again, trying to find a comfortable position. "When I'm at work, I feel so powerless. Nothing I do makes a damn bit of difference. Take a look at what you do, you can help people. A kid gets sick, you give her a shot, *voilà*, she's better. Not me. By the time I meet someone, it's too late, the damage has been done."

Elizabeth looked at Rebecca with compassion. "I think you're too hard on yourself."

Rebecca couldn't get comfortable. She sat up suddenly, clutching the pillow on her lap. "No. I'm just being realistic. In a lot of ways, what I do just adds on another layer of pain. First they're victimized by their perpetrator, then they're victimized by the system I'm sworn to uphold. I don't know how I could have fooled myself for so long into believing that I was doing any good. You know that old saying, 'if you're not part of the solution, you're part of the problem'? Well, I finally realized that I'm not part of the solution, I'm part of the problem. And I'm just sick of it."

Elizabeth wished she had one of those magic shots right now to make it all better for her sister. "Bec, you're doing the best you can," she said, trying to sound comforting.

Rebecca looked hurt, as if the inadequacy of Elizabeth's words of support showed just how hopeless things were. She lowered her head, shaking it sadly. "I don't do shit. You should try sitting in court some day—it'd blow your mind. You get these judges who sit up there on their regal thrones, hiding behind their robes, babbling on about incest being a family problem." Rebecca threw her hands in the air in disgust. "Family problem! No, fighting over the remote is a family problem."

As she spoke, Rebecca's voice rose and was laced with anger and frustration. "I just don't understand how judges can continue to trivialize incest by giving the fathers probation instead of jail time. I don't see any reason why stranger rape should be punished more severely than familial rape. To me, it's worse when you're raped by someone you trusted and loved." She stopped and lowered her head, dejected. She dropped her voice back down. "But what's worse still is that there's nothing I can do or say that's ever going to change things."

"So what you're telling me is that you've never been happier?" Elizabeth asked, trying to lighten the mood.

Rebecca smiled, relieved to know she hadn't ruined the evening with her rantings and also relieved that both of them could still find humor in her situation. "Aren't you glad you asked?"

Actually, yes, Elizabeth thought. "It's okay. If you can't dump on me who can you dump on?"

"And that's another thing," Rebecca said, her voice sounding sadder, more resigned. "I have no one to vent to besides you. Sure, I can still call Tom, but afterward, I feel like an idiot for spilling my guts to him. He's got his own problems, and he doesn't need me dumping on him as well."

"Why would you call Tom, of all people?" Elizabeth hesitated, seeing Rebecca's reaction. Yet she had to speak her mind, even if it wasn't what Rebecca wanted to hear. "Rebecca, I just don't understand you. When relationships end and people say, 'we can still be friends,' nobody means it. You're the only woman I know who considers the person who strung her along and then dumped her to be her best friend. You're a lot more forgiving than I am. You need to lose his number and get on with your life."

"But he really is a good friend," Rebecca protested.

"Look, you know what I think of Tom," Elizabeth said flatly. She remained unconvinced.

"I know, I know. So let's change the subject." Rebecca replaced the pillow on the bed and laid back down. "I did get an interesting call today from a homicide detective."

"A detective called you? Here? How'd he get my number?"

Rebecca raised her hands palms up. "Don't know. Guess that's why they call them detectives. Anyway, he called about that guy I prosecuted a few years ago who was just killed. I told you about him, didn't I?"

"No . . . what did he want to talk to you about?"

"I guess just to get some more background on the guy. Easier than reading his file."

"Were you any help?"

"I suppose." Rebecca propelled herself off the bed. "C'mon, enough about work, let's go stuff ourselves."

"It's about time."

Elizabeth sat at the table, watching as Rebecca brought course after course of tonight's feast. "Are we expecting guests?" she kidded. The dining room table had been set with Elizabeth's formal china, antique white with the pale roses, and the good silver, on an off-white lace tablecloth. Rebecca had even found the matching linen napkins that Elizabeth had assumed were long gone. There was a bouquet of fresh flowers as the centerpiece, and Rebecca had even given up her penchant for rock music tonight, playing one of Elizabeth's classical music CDs instead. Elizabeth figured that Rebecca wouldn't be able to put up with this music for long, so she enjoyed it while she could.

Rebecca looked at the spread, a little embarrassed. "I never get a chance to cook at home, so I guess I got a little carried away. Sit, enjoy." Rebecca gestured for Elizabeth to take her seat at the head of the table and picked up Elizabeth's plate. Tonight she was serving as well. "So tell me, what about you? How come you seem so unhappy?"

"I'm not sure. I guess things are just kinda dull right now."

"Seeing anyone new?" Rebecca asked as she piled on the food.

"Not since you asked me last night."

"Oh."

Elizabeth looked a little melancholy as she set her plate down in front of her. She picked up her wineglass and looked at the light glimmering off the rosé. "I'm in the middle of a ships-passing-in-the-night spell. I'd like to settle into dock, as it were, but so far no luck. Lately, the women I've been meeting all seem intimidated by the fact that I'm a doctor. Half want me to make on-the-spot diagnoses of various maladies, and the other half entertain me with a five-minute lecture on the crisis in the health care system. But so far no one who wants to come home with me wants to stay."

"I'm sure it's just a phase. C'mon, Wendy only moved out a year ago. And you and she'd still be together if you weren't so stubborn about moving."

Elizabeth stopped in midbite. "She moved to fucking Kentucky. No job is important enough to make me move there."

"She did love that country music."

Elizabeth laughed softly, noticing the pang in her heart felt less acute tonight. "Enough about my stalled love life. What about you? When are you going to get back in the hunt?"

"Elizabeth, I'm not like you. I don't think I'm willing to risk being hurt again."

"And you're not willing to risk being loved either?"

Rebecca sighed, took her fork and pierced a piece of lettuce and a slice of tomato, then scooped up a chunk of feta cheese, before putting the mixture into her mouth. Elizabeth watched her, sipping a little wine, and waited for her to answer. "I gave my heart and soul to Tom, I opened up to him like to no one before or since, and where did it get me? The thought of becoming intimate with someone and exposing myself again is scary. So I just put up a wall that no one will try to climb over, and that way I'm protected from being hurt."

"Protected from being happy, too. Why do you have to assume the worst? Why not assume that you'll find someone and have a wonderful relationship?"

Rebecca kept playing with her salad, moving bits around, before finally taking another mouthful. Elizabeth sat patiently waiting for her to finish, not wanting to give Rebecca an excuse to avoid the subject. "It's easier to prepare for the worst. You save yourself a lot of pain."

"Stop saying 'you' when you mean 'me.'" Elizabeth was easily exasperated by Rebecca's cop-out. "Not everyone feels the way you do. Not everyone tries one time and then gives up if it isn't successful. You've gone way beyond 'once bitten, twice shy.' It doesn't make sense. You are a beautiful, intelligent woman who could probably have anyone she wants. Aren't blondes supposed to have more fun?" Elizabeth smiled. "All I know is you're throwing it all away for nothing. You can't give up because of one bad relationship."

"I haven't had just one relationship," Rebecca said with the defiant conviction of a five-year-old.

"Look, dating someone for a couple months in college doesn't count. You've really only been in one serious relationship and it turned out to be bad and now you've decided that relationships don't work and you're not even going to try. I'm no expert about relationships. But I do know that you're cheating yourself if you don't at least try. Mr. Right is out there somewhere just waiting for you to find him. I know it's not easy, nothing worthwhile is. Was law school easy? Did you quit when it got hard?"

"No," Rebecca said softly.

"So don't give up, okay?"

"I noticed you're doing a lot more talking than eating," Rebecca said, finally, pointing to Elizabeth's still full plate.

"Nice try," Elizabeth said as she picked up a phyllo triangle, the epicurean delight tasty enough to derail her lecturing for a moment. As she bit into the spinach-and-cheese filled pastry, she remembered something. "Didn't someone else you prosecuted also get killed recently? Oh, who was that?" Elizabeth wondered aloud, her mouth full.

"Now that's a pleasant subject for dinner conversation."

"I could go back to discussing your love life."

"Eric Penhall," Rebecca said quickly.

"What?"

"That's the other guy who was killed."

"No, I was thinking it was a Mac something." She popped the rest of the pastry in her mouth, giving out an involuntary "mmm" in appreciation.

"Mac? Oh, yeah, Henry MacDonald. That's who you're thinking of. But I never got to take him to trial. Remember when I had appendicitis? I'm out of the office for one week and Ralph lets that pig walk with just probation. But he wasn't a murder, it was suicide. He'd violated probation—he had tried to see his daughter—and we were going back to court to get him thrown in jail. Instead, Mr. MacDonald saved the good citizens of California the expense of incarcerating him." Rebecca took a bite of lamb and thought for a moment. "That's strange you should bring him up. I didn't realize I had mentioned him to you."

"Yeah, you said that it was one less piece of scum you had to worry about," Elizabeth said with a laugh.

Rebecca refilled her wineglass and took a sip. "I've always felt that I was the only one who thought these guys got off too easy. Maybe I wasn't alone after all."

"Apparently not. Three child molesters die within a few months of each other. Sounds fishy to me." Elizabeth reached for seconds. "So was the detective calling you to find out if you have an alibi?"

"Elizabeth!" Rebecca exclaimed. "That's ridiculous."

"Oh, c'mon. Think about it. Who hates these guys more than you?"

Rebecca got up suddenly and walked over to the CD player. She'd had as much culture as she could take for one night and replaced Beethoven with Bush. Maybe Elizabeth could learn to love alternative music, since Rebecca was no closer to embracing classical.

"You've been watching too many cop shops. They're just doing a thorough investigation, getting background information, that sort of thing," Rebecca said as she sat back down, the first notes from the fuzzy guitar running through her like a jolt of electricity.

"Okay, if you say so. Maybe I've lived up here too long, but I say don't trust the cops. With your reputation, it wouldn't surprise me if they're looking into you."

"Well, thanks for the vote of confidence. Remind me not to call you as a character witness."

"I'm sorry. I was just kidding. I didn't mean to get you all worked up."

"I know. Why don't we both just shut up and eat?"

Elizabeth raised her glass in a toast. That was something they could easily agree on.

8

The Saturday night crowd at The Night Watch was starting to thin out, even though there was still an hour till closing time. It was a favorite place for cops and courthouse denizens from the Westside to unwind before heading home and anyone else who wanted a relaxed, friendly place with a good selection of microbrews and an eclectic jukebox filled with tunes from Patsy Cline to Smashing Pumpkins. For Jack it had the added benefit of being only a five-dollar cab ride to his apartment, in the event he was in no condition to find the ignition.

"So, nothing going on tonight, Jack?" the bartender asked. Paunchy and balding, Joe, the bartender, enjoyed his post from behind the bar where he could make small talk with the regulars while watching total strangers form couples night after night. By now, Jack had usually made his love connection for the evening, but this night he was one of the few remaining loners.

"Nah, getting pretty quiet, Joe. One more and I'm

outta here." Jack looked around while Joe poured him another drink. Smoke hung in the air, casting a pale glow in the darkened room, and the roar earlier in the night had settled down to a dull hum of idle chat interrupted every now and then by the scattering of a new rack of pool balls.

Joe slipped Jack another 7&7. Jack figured that made about fifty-six by now, if his math was right. But after the third, he'd lost most of his faculties. "So, Joe, who's the pretty lady down on the end?" he asked, squinting through the fog.

"You know, I'm not really sure," Joe said as he rinsed off a wineglass and hung it overhead to dry. "I've seen her in here before with people from the D.A.'s office."

"I don't think I've ever had sex with a lawyer. What do you think it's like?" Jack slurred.

Joe leaned over to Jack, laughing. "I suppose it's either very good or you get sued."

"Yeah, I can see it now. 'Your honor, how was I supposed to know she wasn't done yet?'" Jack laughed, his eyes heavy-lidded.

"More like, 'Mr. Larson, on count one, assault with a dead weapon, guilty as charged.'" Joe grabbed the towel from his shoulder and cleaned off the bar as he laughed at his joke.

"Oh, very funny. So . . . she alone?"

"I don't know. She came in with a bunch of people, but I guess they all left. She must be waiting for you." Joe patted Jack on the arm with a "go get her."

"Here." Jack reached into his pocket and pulled out a twenty. "What's she drinking?"

"Chardonnay."

"Good, take her one, and tell her it's from the lonely detective on the end."

Jack watched as Diane Covington looked up, surprised by the offer. He waited for the smile and then, getting the signal, sauntered on over, taking a seat next to her.

"Hi. Diane Covington." A firm handshake, maybe a little too firm. "Thank you for the drink." She raised her glass.

"You're more than welcome." Jack tipped his head, then worried he wouldn't be able to straighten it.

She nodded toward the bartender. "So, Joe tells me you're a detective."

"Yup, I'm a dick." Jack grinned broadly.

"Aren't most men?" Diane said as she tried to stop herself from laughing.

Jack looked down, pretending to scan himself for blood. "Missed," he said proudly.

"Well, you left yourself wide open. What's a person to do?" Diane smiled apologetically, then reached over and gently squeezed his hand. "Sorry."

"You should be ashamed of yourself, attacking a defenseless man like that. By the way, I'm Jack Larson."

"You don't look defenseless," Covington quipped as she scanned Jack. "I'd offer to buy you a drink to make it up to you, but it looks like you're taken care of."

"Joe," he called to the bartender, "this pretty lady has offered to buy me a drink. Can I have another one?"

"No, you've had too many," Joe shouted back.

Jack turned back to look at Diane. "He says I can't have another one," he said incredulously.

"He's probably right, you know," she suggested. As she spoke, she took a long manicured finger and slowly circled the top of her glass with it. "You certainly can't drive home in that condition. You could get arrested. I'd hate to have to prosecute you." She dropped her head down so she could look up at Jack from under her eyebrows, the move perfected by Princess Di.

Jack was too drunk to do much flirting, hoping she'd take the fact he was struggling to remain vertical as a sign he was interested. "Joe said you might be a D.A.," he said.

"That is true," Diane nodded, her dark hair falling in layers around her angular face.

"Well, you'd go easy on me, wouldn't you? You'd explain to the judge what a nice guy I am, right?" Jack gave her the big smile, the killer one with both dimples.

Diane raised her eyebrows. "Are you?"

"The nicest, ask anyone. Hey, Joe, aren't I a nice guy?" he shouted across the bar.

"You're one in a million, Jack."

"See? And he doesn't say that just 'cause I carry a gun."

Diane smiled and fiddled with the heart-shaped pendant hanging around her neck. "Okay, you've convinced me. I'd tell the judge you're a prince and he should give you time off for good behavior."

"You know, though, my bad behavior is more fun."

Diane stroked the long stem of her wineglass slowly, suggestively, all with a slight smile on her face. "Oh, really. Is that what Mrs. Larson says?" An obvious ploy, but it was too late in the evening for anything too subtle.

"There is no Mrs. Larson. All I have at home to keep me warm is an old blanket and a bottle of scotch."

Covington turned to face Larson, her drink being ignored. "Not even a dog?" she asked with due concern.

Jack shook his head slowly. "Got run over by a car."

"What about a cat?"

"Allergic to them." Jack threw back the rest of his drink.

"This is so sad," Covington said, pretending to dab tears with her napkin.

"Isn't it though?" Jack sighed deeply. "Nope, it's just me." Jack placed his hand over Diane's and began rubbing it. She responded, moving her fingers to entwine Jack's and offering a seductive smile.

Diane leaned over and whispered in his ear. "I'll tell you what, if you promise to be nice, I'll give you a ride home."

"How nice?"

"Very nice."

"By nice, do you mean hands off?"

"Well, I think we've blown that," Diane said, looking at their knotted fingers.

"Then I think we have a deal."

The ride to Jack's place was quick and filled with some light banter, marginal double entendres, and a little adolescent groping. As they stood outside his apartment, Jack fumbled for his keys, wondering if he'd have as much trouble finding his dick. He needn't have worried. No sooner had the door closed than Diane started peeling him like a grape.

"I can get my own clothes off," he suggested.

Diane slowly removed Jack's belt, then started on his pants. "What fun would that be?"

Jack looked at her with mock suspicion. "You've done this before."

Diane smiled as she slid her hand between Jack's legs. "Now what makes you think that?"

He breathed deeply. "Just a guess." Jack reached out and started unbuttoning Diane's blouse as she slid out of her skirt. There would be no more conversation tonight.

He led her to his bedroom, his movements instinctive, and gently laid her down on the bed, kissing first the side of her neck, then her breasts. He felt her quiver with each kiss. Jack worked his way back up to Diane's ear, gently tugging at her lobe with his teeth, listening to her soft moans. Her legs parted, beckoning Jack as she slowly arched her back. He reached down and began rubbing her, exploring her, feeling her warmth. Diane's breathing quickened. She pulled his face to hers, kissed him feverishly, then reached down and brought him to her. He moved on top of Diane and slowly slid inside her.

Jack closed his eyes and smiled. Apparently he wasn't as drunk as he thought.

He awoke to the annoying sound of Diane's watch alarm. Jack sat up and looked over at the woman lying next to him slowly coming to, and wondered why it never got any easier knowing what to say the morning after, although, "Good morning, your name was . . . ?" clearly was not appropriate. After an awkward few minutes, Diane dressed and left, scribbling her number on a piece of paper before heading out. Jack went to take a shower, knowing that he would never call her, but surprised that for once he felt a fleeting pang of guilt.

"Ste-eve. Wake up. It's the truth fairy. Time to wake uh-up."

"What?" he mumbled sleepily. His eyes, half-open, scanned the darkened room, lit only by the amber glow from his clock radio. When he saw the figure standing at the foot of his bed, he was startled awake, realizing for the first time that when he'd gone to sleep, he was alone. He fumbled for his glasses, instead knocking them to the floor.

He reached down to try and find them but stopped short when he heard a sharp click as the gun's hammer was pulled back. The sound eerily pierced the quiet of the room and left Steve Jaffe paralyzed with fear. "Don't you just love that sound?"

The killer turned on the bedside lamp. "There, that's better, don't you think? It sort of sheds a little light on things."

As the killer paced back and forth, gun pointing at him, Steve struggled to speak. "What are you doing here? What do you want?" he asked, his voice filled with confusion and fear. He squinted toward the figure in front of him.

"I suppose, Steve, if you were the one with the gun, I might be more willing to answer your questions. Bu-ut, since I have the gun, I get to ask the questions. And, if you can believe this, I get to make the rules too. Now, then, rule number one is: you are to keep your mouth shut unless instructed otherwise. Do you understand?"

Steve nodded his head slowly.

"Good. Rule number two, I don't have to explain anything to you. It's late and I have to get up early and I'd rather if this didn't take all night. I could be home now, all tucked in nice and warm like you, but instead I have to come here and see you. So the least you could do is cooperate. Okay, let's get down to business. You wanted to know why I'm here? Why don't you take a guess?"

Steve remained silent, not sure what to do.

"Time's up. You lose."

Steve started shaking. "Is this some kinda joke? What's going on? Why are you doing this?" he cried, his voice booming with false bravado.

The killer stopped pacing and turned toward Steve, looking perplexed. "I'm sorry. Did I give you permission to talk? I don't think so. But to answer your impertinent question, Steve, no, this is not a joke. At least not a joke that you'll get."

The killer studied Steve for a moment—the wide-eyed stare and shallow, rapid breathing, the nervous twitches and contorted, silent mouth—and smiled broadly. "Personally, though, I think it's pretty damn funny. Especially when the sweat starts rolling down your face like that, and you don't know if you should brush it away, 'cause you don't want to make the wrong move, so it just stays on your face looking like a snail walked across you. Now that's funny. Anyway, you wanted to know what this is all about. Well, Steve, it's about your chickens coming to roost. Good chickens will do that, you know."

"What did I ever do to you?" Steve could almost feel the adrenaline pouring into his bloodstream.

"Why don't you think about it? But do it quickly, I don't have all night. And neither do you."

"You're crazy if you think you can get away with this."

"Well, let me look around. Nope. I don't see any-one who's going to stop me. Are you seeing things, Steve? Looks to me like it's just you and me, and I'm the one with the gun. So I've got this sneaking suspicion that I'm going to be able to get away with this."

"You're nuts." Steve looked around the room frantically, his chest heaving with every breath. "You really are."

"Maybe, but that's really not your concern." The killer paused. "You know, Steve, you're looking awfully nervous. This will all be a lot easier if you just settle down. Here, let's play a relaxation game to help you out. This is how it works. You lie perfectly still and the first place that moves, I'll shoot. Okay? Hope you don't get an itch."

Steve lay motionless, staring up at the barrel of the gun. He heard his clock tick off the seconds, each click louder than the last. He concentrated on slowing his breathing, staying as still as he could. As he lay there the gun stayed locked on him, the killer patiently waiting.

A fly buzzed around the room then landed on his

nose. Steve stared at it, immobile, struggling to keep from sneezing or brushing it away. His eyes stayed locked on the fly, willing it to get up and fly away and take the killer with it. Then, without thinking, Steve blinked.

The killer smiled. "Good choice."

9

All last week, it had seemed to Tom that Claire would pick a fight with him just as he was leaving for work. Usually it was his lack of ambition and stubborn refusal to get a better-paying job. Last Friday, however, was the topper. She cornered Tom at the door with tears filling her eyes and demanded to know when he had stopped loving her. Tom was half-tempted to give her the specific date, but he didn't think that would help matters. All he could think to do was continue out the door without answering her. He hoped that would end it. It didn't. She chased him out the door, screaming into the street, "How dare you walk out on me like that!" Tom grabbed Claire by the arms as firmly as he could, looked straight into her wild eyes, and, through gritted teeth, told her to go back inside and try to get a grip. It stopped her only for a moment. As he got into his car, she continued screaming, "Don't you dare drive away!" Tom knew better. He drove away.

Tom spent the weekend at the club—two pleasant days full of racquetball and basketball and no acrimony. He finally had to return home early Monday morning to pick up a suit for work. When he did, Claire apologized, as she always did after one of her episodes, blaming her hormones and joking that he must think that PMS stands for psychotic man-hating shrew. But Tom was long past being able to find the humor in her tirades, so he changed his clothes and headed to the office.

While more peaceful, the office always brought Tom a mix of pleasure and pain. Seeing Rebecca made him happy, yet it was also a painful reminder that but for his own stupidity, Claire would be driving some other poor schmuck crazy and he'd be sharing his morning coffee and newspaper with the only woman he ever truly loved. Oh well, life's a bitch and then you marry one, Tom thought with resignation.

He made an early visit to Rebecca, a combination welcome-back and are-we-still-friends, their last discussion having ended more acrimoniously than he had liked. He popped his head into Rebecca's office and saw her sitting behind her desk, looking rested and radiant in a cobalt blue Ann Taylor suit. "How was the vacation?"

Rebecca looked up from her desk, where she was just starting to wade through the paperwork that had stacked up since she'd left. "Too short. How was your weekend?"

"Too long," he groaned as he collapsed into a chair. He leaned forward and placed his coffee cup on her desk. He looked tired to Rebecca, the crow's-feet around his brown eyes appeared more prominent and his sandy brown hair moved from its usual tousled, if somewhat receding, state to flat-out unkempt.

"Claire?" she asked, knowing the answer.

"Who else?" Tom responded weakly. He quickly shifted the topic. "I did play racquetball with your buddy, Simpson. He told me that you gave him a hard time about Matheson."

"I gave him a hard time? Oh, give me a break," Rebecca exclaimed. "*Your* buddy," she intoned, "sympathizes too much with the people he prosecutes. That's not a good thing for a district attorney to do."

Tom shrugged, knowing Rebecca was right. "Well, just be careful what you say. I understand what you're trying to say, but some people could misinterpret you."

"I appreciate your concern." A smile crossed her face. "I guess then a 'Matheson's dead, let's have pizza' party wouldn't be a good idea?" Tom looked at Rebecca, unsure if she were kidding or not. "C'mon. Free beer. Pin the body part on the autopsy photos? It would be a blast."

Tom just rolled his eyes. "Hey, did Jack call you about Matheson?"

"Oh, so that's how he got the number," she said with a sly smile.

"You're not mad at me, are you?"

"No, that's okay. I'm not sure why he called me, though."

"Maybe he thought you might know something helpful." Tom grabbed a handful of M&M's from the jar on Rebecca's desk, picking out the brown ones first, leaving a brightly colored mix in his hand.

"Even if I did, do you think I'd tell him?"

"Huh?"

"Oh, yeah. Right. Like I'm gonna help him catch Matheson's killer," she said incredulously.

"Hunh. I guess it's a good thing you're not on the murder review committee. You'd probably refuse to file charges." Tom popped the rest of the M&M's in his mouth and followed them up with a black coffee chaser. "Now that's a good breakfast," he said, lifting his cup.

Rebecca ignored the joke. "You know, killing Matheson probably spared some girl having to be his next victim."

"You don't know that."

"Oh, please. These guys give recidivism a bad name. They should all get tattoos that read 'Have penis, will rape.'"

Obviously, she was not going to give an inch, so, as usual, it was up to Tom to call time out. "Look, it's too early in the morning for a fight. You know we never get anywhere debating this. Anyway, I've had enough hostility to last for a while."

Rebecca's face softened as she realized—too late as usual, she noted—that she was alienating the one person she actually considered a friend. "So what's going on with Claire?" she asked gently.

Tom sighed. "Who knows?"

"I'm sorry," Rebecca said. She fiddled with the papers on her desk, not knowing quite the right thing to say. A strained silence passed between them.

He took another sip then put his cup back down on Rebecca's desk. "I just don't understand her."

"Maybe you don't want to," Rebecca said, trying to be of help.

"Maybe she's too irrational to understand." Tom had long ago decided their problems were all Claire's fault and he wasn't up for discussing his contribution.

"I'm sure you guys can work it out." Rebecca had sworn to stay out of Tom's marital problems. She believed in the "you made your bed, now you sleep with her" theory of life. "If this is what married life is all about, then maybe being an old maid isn't so bad after all." Rebecca laughed halfheartedly.

"You're not an old maid. Some guy will be lucky to snap you up. He won't be a jerk like me and let you get away," Tom said.

Rebecca let his words hang in the air. This was unexpected candor from him in an area usually marked off-limits. And she especially liked the part about his being a jerk. "I think we better change subjects, okay?"

"You're probably right." Tom stood up to leave, grabbed his cup, and dropped another handful of M&M's in the coffee to melt. "I'm sorry. I don't want you mad at me too. How about I buy you lunch?"

"Not today. I've got a ton of work to catch up on. I promised myself I won't leave until I can see the top of my desk again. But I'll take a rain check."

Tom nodded. "You got it," he said and headed out of her office. Rebecca sat still, staring out the door long after Tom was gone, suddenly struck by their odd relationship, where Tom flaunted his wretched marriage in front of her as a balm to ease the pain of her own loneliness. She wondered fleetingly whether she'd ever stop needing Tom's misery and he'd ever stop needing to be miserable.

As Rebecca started going through her message slips, she saw one marked urgent—Detective Larson. She caught him as he was returning to the station. "Detective, this is Rebecca Fielding. I noticed a message from you when I got back to the office this morning and didn't know whether this was a new or old message."

"That must have been from last week. There's not much new since we last talked." Jack pulled out the bottom drawer to his desk, leaned back in his chair, and put his feet up on his instant footstool. "So how was San Francisco?"

"Good."

"That's it? Just 'good'?" Jack asked. "I don't think they're going to hire you to do tour promotions."

Rebecca smiled. "Unfortunately, five minutes back

in the office, and I can't even remember being on vacation."

"Yup, I know the feeling. Look, now that you're back in town, I would like to get some more details from you about Matheson, take a look at his case file, that sort of thing."

"Well, I'm here pretty late, so stop by whenever you'd like."

"I hate to discuss homicides on an empty stomach," he joked. "Can I buy you dinner and we can talk then?"

That sounded like a date to Rebecca. Her mouth went dry as she thought back to Elizabeth's comment about getting on with her life. Would saying yes count? She tried to speak, but her cotton mouth permitted only an "uhhh," which dropped off before she could finish with sure, yes, or any other affirmative response. Rebecca took a deep breath and let it out slowly and tried again. "That sounds great."

"How 'bout tomorrow?"

"Sure."

"Ever eaten at Chinois?"

"Not in a long time. But, you know, we don't have to go to such a nice place." With most of their entrées costing more than a small appliance, Rebecca tried to give Larson an easy out.

"Okay, Denny's it is," Jack said brightly.

Rebecca grinned. "Maybe I was being hasty."

"I knew you'd see it my way. Seven o'clock."

"See you then." Rebecca hung up the phone and found herself feeling like a high school girl who had just been asked to a dance. She was unaccustomed to feeling this happy at the office. Maybe the trip to Elizabeth's did some good after all.

✛   ✛   ✛

It was almost a full house for Monday night's group, their first session since Matheson's murder. The empty seat was a focal point for most eyes, almost like the child molesters' version of the missing man formation. Most of the men had called the clinic last week to find out more about what had happened and had been told that they would be updated at their next session. They were anxious to hear something comforting.

Valerie Kingsley entered abruptly and made a blunt announcement. "As you all know, Bill was killed last week after he returned home from group. The two detectives who are investigating the murder would like to speak with all of you. They're waiting outside, so let me bring them in. After they leave, we can conduct the remainder of the session." Valerie's tone of voice and blank expression made it clear she was not asking their permission to bring the police in but was merely informing them as a courtesy. She didn't wait for any questions but turned away quickly to bring in the detectives.

Some courtesy. The men fidgeted noticeably in their chairs, their anxiety level raised another notch. This clearly wasn't what they had in mind for tonight. The last thing any of them wanted to do was talk to the police. They hated the cops as much as they distrusted them and knew that the feeling was more than mutual—that on the evolutionary scale of criminals, child molesters failed to rise to the level of amoeba.

As Larson and Randazzo were led in by Valerie the temperature in the room seemed to spike up precipitously. The matter wasn't helped any by the sight of a female detective. Although the group felt the women at the clinic were pretty tolerant and understanding, most women "out there" seemed too irrational and militant to give child molesters a fair chance.

"Good evening. My name is Detective Larson and this is my partner, Detective Randazzo," Larson began, taking charge of the session. He cautiously sat down, careful not to touch anything. "As I'm sure you all heard, one of your group members, William Matheson, was killed last week. My partner and I are conducting the investigation and we have a few questions for you." Larson matched the men's discomfort, finding it difficult just being in the same room with them. He calmed himself by looking down at his notepad, the empty lines begging to be filled. There was not a sound in the room. He looked up, scanning the room. "First, did any of you see Mr. Matheson after last week's session?"

Eleven heads remained still, each group member wondering for the first time if he was a suspect. The only movement in the room was Randazzo's irritated foot tapping.

"None of you had any contact with Mr. Matheson after your session last week? Maybe grabbing a cup of coffee or something?"

Each eyed the other to see who might speak first. No volunteers tonight, just more throat clearing than the humidity level seemed to warrant. "Nobody?" he stressed.

There was no response from the group. Deafening silence enveloped the room as Valerie sat staring at each of her group members, her face hard, her arms crossed stiffly in front of her, in a display of supreme disappointment at their lack of cooperation.

Larson quickly realized that this approach was going to get him nowhere. "Ms. Kingsley, to save time, would you mind speaking with Detective Randazzo in another office? She has a few questions for you. I'll finish up in here." Valerie looked momentarily flustered before consenting hesitantly. She stood up and followed Randazzo out the door.

Randazzo was more than happy to get out of there. She felt the urge to get their attention with a few kicks to the groin. Better that she talk with Valerie and leave the deviants to Larson.

After the women left, Larson shifted mode. He leaned forward and scowled, dropping any pretense of affability. "Listen," he snarled, "I didn't come here for my health. You guys may have, but I didn't. We can either do this the easy way or I can drag each one of you down to the station."

His change of tone and his mere mention of "the station" caused the men to drop their pretense of uninterest. "Now, let's start over," Larson continued. "First, why don't we go around the room and each of you can give me your names. That way if I need to follow up with any of you, I don't have to tie up the whole group." After drawing an oval in his notepad and penciling in everyone's name, he began again. "Did any of you see Matheson after your meeting last week?" He looked around the room, and every eye avoided his.

"None of you ever got together after your sessions, to hang out, bullshit a little, nothing like that? Oh, come on." Larson was clearly annoyed. "Who here ever talked to Matheson outside of this place?"

Larry sat forward, 250 pounds focused directly on Larson. "Look, you can't make us talk to you."

Larson grinned, as if amused that anyone would seek to take him on. "That's right, I can't. But I can sure make you wish you had. Now, is there anything else you want to add, smart-ass?"

Larry leaned back in his chair. "Why do all cops think they own the world?" he mumbled under his breath, a little too loudly.

"Maybe you didn't understand me," Larson challenged.

Larry sat back up. "And maybe you don't understand me," he countered brazenly, suddenly emboldened by the strength-in-numbers adage. "We don't
have anything to say to you."

Larson did not share Larry's belief in the distribu-
tion of power. "I'll tell you what I do understand,
big mouth. I understand that you're not man
enough to fuck someone your own age. Now if you
don't shut your mouth, I'll be happy to shut it for
you," he said matter-of-factly, putting an end to any
further show of bravado.

"This isn't getting anywhere," Ray chimed in, taking on the role of mediator. One thing Ray, a tall,
thin man with round wire-rimmed glasses, hated
was confrontation. One thing he liked was pre-
pubescent girls, a significant problem for a sixth-
grade teacher. "I spoke with him sometimes outside
of group, just to shoot the breeze. He liked to hear
himself talk. It was just bullshit, nothing important."

"Yeah, same with me," Roberto interjected, assuming the quickest way to end this was to give the
detective something. "Nothing heavy, like Ray said.
Mostly Bill'd be crabbin' about something. Sometimes he'd talk about tryin' to get laid, how hard it
was to get any when you're broke. I could relate," he
added with a knowing snort, cut short by Larson's
irritated glare.

"Did he seem to change recently? Did anything
seem to be on his mind, some new problem?" Larson
asked.

"No. In fact, he seemed pretty happy. He was
counting down the days until he was off probation,
calling himself a short-timer and talking about how
great it was going to be to have Monday nights free
to watch football," answered Ray.

Frank leaned forward and cleared his throat, signaling his entrée into the conversation. "You know,

Detective, far be it from me to gossip"—Frank ignored the chortling coming from Larry's direction—"but Bill was in a pile of shit during last week's session. Kingsley was all over him like a cheap suit, giving him a real hard time about screwing up that family session she'd set up. But then, as usual, she just let him get away with his bullshit 'I'm sorry, Valerie' and he tap-danced right out of trouble. So when he turned up dead, it was, like, cosmic. Here he'd left here so cocky and smug, then wham! Instant karma slapped him right in the head."

Jack looked at Frank, not sure what to make of him, with his exaggerated flouncy gestures and pronounced lisp. Jack couldn't tell if his overstated foppishness was an act or not. "Well, uh, instant karma certainly is an interesting theory, Frank," Larson said as he turned toward the other group members, still trying to pull something useful out of them. "So, did Matheson mention anyone outside of the group he was having problems with? A new girlfriend with an angry husband, someone he'd pissed off at work, anything like that?"

"Not that I'd ever heard of," answered Ray, shaking his head and looking around the room for agreement. Shrugged shoulders and bored looks were exchanged.

"I can't imagine anyone having anything to do with him. He was more of a prick than a porcupine in heat," Frank said as he smiled at Larson.

"Yeah, you wish he was," Larry sneered. "Oh, I forgot. It's the little pricks you prefer."

Before Frank could respond, Ray put his hands up and interjected, "Enough, gentlemen, please," his voice filled with exasperation over the unseemly display.

"Frank, you were saying?" said Larson, irritated with the adolescent sniping.

Frank looked disdainfully at Larry before cocking

his head toward Larson. "Bill was a major attitude problem around here. As you can see, we have a few of them." Frank smiled at Larson, oblivious to the dirty looks sent his way from the guys in the group. "Anyway, you're not gonna see me shed any tears over him."

"Was he enough of a jerk for someone to want to kill him?"

Frank threw his hands palms up and shrugged with an exaggerated gesture. "Who's to say? I'm not saying he deserved to die, or anything like that," Frank said. "He was just another asshole in group. Now he's dead. Big fucking deal. Life goes on."

Larson still couldn't tell if Frank was for real or not. He made a note to pull his case file, it was sure to be delightful reading. "I see a handful of guys doing all the talking and the rest of you sitting there not saying shit. What about the rest of you? You guys are supposed to share all your most personal crap in here. You mean to tell me Matheson never mentioned anything about any fights with anyone, anyone he was worried about, anyone he owed money to, nothing like that?"

One of the group members called out, "The only thing Bill ever shared was his odor," and the group erupted in laughter. When it subsided, Frank spoke up. "Sorry, Detective, that sharing crap is all TV. Here, we say a few of the buzz words, get our little gold star for the day, and then go on our merry way."

Larson was surprised at the admission. Apparently Velma was right and Hillerman's version of the Oakwood existed only in its shiny brochure.

Ray shifted forward in his chair. "Yeah, really, the only thing we ever heard about was that meeting with the ex. The one Kingsley got on him about. That's why I figured it had to be the ex—seems he'd really pissed her off."

"Obviously Ray was wrong, right, Detective?" Frank said proudly. "I mean, if it was his ex you wouldn't be here. She'd already be arrested, case closed. So you must think it has something to do with us." Frank started rubbing his chin with his thumb and index finger. "Now who here could have done it?" Frank looked around the group and then back at Larson. "That's what you're wondering, isn't it, Detective?"

Larson figured that this wasn't going anywhere and he didn't want to engage in a question-and-answer session with Frank, so he stood up to leave. "Well, I'd like to say it's been fun. You guys are really something else. One of your own gets killed after leaving here, and none of you has anything worthwhile to offer?" He really didn't expect a response. "Well, if there is anything else you can think of, you can reach me at the East Valley station. I'll leave some business cards on the table over by the door." As he walked out, Larson resisted the temptation to coldcock Larry. Instead, he merely leaned over and whispered in his ear, "If nothing else, I learned that I don't like you—and you shouldn't consider that a good thing."

"I need a shower," Larson said to Randazzo as they walked out of Oakwood.

"Too much for you?"

"You said it. I mean, they all look normal enough. Walking down the street you could pass any of them and not know. But they sure as hell give me the creeps. They're like regular guys, with this disgusting little secret."

"I know what you mean," Randazzo agreed. "I was so glad to get out of there. I don't know how their therapists can stand being in the same room with them. Kingsley gave me the rundown on the group. She said they were just 'garden variety' child molesters."

Larson hurried down the stairs, eager to get a little distance from the place. "Just be glad you didn't have to sit in the middle of the garden. It made me wish I had a Weedwacker."

Randazzo laughed. "Yeah, but I had to spend my time with Miss Bleeding Heart, hearing a replay of Hillerman's speech about all the wonderful work that they do at the Oakwood. She's a big fan of therapy and how it can solve all the world's ills. Apparently she comes from a long line of shrinks —her father's some big-shot child psychiatrist—and I guess she's got this help-your-fellow-man stuff in her blood."

Larson stopped at the bottom step and turned to Randazzo. "You're the psych major, didn't you once believe in better living through psychotherapy?"

"I may have studied psychology, but at least I got out before it was too late and I was brainwashed like the rest of them. Counseling is not the answer to all problems. Some people are just beyond therapy. And no question in my mind, pedophiles are in that group. Chemical castration I can see, but talking therapy, forget it." Randazzo shook her head. "I just don't know how she can do it."

"I guess you get used to it."

"I don't see how. I never could." Randazzo felt a shiver of repulsion. "I'll tell you one thing, sitting there looking at those guys all I could think was it was sure a shame that God saw fit to trust them with a penis."

"How did the meeting go with the police?" Hillerman asked from behind his desk. Valerie paced nervously in front of him till she picked up his signal to take her seat.

"Fine, I guess." She sat down across from him and began to pick at her nail polish, avoiding his gaze.

Hillerman raised his eyebrow. "You guess?"

"Well, the men were a little hesitant to talk in front of me, so the detectives suggested I step out and—"

"You left the men in there alone with the detectives?" The edge in his voice was clearly recognizable to Valerie. "I specifically told you to monitor everything that was said to the police. Why do you think I prepared you all morning?" Hillerman stormed.

"I'm sorry, Dr. Hillerman, I didn't think there would be a problem," Valerie said defensively. She looked away, focusing on a point over his shoulder, the gold seal on one of his diplomas.

"You didn't think there would be a problem?" he scoffed.

Valerie glanced at Hillerman and saw that vein pop out on his head again, the blue line flagging his ire with impeccable accuracy. She swallowed hard, not having enough saliva to send down. "Well, no, Dr. Hillerman. I think I know my guys pretty well, and they have no interest in telling anything to the police. I checked with them afterward. They told me nothing happened." She tried to keep her voice steady as she spoke, belying her fear.

Hillerman studied her for a moment. "You'd better be right. I have come too far and worked far too long to lose everything. This is a crucial juncture in the center's future. Do you understand?"

Valerie could feel her heart pounding against her chest with the full knowledge that she was coming dangerously close to being fired. "I do, Dr. Hillerman," she said evenly. "You can't possibly doubt my commitment to the clinic."

Hillerman got up and walked over to where Valerie sat, put his hand up and cupped her cheek. He flashed a disarming smile, and Valerie visibly relaxed. "Good. That's what I like to hear."

10

Jack avoided the valet and parked around the corner. Aside from saving $3.50, he got the pleasure of walking down Main Street in Santa Monica and perusing its eclectic antique stores and elitist art galleries. He arrived at Chinois before Rebecca did. Punctuality ordinarily wasn't his strong suit, but he wanted to get at least one drink in him before she arrived. For an old pro, he was surprisingly nervous. It was technically a working dinner, but his pulse told him it might be more.

He had just started to relax, a few rushed gulps helping the process, when he spotted Rebecca walk in. She was drop-dead gorgeous in a simple black dress, fitted to her small waist and flared out just above the knee. She wore no jewelry, and yet she seemed to sparkle. Jack didn't know where to stare first, but her walk from the door to the bar gave him the time to decide.

He hopped down off his stool as Rebecca extended her hand. "Detective, nice to officially meet you," she said. She had a firm grip for someone with such soft skin and delicate hands. "After hearing Tom talk about you for years, I feel as if I know you already."

"It's nice to meet you too." Jack, an incorrigible Boy Scout, pulled out a stool for her then sat back down. The bartender came over to take Rebecca's order—Chardonnay—which left Jack wondering if that was the official bar drink for women. "Actually, you probably don't remember, but I met you a couple times back when you and Tom were dating. In fact, weren't you at his big birthday bash?"

"Yeah. I didn't realize you remembered me from there." Rebecca tilted her head as she spoke, the lights from behind the bar shimmering on her hair as it moved. The bartender returned with her drink before they even realized he had gone.

"How could I forget?" Jack said, flashing a rakish smile. Rebecca took a quick sip as she looked away a little shyly, then pondered the aquarium behind the bar.

The hostess broke Rebecca's embarrassed silence with a "We can seat you now," and escorted them to a small black marble table along the wall so that they could hear each other over the din of the restaurant.

Once seated, Rebecca set her menu unopened on the table and looked across at Jack. "You and Tom go back quite a ways, don't you?"

"Yep. We went through the academy together. Boy, were we young," Jack said with a melancholy grin as he cradled his V.O. and 7, tonight's version of his usual drink. "You know, Tom was my first partner. I'm sure you know the rest of the story."

"Not really. Tom never liked to talk about his time on the force. And I never wanted to push."

"Well, it was brief, but it was ugly." Jack quickly finished the rest of his drink. "We'd only been out of the academy a couple of months. Real wet behind the ears. We got a call, domestic disturbance. When we get there, the guy is threatening his wife with a butcher knife, she's screaming, the kids are crying, his mother's hollering her head off. Too much commotion. Tom thinks he can reason with the husband, starts moving toward him, you know, 'Give me the knife, let's work this out,' while I move the rest of the family away. Suddenly the guy charges at Tom. Tom froze, I guess he didn't want to shoot 'cause the rest of the family was watching or was too close. I don't know. He never told me. Anyhow, the guy lunges at him with the knife, misses his heart by a hair. Not that I knew that at the time—I thought for sure he was dead. I turn around, see Tom falling, blood spurting, and the husband coming toward me. I emptied my revolver into him."

Jack paused, fidgeting with his empty glass, spinning the ice around in circles. Rebecca looked at him earnestly, seeing how hard this was for him even now.

Jack shook his head at the memory. "It was bizarre. There I was, trying to give Tom CPR and the guy's wife is pummeling me for shooting her husband. It was a nightmare. Anyway, Tom was never one hundred percent after that. I think he wondered whether he could shoot if he had to. The department switched him to desk duties. Well, I wasn't going to let him become some desk jockey, feeling sorry for himself and drinking himself to an early grave. He'd always talked about going to law school, so I called his bluff. I picked up an application for him and told him to fill it out. The rest you know. It seems to have worked out pretty well for him. I don't think he misses being a cop."

"Yeah, he seems pretty happy at the D.A.'s office," Rebecca offered.

"But not so happy at home," Jack said, not as a

question but a statement of fact. "I know this is none of my business. And I know Tom's a big boy who can make his own decisions. But, for the record, I never understood why he married Miss Clarabel."

"Ooh, not a big fan of Mrs. Baldwin?" She and Jack already had something in common.

"Not really. I can't remember the last time she let him go to a game or play poker or meet me for a drink. It's like she's determined not to let him have any fun. But, then, it's his life, right? I should just keep my nose out of it."

"No, you're just being a good friend. I think that's sweet." Rebecca cocked her head and smiled at Jack, then picked up her wineglass and studied it for a moment before her smile slowly faded. She sighed, then took another sip. "Unfortunately, it's too late for any of us to save Tom from his own mistakes."

The arrival of the black-clad waiter broke Rebecca's melancholy, moving her focus to the more pleasant—though difficult—task of choosing among many inviting items on the varied, quasi-Asian, quasi-French, all-enticing menu. After some great indecision, she settled on lobster tempura as her appetizer and Szechuan beef for a main course. As the words left her mouth, Rebecca could have kicked herself. She'd become a stereotype, the girl who orders lobster on the first date—assuming this was a date, that is. Rebecca considered changing her order, but her taste buds won the battle for her soul. Jack, knowing his bank account wouldn't allow for another visit here all year, was similarly vexed by having to choose among all of the culinary wonders that Chinois had to offer. He decided on the yellowtail sashimi and the fried catfish, two items as far from his usual burger fare as he could find. That job completed, they relaxed, and Jack poured Rebecca a room-temperature Pellegrino.

Rebecca, remembering the ostensible reason for the dinner, said, "I brought this," as she handed Jack a large envelope. "I had our file on Matheson copied for you. I looked it over this afternoon and I did notice something I had forgotten to mention. Matheson's prior girlfriend had filed a complaint against him when they were dating, claiming that he had fondled her ten-year-old daughter. The charges were dropped for insufficient evidence. I had interviewed the girlfriend and she had agreed to testify at our case, but the judge excluded her testimony. Her name's in the file along with her statement to me."

"So this wasn't a one-time deal with the guy? Sounds like he would have done it again."

"Well, that's not a concern anymore," Rebecca said. A little too brightly, Jack thought. "So, do you have any idea who may have killed him?" she asked.

"Not really. I have some suspicions. The press is sure playing up the vigilante angle because another child molester was killed just a few weeks ago. But right now, I'd say Ann or Laurie is the most logical suspect, although we have nothing tying them to the scene. You must have spent a lot of time with them at the time of the trial. Would you say either was capable of murder?"

"Aren't you assuming something?" Rebecca asked. "What?"

"Well, if they killed Matheson, who's to say it was murder? How 'bout justifiable homicide?"

Jack was caught off guard and pondered the question. "I guess what you're asking is whether molesting Laurie gives them the right to kill him?"

Rebecca looked around the dimly lit restaurant at the small tables—some crammed with businessmen on power dinners, others where couples engaged in light conversation. She watched the waiters maneuver effortlessly around the tables, through the narrow maze leading to the open kitchen in the back, and sighed. She doubted any of them would understand what she was about to say. Would Jack? she wondered. "Well, that's not entirely the question. He did more than molest her. Have you ever looked up the word *molest* in the dictionary? It means 'to annoy.' When a man sexually abuses a child, he's not being annoying. He's a rapist. How are we ever going to take the crime seriously if we describe it with euphemisms?"

Jack smiled. "I noticed you didn't answer my question."

No skating around with this one, Rebecca thought. She shifted forward in her seat, resting her arms on the table. "Okay. I think parents have a right—no, a duty—to kill the man who rapes their child. Parents are supposed to protect their children. If Ann had killed Matheson, it could have been her way of apologizing to Laurie for not believing in her sooner. It would have been a way to say 'this is what he deserved all along.' I would applaud that as justifiable homicide. It's certainly not murder in my book." Rebecca paused for a beat, then quipped, "Does that answer the question?"

The waiter hid well the fact that he'd been standing there for minutes. Now that Rebecca had finally come up for air, he quickly served the appetizers and departed. Unobtrusive but efficient service was clearly going to be the key to a large tip this evening.

"So you condone killing child molesters?" Jack asked, more amused by Rebecca's tirade than put off. He felt a little guilty as he thought, *She's cute when she gets all worked up.*

"Yes. And not just by the parents either. I can truly understand if a victim wanted to strike back at her abuser. It's not like victims can look to the courts to get justice anymore."

Jack started in on his appetizer, spearing a piece of sashimi with one chopstick rather than using both to pick it up. Why risk dropping food in his lap? He wondered why everyone didn't just use one chopstick—two seemed unnecessarily difficult. "I know what you're saying, and my partner would say that you and I think alike. But, I've got to tell you, as a cop, vigilantism is not something I want to deal with. We need people to trust the system."

"I hate to sound like I'm on a soapbox"—even though I am, Rebecca thought to herself—"but I'm not so sure the system deserves our trust anymore." She leaned forward as she spoke. "Look at how inadequately we punish child molesters. They do so little time and yet they do such great damage—permanent damage. Maybe I wouldn't be so intrigued by someone taking justice into their own hands if I knew the system was prepared to lock child molesters away for good. But that's never going to happen. Now," she said, emphasizing her point with a piece of tempura broccoli trapped between two chopsticks, as if to show Jack how it was done, "they had the right idea in Washington."

"What's that?"

"A state with lots of rain. But that's not important," Rebecca deadpanned.

"Very funny, you know what I mean."

Rebecca smiled, a little embarrassed by how intense the conversation had turned. She didn't want to turn Jack off, yet he seemed genuinely interested in what she had to say—something she was unaccustomed to. "Sorry, I thought I was getting too serious for you. I noticed you weren't eating much, so I figured it must be the topic."

Jack couldn't tell Rebecca that the real reason for his distraction was he'd been trying to figure out if her sparkling eyes were gray, green, or hazel because their color changed as the candle on their table flickered. "No, I want to hear what you have to say. It's nice when people believe in something so strongly. I'm always envious of people like that. I've never really been able to develop a strong passion for any one particular thing."

"Maybe you're better off that way. Passions can make you crazy."

"Or make you very happy," Jack said, dipping his sashimi into the fiery wasabi. "So tell me about Washington."

"It was the first state that tried locking up sex offenders and throwing away the keys, even beyond their sentence."

"How'd they do that?" he asked between a string of gasps as the hot horseradish started burning his throat.

"Take it easy, that stuff'll kill you."

"Thanks for the warning," he managed between coughs and useless gulps of water. "I'm fine, really. You were saying?" he finally choked out.

Rebecca laughed as Jack struggled to regain his composure. "You'll signal if you need CPR, right?" Jack nodded. Rebecca smiled to herself—he looked so helpless and vulnerable, the big cop brought down by a little green dollop. "Okay, in Washington they passed a law so that you could keep a sex offender in prison even after he'd served his sentence if it was likely he would offend again. It's called the sexual predator law. It wasn't perfect—it only applied to repeat, violent offenders, so the typical incest offender couldn't be held under the law—but it was definitely a good start."

"Didn't we pass a similar law here last year?"

"Yep. That's the one. It was first enacted in Washington after this guy, who'd been arrested, jailed, and released repeatedly, molested and then killed a little boy. The belief is that if you can't cure sexual offenders—and you can't—then the only reasonable solution is to keep them segregated from society. It made sense to me."

"But if we have the same law here, you should be happy," Jack said. The fire had subsided and his voice was once again strong, although his pride was somewhat damaged.

Rebecca looked more resigned than happy. "It didn't last in Washington, and I'm not confident it'll last here. In the long run, laws like that get shot down. You get all these ACLU lawyers and the defense bar wrapping themselves in the Constitution and carrying on about the rights of the accused. They had the Washington law overturned as unconstitutional, and already judges here have been refusing to enforce it on the same grounds. It's probably just a matter of time before it gets thrown out here as well. Evidently, it's okay to deprive the victims of their right to be safe from rapists, but God forbid we set a finger on the rights of the rapist."

"You don't have to tell me. I deal with that every day. It's almost funny to see criminals who don't even know who the president is spout off about their constitutional rights," Jack said, shaking his head. "So how's your tempura?"

"Terrific."

"You know, if you don't overdo it on the hot stuff, the sashimi is great. Here, try some."

Rebecca offered Jack a bite of lobster and then had what looked like a religious experience with a slice of his sashimi. "Fantastic. The food here is just incredible. I was surprised you knew about it. I thought you guys ate only hamburgers and donuts."

"Not a bad idea. We'll do that next time."

Next time? Well, my diatribe apparently didn't

scare him away, she thought. Rebecca felt an unexpected excitement rush over her as her cheeks
flushed red.

Jack stared at Rebecca, pondering her with a
quizzical look on his face. "So let me get this straight.
You, as a district attorney, actually believe that the
courts should condone murder for revenge?"

"Well, no more than the courts should condone
incest for sport." Rebecca winced inwardly as soon
as she had said it. Jack deserved better than a quick
comeback. "I'm sorry, but until the courts take this
crime seriously, I'm not sure that we can blame victims for reacting out of anger and frustration."

Larson let her words sink in, trying to better
understand the person who spoke them. "You must
have been angry as hell that Matheson didn't do any
time," he said finally.

"You're damned right, I was." Her answer came
fast, laden with the memory of the years-old anger.
Then, her face softened, as did her tone. Resignation
replaced the anger. "I was young and naive back
then."

"So why do you still do it?"

Rebecca had answered that question dozens of
times and never felt comfortable with the answer. The
real answer was that she had to, but she gave him the
answer that was easier to hear. "Better me than someone who doesn't care about the kids, right? At least
the kids I represent leave knowing that they weren't
just some case on the docket, but that someone took
the time to listen and to be there for them."

"But it must get frustrating."

"I'd be lying if I said it wasn't," Rebecca said, a little sad.

Jack offered a supportive smile. "I think the kids
are lucky to have you in their corner."

Rebecca thought that was about the nicest thing

anyone had said to her about her work and yet felt unworthy of the compliment. "I just wish I could do more." She took a long sip of water and shifted in her seat. "What about you? Why did you become a cop?"

Jack spotted the waiter, picked up his empty glass, and motioned for a refill. "Maybe I watched one too many cop shows when I was growing up. The police were still the guys in the white hats back then, catching the bad guys and helping keep the streets safe. Who wouldn't want to do that? But now, I'm not so sure. Too many people think we're the enemy."

"Do you think you'll take early retirement?"

"I don't think so. What would I do, move to Idaho and run a bar? I'd end up drinking all the profits, I'd be so bored. And I can't imagine doing anything else for a living. I can't picture ever having a nine-to-five job like my old man. My ex wanted me to do that, something safe and dependable. I just couldn't do it. I needed the freedom."

"You were married?" Rebecca tried to say it nonchalantly, but it came out sounding as if she were taking his deposition.

It was a good time for Jack's refill to appear, the waiter moving in so smoothly that the glass seemed to place itself down on the napkin. "Yeah. We were young, just out of high school. I think she was looking for the picket fence and dinner for six at six and I wasn't ready for that." The busboy came over and swiftly whisked away the empty appetizer plates. "What about you? Ever tied the knot?"

"Nope. I've managed to avoid marriage altogether so far. You must have read about it, the women's movement? I bought it. Get the degree, get the job, don't wait for Prince Charming to come along on his white horse. Then suddenly I look around and all my friends are saying, oops, maybe we were wrong. I've never been to so many weddings and baby showers as in the last couple of years."

"Well, at least you've still got time. If I don't get started soon, I'm gonna be collecting my pension before my kids are out of diapers. Heck, if I wait too much longer, we can be in diapers at the same time," Jack quipped.

Rebecca smiled at the thought. She and Jack sat quietly for a minute, both seemingly drained of conversation. They stared at each other, wondering whether this was still a business meeting. The waiter moved in and laid in front of them two large black platters decorated with splashes of reds and greens. Rebecca was startled when she looked down to find Jack's catfish staring straight at her. "Could you move that?"

"Move what?"

"That!" Rebecca said, gesturing wildly at the fish—only partially for effect. "It's staring at me."

"And for good reason." After Jack stopped laughing, he gladly obliged. He didn't want the dinner ruined by some leering fish. "You know, I've never had my dinner offend anyone before."

"How often does your dinner have eyes and whiskers?"

"Good point."

They shared a smile, then many more, before the night was done.

11

Randazzo came in early to organize her desk, messages to be returned on one side, files of open cases stacked on the other side, and a brand-new notepad in the middle. Despite her fellow officers' excessive kidding about her meticulous organization, Randazzo saw no reason to join the ranks of the scattered and confused, as she called them. As she sat back to admire her handiwork, Larson strolled in and sat down behind a cluttered mountain of paper. He sat humming and grinning slightly, flipping through his mail, pretending not to notice Randazzo. She watched him and waited until she couldn't stand it anymore.

"Okay, who was she? Or should I ask, how was she?"

He looked aghast. "Ms. Randazzo, where are your manners?"

"C'mon, the bird feather is practically dangling from your lips. So go ahead, tell me all about it." Randazzo leaned back, waiting for the details.

Larson smiled noncommittally, then stood up

without answering and walked down the hall to get his morning coffee. Randazzo trailed him like a bloodhound, on the scent of her prey. "All right," he said, having made her wait long enough, "little Miss Nosy, if you must know, I took the stunning Ms. Fielding to dinner last night."

"And how did she enjoy her hot dog?" she said sarcastically.

"Oh no, my dear. We ate at Chinois, followed by lattes at Starbucks and a leisurely stroll down Ocean Avenue. And to answer your next question, yes, I paid."

Randazzo's jaw dropped. "You had a date, and an expensive one at that, with Rebecca Fielding?" She was stunned that Larson would buy dinner for a woman whose IQ was larger than her bra size.

"Well, yes and no." He filled his cup and headed back to his desk, Randazzo following close on his heels, lest she miss anything good. "It was supposed to be a working dinner. She was going to give me more information about Matheson, but I thought I'd take the opportunity to—"

"Get laid?"

"Is that all you think I'm interested in?"

Randazzo's facial expression roughly translated to "Oh, please, I know that's all you're interested in."

Larson sat back down and propped his size elevens up on his desk, knocking his cup enough to leave yet another coffee ring on his desk. "Well, you're wrong," he said, taking a leisurely sip of coffee.

"No, I'm not." Randazzo rolled her chair over to his desk. "So, did you do it?"

"No. We just had a very enjoyable evening."

"That's it?"

"That's it."

She squinted in disbelief. Perhaps aliens had

taken over Jack's body during the night. "You didn't do it?"

"Sorry, not even a peck on the cheek. I'm a gentleman."

Now Randazzo knew this wasn't Jack Larson. "Since when?"

"Since about ten o'clock last night." Jack dropped his feet back on the ground and sat back up, pulling a piece of paper from out of the breast pocket of his gray serge jacket. "I did, however, get us a little more background on Matheson. Turns out he had tried to molest a girlfriend's daughter a few years before he molested Laurie. So we need to check out the ex-girlfriend."

Randazzo took the piece of paper and pushed herself back to her desk. She pulled open the Matheson file and put Larson's notes in their proper place. "Great, so instead of narrowing down the list of suspects, you've increased it, and with someone rather remote at that."

"So what have you been up to today?" he said matter-of-factly.

"Getting the forensic reports from the lab. The fibers recovered from Matheson's door are from hundred percent virgin wool, dyed navy blue, common in both men's and ladies' jackets. Some partial shoe prints in the carpet leading out the door—I don't know how useful they'll be, but I've sent them off to the FBI. Maybe they'll see something. We've got a few hairs, long and blonde—natural hair, but that doesn't tell us much. Could still be from a wig—we didn't get any roots. We also recovered some short brown ones. The bullets were all hollow nosed. They were distorted by the trip through Mr. Matheson, so no ballistics, but the lab was able to identify them as .22 caliber. All the blood at the scene belonged to the deceased."

"So, in other words, we're no further along."

"Right." Randazzo looked down at her notes. "Oh, and there was a latent palm print on the outside of the door. Not enough to run, though. It doesn't match Matheson or the apartment manager. But there's no way of telling how old the print is."

"It's better than nothing. If we get close to someone, the print might be useful. We can use all the help we can get."

Randazzo tapped her pen on her notepad, wishing she had more to write. "It's not good if the best you can say for our evidence is it's better than nothing. Talk about a cold trail."

Rebecca refused to sit, pacing the small waiting room, trying to remain calm. As she looked around she couldn't help but fume over the fact that this was most judges' idea of appropriate punishment for child molesters, coming in here, sitting through a couple hours of psychobabble, and going home again. Elena interrupted her building rage with a sunny "Ms. Fielding, you can go on back now."

Hillerman rose from behind his desk and extended his hand, a warm smile spread a bit too broadly across his face. "Ms. Fielding, thank you for coming by. Please, have a seat." He looked handsome, trustworthy, and respectable—almost Ivy League—in a navy suit, red and blue striped tie, and crisp white pocket square. He couldn't have appeared more gracious had she been here to present him with a check from the Publishers Clearing House.

He cleared his throat and, after adding a slight exaggeration to his well-studied Boston accent, began. "Well, I'm sure you're wondering why I asked you to come down here."

"No, I think I know." Subtlety was never one of Rebecca's traits. "Apparently my interest in your clinic hasn't gone unnoticed by you. Frankly, I'm surprised you haven't asked to meet with me sooner to make nice-nice."

Rebecca's self-satisfied smile irked Hillerman, but he was careful to betray no irritation. "Yes, you have been busy." He tried for a lighthearted laugh, but it came out forced. "It was your last letter to the board that caught my attention in particular." Hillerman swiveled in his chair, crossed his legs, and leaned back. "Frankly, I must admit I was somewhat taken aback by your hostile attitude toward us and, well, I thought it might do us good to talk." He uncrossed his legs and leaned forward, his elbows resting on the desk, his face sincere. "I'd really like to clear the air between us."

Rebecca sat straight, staring at Hillerman with a touch of amusement, her weapon against his obvious brownnosing. "Well, I'm here. What is it you have to say? Let's cut to the chase, as they say."

Hillerman was unaccustomed to relinquishing control and wanted to tell her in no uncertain terms that she wasn't going to set the agenda, but he thought it best to continue in as amicable a posture as he could stomach. "Well, I think that part of the difficulty you and I are having is that you are misinformed about what we do here."

"Quite the contrary, Doctor. I know exactly what you do here. But more importantly, I know exactly what you don't do here." Rebecca settled back comfortably and crossed her arms in front of her. She wasn't buying whatever he was selling.

Hillerman had a fleeting thought that not even the future of the Oakwood was important enough to continue sitting in the same room with this woman, but he decided instead to consider this discussion as a test of his inner strength. "Really, Ms. Fielding, there is no need for that kind of insinuation. You needn't assume we are in an adversarial relationship. We are on the same side. We all want the same thing. Maybe we have a different idea of how to achieve our goals, but deep down I'm certain we agree on what those goals are."

Rebecca had enjoyed the serve and volley but decided to shake things up with an overhead slam. "Well, let's see. My goal is to shut you down so that the courts don't have the option to send molesters here. Is that one of the goals we can agree upon?" She looked at Hillerman, waiting for his retort. Instead, he methodically filled and then lit up a pipe, slowing down the exchange. He sent a few wispy gray swirls up around his head while sizing her up.

"Ms. Fielding, I would hope that you could put aside your personal views and embrace a more enlightened approach to the treatment of sex offenders." Hillerman swiveled his chair to the side and continued speaking. "Clinics such as mine seek to humanely treat and rehabilitate these deeply troubled men. If you're opposed to this, there's not much I can say to you except that you are being short-sighted. It troubles me that you do not see how dangerous your campaign against me is. Because if we simply punish and warehouse these men, they will be no different than they were when they committed their crimes. But if you continue to send them here, we can help them."

Rebecca dropped the amused expression, her face turning earnest. "If I believed that, I'd be happy to see the men sent here. But I don't believe you do anything useful."

Hillerman turned back toward Rebecca and put up his hand. "Let me stop you there. That's where I think your problem—uh, that is—our problem lies. I think we should try to work together toward the greater good. From now on, if you have concerns about us, please feel free to contact me directly. It isn't necessary for you to go through such formal channels as writing to the board. They are, after all, just bureaucrats. They lack the necessary hands-on experience with this population, so to involve them really is a mistake." Hillerman relit his pipe and sent another cloud skyward. The smell was starting to permeate the room.

"They're your licensing board, so I assume they are in a better position than I am to ensure that you're doing your job. My job is to alert them to my concerns and allow them to investigate as they see fit." Rebecca looked out the window and shook her head slowly. "The fact that defense attorneys consider having their clients sent here as a win doesn't fill me with confidence that therapy does much good. But then, I think these men should be punished for their crimes and I fail to see how therapy is punishment."

Hillerman maintained his cordial pose. He leaned back and smiled. "Well, again, you've just highlighted the problem you and I seem to be having. Your focus seems to be only on punishing. You see, I want to help these men understand why they committed their offenses and to help them so that they won't reoffend. Our goal here isn't to punish, but to help."

Rebecca thought back to the debate in her criminal law class whether the goal of the law should be to punish or to rehabilitate. Hillerman's noble speech did nothing to change Rebecca's long-standing opinion that only Pollyannas believed in rehabilitation. "Fine. You want to help. Then you tell me that you can guarantee that your clients won't reoffend when they leave here." Hillerman stared at her with an incredulous look on his face but said nothing. Rebecca knew why. "That's what I thought." She leaned forward. "I'm not convinced you do anything here other than collect fees and issue worthless status reports."

Hillerman felt his face flush red and took a deep breath to calm himself. "Ms. Fielding, with all due respect, it isn't you that we need to convince. The judges who send the defendants here, and the probation department which oversees our work, have been more than satisfied with us." Hillerman puffed furiously on his pipe. The room by now was filled with a low fog.

"And maybe, Dr. Hillerman, that's the problem. Maybe they're too eager to have the problem 'handled' so that they don't have to worry about it. They can say these men are getting treatment and then go on with their business without ever checking to see if you really are rehabilitating anything beyond your pocketbook. The judges who sentence sex offenders to counseling can just wash their hands of the whole problem and be pleased with themselves that they're doing something, without ever asking the question 'Does it work?' Well, I'm here, and I'm asking that question, and I'm not going away till I get an answer."

Hillerman studied Rebecca. This was not going to be resolved today, that was clear. "Ms. Fielding, you have a right to your opinion as, I would hope you would agree, we have a right to ours. What I had hoped to accomplish in this meeting was to open a dialogue between us. I don't think either of us will be able to change the other's opinion, but we can respect each other's right to hold that opinion. Don't you agree?" He stood up and extended his hand to Rebecca.

"Certainly, Dr. Hillerman," Rebecca said, smiling

sweetly as she leaned over to pick up her purse. "I doubt there are enough words in the dictionary for either of us ever to change the other's opinion. We should merely agree to disagree." Rebecca stood up, and turned for the door, waving her arm as she went, as if to cut a path through the smoke.

"Stan, take me off the speakerphone."

"Bob? You sound upset. What is it?"

"That goddamned bitch Fielding—we've got to do—I don't know—something," Hillerman sputtered.

Stan couldn't help but ask the obvious. "The meeting didn't go well?"

"You tell me. She breezes in here telling me that she's going to have us shut down. She states it as an absolute fact, like the sun coming up tomorrow. I don't need this, Stan. It was bad enough having to deal with the problems that Rubin is causing us. Now I have to deal with this one trying to put me out of business altogether."

"Look, don't worry about her. She's not going to be able to do that."

"Oh no? You haven't been right about too much so far. You thought this would all blow over without us having to do anything. Wrong. You thought the board wouldn't get involved. Wrong. You thought no one would listen to her. Wrong again. At least you have consistency on your side."

"Bob, I told you that the clinic will withstand this attack, and I still believe that." Stan knew that inertia was on Hillerman's side and that closing the Oakwood meant making many changes no one was prepared to make, but Hillerman wasn't as convinced. "I think you're worrying needlessly. First of all, we have the situation with Rubin under control." Stan didn't believe it but hoped he sounded convincing. He didn't have the nerve to tell Hillerman just how volatile the situation was. Spurned ex-lovers are always problematic, even more so when they were Hillerman's. "As for Fielding, let's get the accreditation taken care of, get whatever data you need together to show how well the clinic's treatment approach works, and that'll be that. Everything will go back to normal."

Hillerman sat quietly, thinking about the meeting with Fielding. If she could be silenced, his problems would disappear and everything would go back to the way it was. But the woman who just left his office didn't seem likely to be silenced easily. Hell, she wouldn't even shake his hand.

"Goddammit, Stan, this whole thing is going to blow up because you fail to appreciate what a real threat Ms. Fielding is to the future of this clinic. She's on a crusade," Hillerman seethed. "And people on crusades seldom stop until they get what they want, and she wants me shut down. You've got to get her off my back."

"Now, Bob, I really think you are worrying about nothing. You have the expertise, you have the experience, she has nothing. But to put your mind at ease, I'll make sure that our people stay on track. If it becomes necessary, we can ruin her."

"You better be right. Don't let me down."

Stan lowered his head and began rubbing his temples. "I haven't yet."

His comment was met by a click on the other end. Stan marveled at how even Hillerman's phone seemed to have an attitude.

12

Six o'clock in the San Fernando Valley. Businesses were closing for the night, preparing to turn the streets over to the gangbangers who ruled after dark. The Whole Health Acupuncture Institute of Encino was ushering out its last customer, Bradley Knight, a Friday night regular. Knight had just written his umpteenth rubber check to the Institute and was ready to go home for an exciting microwaved burrito—a staple of his diet. Ever since the divorce, Knight was barely making it from paycheck to paycheck. He had long since maxed out his credit cards, and he owed thousands of dollars in back child support and hundreds of dollars for worthless group therapy. The bottom line was that Knight owed more money than he could ever hope to save and spent more money than he could ever possibly earn. But what did he care? Life was a piece of shit, and he was getting used to having his nose rubbed in it.

The parking lot was deserted as Knight hopped into his van. It was starting to get dark, and the streetlights hadn't yet come on. He was feeling relaxed and rested. Nothing worked better on his headaches than the skilled hands of his acupuncturist. To most people, including the guys in his group, the thought of getting stuck with needles seemed far worse than any headache. Knight disagreed. He leaned back, closed his eyes, and reveled in supreme relaxation.

"So you like needles?"

Knight was startled by the voice from behind his seat. Before he could speak, he felt a sharp stab in his neck and then heard laughter as he quickly drifted asleep.

When he awoke, he was disoriented but sensed that something was very wrong. From the faint trace of marijuana and the odor of his gym bag, he assumed that he was still in his van. As he checked his senses in stages, his fear spread. He couldn't see, he couldn't move, he couldn't scream. He was flat on his back—tied up, blindfolded and gagged. Vulnerable, and scared.

"Bradley, so nice of you to wake up. I was getting bored with just killing time. I suppose we can now do what we have to do."

His mind raced. What's going on? He tried to speak, but that was impossible. Even without the gag, his fear would not permit speech.

"Do you know why I'm here?"

Knight stayed still, not knowing what to do. The voice, so menacing, cut through the darkness as his only connection to reality.

"I asked you a question, Bradley. Now, do you know why I'm here?"

He slowly shook his head from side to side.

"Well, let's see if you can figure it out. I'll give you a hint. I'm like Santa Claus, only everyone on my list has been naughty, not nice. Does that help?"

Knight brought his head up, straining to see

through the darkness. The voice was vaguely familiar.

"Here's your next clue." The scarf was pulled off his eyes. Before he could focus in the dark, he felt a sharp piercing pain as a short, thin knife punctured his left eye. His eye burst like a grape and blood ran down his face. From deep within him came the sound of a pain he hadn't experienced before, intense and relentless.

"Wasn't that fun? You know, I sharpened the knife before I came here. It was so dull. Just like you." Knight moaned in agony, the sound muffled but undeniable. "Hey, that was a joke. I'd appreciate a little feedback here. I understand it may be hard to laugh with all that blood in your mouth, but you could at least manage a little smile. Would it kill you?"

Knight's head jerked violently from side to side, his screams distorted and muffled as his mouth struggled against the gag.

"So, have you figured it out yet? What I'm doing here, that is? No? Well, Brad, payback is hell, as they say. And, yes, you are the next contestant on the Price Is Life. Johnny, please tell Mr. Knight what he has won." The voice was charged with game show enthusiasm. "You have won a pine box. What would you like to put in it?" A pause, but no answer. "If you can't think of anything, I can. Just think, your death—the gift that keeps on giving."

The knife stabbed Knight's other eye. "Now you're as blind as justice. Get it? God, I hope so. I hate when I have to explain my jokes."

Knight entered total darkness, his head filled with searing pain. He tried to grab his face, his arms instinctively pulled toward his eyes to push back the pain, but the handcuffs restrained him. His sobbing subsided to a rhythmic moaning.

"Why are you crying? I'm trying to be therapeutic.

This is my special brand of holistic medicine. The more holes I make in you, the better I feel."

Knight felt a sharp, burning sensation as the knife was plunged first into his stomach, then into his chest. The blood felt warm as it ran down his body. And yet he couldn't stop his shivering. Knight heard his attacker groan from the effort of each new stab of the knife, an odd percussive sound. The groan was followed by the squishing sound of the knife tearing through the skin and punctuated by Knight's corresponding moans of agony. Then the stabbing and the strange music stopped.

Knight shuddered into death, barely missing the final gesture as the knife was plunged up his ass. "Boy, you didn't seem to enjoy that very much. Oh, well. Toodles."

Jack was irritated with the guy singing on the radio. He didn't need to be reminded that he was alone on a Saturday night. Leaning back on his couch, he looked through the window of his apartment at the boats in the marina, some rocking gently at the dock, others gliding slowly along the smooth waters, and nursed a Guinness. Not quite the companion he had hoped for tonight.

It didn't have to be this way. He had meant to call Rebecca all week, but he never got around to it. Must be getting old, he thought. Never used to let work get in the way of his social life. It was even more pathetic, since a week's worth of good old-fashioned investigating had turned up nothing, zippo. So here he sat, with no leads and no company but the strangers out on the water.

Across town, in an apartment that was too small, his partner was not faring much better. Jennifer was rereading the same *People* magazine for the fourth time while Ben faded in and out of consciousness next to her on the couch. Between Law Review and studying, Ben was near exhaustion. So even when he was home, it was only to eat and sleep, and sometimes he was even too tired to eat. Jennifer tried to be patient because she loved Ben more than life itself and knew this would be over before they knew it. Still, she often joked that if she'd wanted to go three years without sex, she'd have joined the convent like her Aunt Sophie. Jennifer decided to ring up Jack, hoping at least to have a stimulating discussion with his answering machine. She was surprised instead by the live version.

"What are you doing home?" she asked.

"What are you, my mother?"

"Someone has to be," Randazzo kidded.

Jack sighed, bored. "I was watching the Kings, but I turned it off at three-zip. So what's up with you?"

"I was thinking about the case, and I had an idea. Maybe we're ignoring some obvious suspects. Maybe—"

"Jen," Jack interrupted, "it's Saturday night. My brain is closed for the weekend. I'll leave it a message and have it call you on Monday." Jack made it a policy never to work when he was off duty. Nothing good ever came of it, and the brass never thanked you for it.

"C'mon, just hear me out."

"What's really going on? You must be pretty bored to call me on a Saturday night. It's bad enough for my reputation that you found me here. It's even worse that you expected to find me here."

"I guess I just wanted to talk to a person who wasn't snoring."

Jack looked over at his clock. "Awfully early for Ben to be asleep. Why don't you try dancing naked in front of him? I'll bet he pops right up."

"Very funny."

"I'm being serious. Sometimes us guys need a little help." Jack figured just because he wasn't getting any tonight, no reason he couldn't help his fellow man. As he saw it, the sexual experience of any of his brothers enriches us all.

"So what's your excuse for being home tonight instead of out with Rebecca? I thought the first date went so well?"

"It did. I just forgot to call until it was too late."

"That's silly. Come on, one of us should have some fun tonight. Give her a call. It's not too late. Maybe she's at home wondering why you haven't called. She probably thinks you're a jerk."

Larson thought a moment. Well, Randazzo was of the female persuasion. Maybe she knew something he didn't. "All right, I'll give her a call. But now I've got some advice for you. Go take your clothes off and then wake Ben up. I'm sure your only problem is timing. Okay?"

"Thanks, partner."

He hung up on Randazzo, then dialed Rebecca's number quickly. She picked up on the third ring. He actually felt a rush of excitement.

"Hello?"

"Hi, it's Jack. I hope this isn't a bad time."

"No, I was just watching the hockey game," Rebecca said, as she turned the sound off the television.

Oh, my God. She is the perfect woman, he thought. "Can I tear you away from the game? If you're not doing anything, maybe we could catch a late dinner. I know this isn't much notice. I was planning on asking you out, but the week just flew by and before I knew it, it was Saturday. I'll come out your way if you want." Jack hoped he didn't sound desperate, it wouldn't do his reputation much good. But he also knew he didn't feel much like being alone tonight.

"Okay, sure. That'd be great," she said enthusiastically. "But we already did my area. Do you like Benihana's? It's my treat." Rebecca devilishly suggested a restaurant that would once again test Jack's questionable skills with chopsticks. But he caught on in time.

"Yeah, but there's no privacy there. Besides, I get too much violence at work to watch someone take a cleaver to some helpless food. How 'bout the Beachhouse? I've heard good things about it." Dark interior, good view of the water, great drinks, pretty much all Jack looked for in a restaurant.

"Sounds good to me."

Jack sat up. "One hour?"

"One hour it is. See you there."

Larson hung up, guzzled the rest of his beer, and quickly dialed Randazzo to thank her for the good advice. Her machine answered, so he left a message. "Hey, Jennifer. Thanks for a great idea. Hope you took my suggestion too."

Randazzo didn't pick up, but whispered, "I sure did."

"You sure did what?" Ben asked in between nibbles on her ear.

"I sure did marry a great guy," she replied.

Thanks to the street vendors who along with the entrepreneurial homeless seemed to stake out every corner and freeway off ramp in Los Angeles, Jack had no trouble finding flowers to bring to the restaurant. He knew it was a little hokey, but sometimes the tried and true works best. Rebecca's smile and slight blush let him know he had been right.

They sat in a small booth facing out over the

water, the view of thin strands of light dancing across the rippling sea more than compensating for the mediocre meal. But Jack and Rebecca were too transfixed on each other to notice the view or the food or anything else, including the thinning of the restaurant, until the waitress hesitantly suggested they might want to forgo another coffee refill. They had talked about sports, music, politics, everything but work. They found themselves amazingly compatible, down to the most obscure of details, including both picking Kirk Gibson's home run in the 1988 World Series as their greatest sports moment, *Taxi* as their favorite TV show, and REM as their favorite band. It was more of a first date than their first dinner, with its attendant excitement and anxiety, and yet they felt surprisingly comfortable with each other.

"I'm so glad you weren't busy tonight," said Jack, reaching for Rebecca's hand as they walked out along the sand. Jack could feel her softness in his hand. "You know, I'd wanted to call you all week, but I'm just swamped right now. I'm so glad you were free."

"Me too." Rebecca knew that she was supposed to have said "no" to a last-minute date—the dating game demands that you're not supposed to let on that you have no other prospects, especially on a Saturday night. But she was never much for games and, anyway, being herself hadn't hurt so far. After all, he had asked her out again, albeit on pretty short notice. And now, walking with him under the moonlit sky, she was glad she had said yes.

She smiled up at him. Usually, Jack would have taken this as a sign that it was time for the first move. But something told him to wait.

"I know how work can get," she said. "Sometimes I get so bogged down, the weeks just blur together. Especially this week. But, I'm glad you called. Even if it was the last minute," she added with a playful dig.

Jack nodded. He knew he deserved it. But it was worth it, because he'd rather be here, being teased, then home by himself. "You know, when we had dinner last week, I wasn't entirely sure if it was business or pleasure. I mean, the dinner was a pleasure. I didn't mean that it was just all business. I mean— Oh, I don't know what I mean," Jack said, sighing helplessly.

Rebecca laughed. "It's okay, I think I know what you mean. I had a good time, despite the subject matter. But this was nicer tonight. No talk about work." Rebecca sighed, feeling relaxed, as if work were a lifetime away. "But, you know, you should have let me pay for dinner this time. I do have a job, you know."

"I guess I'm just a gentleman at heart," he said. "That's what they call me, gentleman Jack."

"That's not what Tom used to say," Rebecca said teasingly. "It was more like love-'em-and-leave-'em Jack."

"When did he say that? I'll sue him. How could Tom say such a scurrilous thing about me?" he protested. "I'm just a lonely old man grateful to have a little company."

Rebecca laughed softly. "So I take it you're not seeing anyone?"

"Ahh, just my partner. But her husband won't let her date, so I don't think it counts. What about you? Is there anyone special in your life? I guess I should have asked before."

"No, no one. Unless you count the guy who delivers pizza. He comes to my house pretty regularly."

"Well," he said, scanning Rebecca, "it doesn't show." He winced at his automatic retreat into a typical male reaction, but he couldn't help himself. How was he supposed to ignore the fact that she had a great body?

"Thanks," Rebecca said. Hey, she didn't go to the gym four times a week for nothing. "You know, it's hard finding time to get to know someone when work takes up so much of your time. I think, especially for women, you have to make a choice between work and play. I'm not sure you really can have it all."

"I don't know. I'd like to think you can have it all. Why not shoot for the moon?"

Rebecca stopped walking, looked up at the bright face of the full moon and let out a deep sigh. "But the moon is always out of reach. It looks so close, like you can just reach up and grab it, but it's just too far away. That's what makes it special." Rebecca shook her head and looked back down. "I tried for it once, with Tom. After we broke up, I just didn't have it in me to try again. Don't get me wrong. I do go out now and then. It's just—maybe I'm a romantic at heart—but I'm not interested in casual dating. I'd really like to be in a relationship again, but it's hard to trust someone enough to make that kind of commitment. You know, it's the old 'Fool me once, shame on you. Fool me twice, shame on me.' I don't want to be fooled again."

"I know what you're saying, I've been there." Jack paused, looking back out at the water. "Remember how I told you I was married before?" he asked slowly.

She looked at him apprehensively. "Yeah?"

"Well, I was married after before, too."

"So you do love 'em and leave 'em," she said, laughing.

"I think it's more like I love 'em and they leave me. My ex—the first Mrs. Larson—I really loved her and it hurt when I found out she didn't feel the same. At least not enough to accept me for who I

was and what I wanted to be. Number two? She built
me up with all that 'I want only you, I love only you.'
I needed to hear it, so I fell for it. She forgot to mention, however, that it only applied if I was actually in
the room at the time. Unfortunately, she loved everyone, the cable guy, the plumber, the paperboy.
Anyway, after that, having superficial relationships
suited me just fine. But lately, I've been thinking
about trying again. Plus, I'd like to be a dad. Little
League games and trips to Disneyland. Modern
medicine hasn't quite made it to the point where I
can do it by myself." Jack smiled gently. "But enough
about my middle-aged crisis."

"You're not exactly middle-aged. And there's
nothing wrong with still hoping to find someone special," she added softly.

Maybe I've already found her, Jack thought to
himself. He put his arm around Rebecca as they
walked on, trying to shield her from the cold wind
coming in across the water. "You're freezing."

Rebecca smiled. "No, I'm okay. I always forget
how cold it gets out here."

"Yeah, but I don't want you to catch pneumonia.
Maybe we should start heading back."

"I guess it is getting kinda late." Rebecca started
to turn back.

"Wait." Jack leaned down and kissed her. The tension of the moment gave way to a fire of passion as
their mouths met for the first time. Rebecca felt her
body tingle with his touch, a sensation she had
thought died long ago. The calming of Jack's gentle
embrace gave her the moment she needed to steady
herself.

Jack lingered until the pressure of the next move
caused him to slow down. This was not something to
rush, no matter how beautiful she looked, no matter
how magical she felt. He took her hands and stared

into her eyes for what seemed like an eternity. "You're very special, Rebecca. I would love nothing more than to hold you all night. But I think if I don't go home right now, I'll have a coronary from the stress of trying to remain a gentleman."

"I think that's the best compliment I've ever had." Rebecca looked down at their joined hands. "You're an amazing guy, Jack."

After holding time still for as long as they could, they returned to their empty cars, kissed good-bye, and drove home. Without having said a word, they both were struck by the same thought tonight—how their long search for that special someone might be over. It wasn't something they knew, it was something they felt—that they belonged together, that it was all meant to be. And yet neither was willing to run headfirst into romance, preferring small, tentative steps into what they each hoped would be their future together.

13

Larson had just stepped out of the shower when he heard the phone ringing. He ran dripping to grab it before the machine clicked on. "Hello."

"We're running a bit late, aren't we?" an energetic voice teased.

Larson never understood how Randazzo could sound so chipper in the morning. She gave perky a bad name. He glanced at the clock on the dresser, 8:46. Okay, so maybe it wasn't that early. "Hey, go easy on me. At my age I'm lucky I can get out of bed without help. So, what's up?" he said, not wanting to give her the satisfaction of knowing that a puddle was forming at his feet.

"I'm coming to pick you up. We've got two more."

"You're shitting me!"

"No, sir." Randazzo enthusiastically ticked off the details for him, reading from her notes. "The first is Bradley Knight. He was found in his van tucked away in a parking garage behind some large Dumpsters. A uniformed shone his light through the window, probably hoping to catch some young lovers in the act, but instead found one very dead young man. Apparently it looked like a slaughterhouse in there—the guy'd been dead a couple days. A homicide team from East Valley did the scene, but when they made him as a two eighty-eight felon, they thought he might be one of ours."

"And the other one?"

"Steven Jaffe. He was found in a little shack up in Topanga. No job, apparently few friends who gave a shit about him, 'cause he'd been dead so long he had his own little maggot farm. Anyway, same background, a two eighty-eight out on probation. There's no doubt about it now. We've got a vigilante on our hands."

"I can't believe it."

"Believe it. I'll pick you up in an hour."

"Right, boss."

Larson put the phone down, then stood naked and cold, momentarily stalled by shock. Randazzo was right. They were now sitting on top of a major multiple murder case—and the thought actually intrigued Larson, who had grown bored with the routine nature of most homicide investigations. He dressed quickly and waited out front for Randazzo. The brisk air blew in off the marina, invigorating him like a briny cold cup of coffee. He thought about the case, how complicated a simple little murder had suddenly become. And wondered how many more there'd be.

"Where are we going?" Larson asked as Randazzo pulled the car onto the street. She caught the 90 freeway just around the corner from his apartment and headed east to catch the 405 north, which would take them over the hill to the Valley.

"First I want to head over to where Knight was found. I'm not looking forward to Jaffe's place. I'd rather wait for the stench to blow out. Then we can go to the morgue, see how far along they are. You know, we've got to get word out that any male murder victim, we've got to be called immediately. By the time they run 'em and find their record, the scene's been tromped all over, everything's already done."

"Jen, do you know how many guys get killed every day? If they call us on all of them, how'm I ever gonna get my beauty sleep?"

"So sorry. I wouldn't want to ruin your nights with anything as trivial as work."

"Good, keep it that way. So what do we know about these two?"

Randazzo was flying along the overpass from the 90 to the 405 and had to slam on her brakes when she saw the bottleneck in front of her. She checked her clock—rush hour was officially over—and wondered why the freeways never seemed to thin out, even after everyone in the city was supposedly at their jobs. She cranked her head out her window, hoping to see the reason for the standstill. As they crept along slowly, she turned to Jack, "There better be dead bodies up there."

Larson wasn't one to let a little thing like traffic get him down. Especially since he wasn't driving. "Hey, it gives us more time to talk. And you know how precious our time together is." Randazzo shot him one of her patented incredulous stares. "What? I'm wrong?"

Randazzo banged on her horn. "What's with these idiots?"

"Honking isn't going to get us there any faster. Only people from New York think that. So, why don't you just relax and tell me more about the murders."

"All right." Randazzo blew her curly bangs off her forehead. "Jaffe's was a lot like Matheson's. He lived alone, was killed at home, and he was near the end of his probation. Now, things get a little more complicated with Knight. He was stabbed to death, not shot, and he was killed in his car instead of at home, but I'm not sure that those are major differences. One other difference—we have the murder weapon this time, which the killer was kind enough to leave behind, pun intended."

"Huh?" Confused, Larson looked over at Randazzo.

"Too early for sick jokes? The knife was found in his butt. Poetic, don't you think?"

Larson winced. "Nice. So our killer has a sense of humor?"

"I don't think Mr. Knight found it funny." Randazzo changed lanes, hoping that it would do some good. It didn't.

"Well, it seems to me like our killer is starting to have a little too much fun. Using a knife is a lot more up close and personal too. Not like shooting 'em."

"It does look that way. Anyway—huge surprise—I'm told no witnesses at either locale. Now the lab guys were all over the van, and they told me they don't think they'll have much for us, so far just some long blonde hairs in the van, which may belong to the killer."

"Or to a past date of our victim," he added with a shrug. "So were they both being treated at the Oakwood?"

Randazzo was pleased that Larson knew she'd already have checked into this. Her reputation for thoroughness had been permanently established. "Jaffe was, Knight wasn't."

"Where was Knight?"

"Our friend Velma said he was being seen at Elmhurst. It's also in the Valley. It was started by Andrea Rubin, a therapist who used to be at the Oakwood. She was Matheson's first therapist, it turns out. Anyway, she apparently had a falling out with Hillerman and decided to go into competition with him. Velma thinks there may have been a romantic aspect to this falling out. She also thinks they hate each other now."

"Velma is quite the talker," Larson said.

"She's pretty upset about her probationers being killed."

"You'd think she'd be happy to have her caseload thinned out a bit."

Randazzo looked up ahead and saw a jackknifed truck, which had scattered its load of lettuce across four lanes of traffic—on the other side of the freeway. "I can't believe we're at a crawl so everyone can get a good look at a dead truck surrounded by a tossed salad. What is wrong with these people?"

"Hey, we've got bigger problems than annoying drivers."

Randazzo failed to see Jack's point. "Not right now we don't."

The coroner's office had its usual backlog. Understaffed and overworked thanks to the skyrocketing murder rates and declining tax rates, they were running out of room to stash the bodies. Randazzo and Larson didn't have a prayer that the Jaffe and Knight autopsies would be completed today, but at least they might be able to get some preliminary information. From what they had just seen at Knight's van, they imagined he'd look like hamburger meat but hoped the coroner could make sense of it all.

They were greeted by Dr. Sherman, the examiner in charge. A thin, fidgety man, whose lack of bedside manner obviously didn't concern his patients, Dr. Sherman extended toward the detectives a nail-bitten hand that held two masks for them to wear. "You're here for . . . ?"

"Steven Jaffe and Bradley Knight," answered Randazzo.

"Right, right. Over here." He walked the detectives over to where Knight's body was stored and slid open the drawer. The acrid smell that hung in the air was barely dulled by the cotton masks the detectives had quickly donned, but obviously Dr. Sherman was all too used to it. "Let's see what we've got. Okay, nonfatal stab wounds to each eye. The deceased was alive when those wounds were inflicted, causing a fair amount of bleeding. Multiple stab wounds, primarily concentrated in the torso. We counted at least twenty-five discernible separate wounds, not counting the coup de grace. He probably drowned in his own blood. From his color it looks like he may have suffocated when the knife collapsed his lungs, but until we complete the autopsy, we won't know for sure."

Larson studied Knight's body. The blood had been cleaned away, leaving behind a startling, chalky fright mask, his face contorted, eye sockets gaping holes filled with a mushy mass of blood and tissue. His torso bore the scars of overkill, dozens of deceptively thin puncture marks dotting his trunk. Larson politely declined Dr. Sherman's offer to turn Mr. Knight over to view the rest of the carnage.

"What else can you tell us?" Randazzo asked.

"As you can see, there are marks on his wrists—he'd probably been handcuffed." Dr. Sherman pointed to Mr. Knight's extremities. "No evidence of a struggle, so I doubt we'll find the killer's skin or blood under his fingernails. But I ordered a scraping anyway. Aside from that, nothing else too exciting."

He scanned the corpse, thinking he'd forgotten something. He tapped his forehead with his fingers, until it came to him. "Oh, wait, there was a puncture mark in the back of the neck, possibly from a needle.

You see, I think he was drugged first, then cuffed, before he was killed. That's why there are no bruises or abrasions. He must have been pretty compliant." Larson and Randazzo were surprised by the new detail. The killer seemed not only to be finding more enjoyment in the murders but also to be more premeditated in planning them. "There's not much more to tell until we get the report from toxicology. That should take a couple of days, a week at the most. That's about all we can tell you now. We'll send over the full report when the autopsy's completed." Dr. Sherman slid the drawer closed.

"Great. How 'bout Jaffe?" Larson asked.

Dr. Sherman led the detectives down along the wall of stored bodies. "He's over here. He must have been dead a week, he's pretty badly decomposed." As he slid open the drawer, the truth of Dr. Sherman's statement became only too apparent.

As Randazzo looked at the unrecognizable form, she wondered how long ago it still resembled a human. "Doesn't look like his body will tell us much."

"Nope. We won't be able to detect any injuries that were only skin deep, for obvious reasons. We found two bullets still lodged at the base of his skull—the entrance wounds seem like the eyes. Just like that other guy," Dr. Sherman said, nodding back toward the drawer containing Knight. "The biggest question on this one, though, is how long he was like that and the best I think we'll be able to give you is about a week. Other than that, I don't think he'll give us much more to work with. Sorry. But we'll let you know as soon as we can."

"Well, whatever you can do. I can see you're swamped," said Larson.

"Yeah, business is booming," said Dr. Sherman as he closed the drawer on Mr. Jaffe. "Los Angeles is a good town to have a morgue in."

Larson and Randazzo pulled off their masks and dropped them off at the door.

"Thanks for your time, Doc."

"You're welcome," Dr. Sherman shouted back. "Hey, and be sure to stop by our new gift shop."

Larson and Randazzo looked at each other and laughed—they'd never checked it out before, but this time their curiosity got the best of them. They walked over to the morgue gift shop, a macabre boutique that was providing the coroner's department with a surprising source of income earmarked for charity from its bizarre, official souvenirs. Larson picked up a black travel coffee mug as Randazzo thumbed through T-shirts, looking for Ben's size.

"You know, if Knight wasn't a child molester, there's no way you'd connect him to the others," Larson said. "Different murder weapon, different locations, the hypodermic. The other three were killed quickly, ambushed and then boom, you're dead. But Knight, the killer went through a lot of trouble to kill him."

"Yeah, but the wounds to the eyes. Both of them and Matheson. That's as close to a calling card as you can get." Randazzo picked out a T-shirt emblazoned with the chalk outline of a dead body and the coroner's logo in red print on a black background, then showed it to Larson.

"Lovely," he remarked. "So if the wounds to the eyes is the signature, how does that explain Penhall? He was shot in the chest."

Randazzo shrugged. "Maybe he was a car jacking attempt and his death gave someone the idea to kill child molesters. Or maybe the killer just got the idea of the eyes after Matheson and decided to use it for the others or maybe somebody wants it to look like a signature to confuse us. How should I know?"

Larson thought for a moment. "No. The same person

killed all four—you just can't ignore the fact that all four were convicted child molesters." Larson paused. "Someone doesn't like these guys."

"Nobody likes these guys."

"Yeah, but someone hates them enough to kill them. A lot of them. Let's check out the details of Knight's offense. The knife up the ass was a nice touch, especially if he'd been charged with sodomy. Sort of punishment fitting the crime." Randazzo put down the mug. "I'd like to know how the eyes figure in. I'm sure it's got some meaning—to the killer anyway. I just don't know what it is." She walked around looking at the other items—playing cards, watches, notepads, paperweights, calendars, towels, and clothes, all festooned with the coroner's logo, then stopped suddenly and turned toward Larson, exasperated. "I can't work like this. There needs to be some organization. We need to plug in Jaffe's and Knight's data with that of the other victims—their therapists, their group members, their probation officers, everyone who knew all four and who might want to see them dead—put all the factors up on the blackboard so we can see where the connections are."

"Hmmm. Organization." Larson scratched his chin then pointed at Randazzo. "That sounds like your kind of thing. But I'd like to see it when you're done."

Randazzo smiled. She took the T-shirt over to pay for it. "I wonder if the killer followed Knight, or knew his routine enough to know he'd be there. You never told me, did the acupuncturist know anything?" At the scene of Knight's murder, Randazzo had taken some extra pictures and measurements while Larson chatted with the owner of the Whole Earth.

Larson considered a toe tag key chain—a little too macabre even for him. "He said Knight was a regular.

He had a standing appointment there for over a year. Never missed a one. So someone who knew his schedule might have known he'd be there."

"Maybe." Randazzo took her package from the clerk, who also handed Larson a brochure for mail orders in case he changed his mind. "Did he see anyone in the vicinity, any cars he didn't recognize?"

"No," he said as they walked out of the gift shop. "He told me Knight usually parked in the back. He didn't even see him get into the van. Knight's his last patient of the evening, so he usually hurries out."

"Wonderful. God forbid he should peek out the window and maybe see something." Randazzo squinted in the morning sun and rummaged through her large handbag looking for her sunglasses. She found her wallet, her keys, her notepad, and a week's worth of empty candy wrappers, but no shades. She continued walking to the parking lot, hoping her glasses were still in the car.

"So, about all we have are the hairs, just like at Matheson's," Randazzo said as they walked. "Well, we know the killer must drive to and away from the scene of the murders. The van was left just a few blocks away, so the killer could have parked somewhere nearby. I've ordered the traffic reports in the area to see if any cars were seen that didn't belong there. Maybe we'll have some luck tracking down the hypodermic found in the van or the knife. Maybe there'll be something there." Randazzo stopped walking and looked up at Larson, shading her eyes as she spoke. "So what do you think? Is our killer a man or a woman? If it's a guy, what's with the long hairs?"

"Well, could be a surfer or a Fabio wannabe. Or maybe it's a transvestite. Now, the killer tends to kill them where they're found. Maybe because the killer isn't big enough to transport them. That would seem to indicate that the killer might be a woman." Larson thought for a moment, then wondered aloud. "Although women just don't do this kind of stuff."

"Women can be multiple murderers too," Randazzo implored.

"Hmm—funny, but I don't remember that being one of the slogans of the women's movement."

The Elmhurst Center prided itself first and foremost on the fact that it was not the Oakwood, which it considered nothing more than a glorified adjunct to the probation department. While still wanting the Oakwood's lucrative referrals, Elmhurst strived to be accepted as a true therapeutic clinic, with an ambience befitting a Beverly Hills counseling office, right down to the de rigueur espresso machine in the waiting area. Dr. Rubin, the founder of Elmhurst, had great expectations for her center as an alternative to the Oakwood, and for herself as an alternative to Dr. Hillerman.

She greeted the detectives at the door to her office with a warm handshake. Dr. Rubin was an attractive woman in her early forties with sharp, well-defined features and large dark eyes, smartly dressed in a wine-colored Chanel suit. Her blonde hair was pulled straight back off her face in a tight bun at the nape of her neck. "Nice to meet you, Detectives," she said, flashing an impeccable smile.

"Dr. Rubin, thank you for seeing us," Randazzo said as she and Larson took their seats.

Dr. Rubin sat down in her high-back leather chair, which looked as if it cost more than all of Randazzo's furniture combined. Rubin's high-rise office in the more affluent Encino area of the Valley looked out at the hills, visible only on smog-free days. "Whatever I can do to help, Detectives. Although, I can't imagine what help I can offer. As you might imagine, I was somewhat surprised to receive your call. I certainly never thought that Dr. Hillerman's problems would extend over here. I guess that's what happens when you take on one of his patients. He's lost, what, three patients now? I guess four if you consider that Mr. Knight was primarily treated at Oakwood."

Larson raised an eyebrow, having never considered the other murders to be Hillerman's "problem." "How long ago did Mr. Knight start coming here?" he asked.

"I'd say just about four, five months ago. He'd been at Oakwood for over five years but for some reason preferred to finish up here."

"Do you know why he switched?" he asked as he scanned the room. He recognized some of the titles from Hillerman's office: *The Incest Perpetrator, Child Sexual Abuse, Treating Incest, Adult Sexual Interest in Children.* They must go to the same deviant bookstore, he thought.

"Well, I have my suspicions." Rubin leaned forward and lowered her head slightly, as if about to impart a confidence. "As I'm sure you know, the Oakwood is not the same as it used to be. I've heard some people say the groups there have become too antagonistic and you end up with a lot of personality squabbles. Plus, therapist turnover there has been too high. The therapeutic process has just flown out the window." Rubin sat back, seemingly amused by all this. "But, no, he never really said in so many words if that's why he left. I guess I'm actually more surprised that so many stay," she added with a laugh. It occurred to Larson that Rubin was like a divorcée wondering why anyone would have anything to do with her ex.

"Did he mention any group members or therapists

by name he might have been having problems with?"
Randazzo asked.

Rubin shook her head slowly as she thought for a
moment. "No, no one in particular. As I said, it was
just an assumption on my part. I've gotten the sense
that some of the tensions at the clinic are filtering
down to the staff and the patients."

"Have these tensions, as you call them, caused
many of Oakwood's patients to switch to your
clinic?" Larson asked.

"Well, not that many, yet. But, hopefully, word of
mouth will spread and we'll see more transfers.
We're still pretty new, and people are still learning
about us. We've been focusing our efforts on getting
the probation department to refer more patients to us
instead of to Oakwood. I'm hoping that a year from
now we'll be the preeminent clinic and Oakwood the
dinosaur on its way to extinction." A self-satisfied
grin moved across her face. "We're well on our way
to that goal."

Larson and Randazzo each noted the intensity
behind the smile. "I understand you used to work
with Dr. Hillerman," Randazzo said casually.

"Uh, yes," Dr. Rubin said, sputtering slightly. "I
trained under Dr. Hillerman, but we parted company
a while ago over . . . let's just say, methodology."

What, you liked missionary and he liked doggy
style? Larson thought, not letting on that he knew
the real reason. "And is your 'methodology' proving
any more successful than Dr. Hillerman's?" he
asked.

"Well, I certainly think so. Just in the short time
we've been up and running, I've seen our approach
work quite well. I tend to challenge the men here
more, demand more from them, not let them get
away with just showing up and not really working
hard to change, and I believe that gets more from

them. I utilize role-playing and crime reenactments here, which I think are very successful in rehabilitation. But I guess Dr. Hillerman would tell you otherwise. But then, he doesn't take well to competition."

Larson thought he could read her pretty well and wasn't going out on a limb with his next statement. "I take it that you and Dr. Hillerman don't see eye to eye on too many things."

Dr. Rubin managed an icy smile. "That's what makes a horse race, isn't it, Detective?"

"I suppose," Larson added slowly. "So is it fair to say that you're not impressed with the work they do there?"

"Not anymore. There may have been a time when Dr. Hillerman did good work. I certainly would like to think that when I was there, we did good work." Rubin tilted her head up regally. "I take a certain pride in that fact. While I was at Oakwood, I was in charge of supervising and training the therapists, and I took a real hands-on approach. But since I left, my sense is that the quality of the work has deteriorated significantly. There's simply no one there who has taken on that responsibility, and without proper training, the therapists can't do their job adequately." Rubin fiddled with a diamond tennis bracelet on her delicate wrist. "Dr. Hillerman doesn't do that, and he hasn't found anyone to replace me yet. At least not in that role," she added with a sarcastic laugh.

Larson and Randazzo cast each other a quick glance, noting her comment and tone. "What did Dr. Hillerman say when Mr. Knight decided to change clinics?"

"I don't know. I guess you'd have to ask him," Dr. Rubin said coolly.

"Dr. Rubin, if you wouldn't mind, we're due at the lab shortly. Could we take your files on Mr. Knight and then set up a follow-up at a later time?"

"Oh, sure. Just call if I can be of any further help," she said indifferently.

As they walked down the corridor leading to the exit, Randazzo whispered to Larson, "What do they say about a woman scorned?"

Larson leaned down, to keep his voice low. "Something like—she'll go into competition with you and drive you out of business."

14

Randazzo stormed in and threw the memo on Larson's desk. "Did you see this?"

Larson looked up from the sports page to find a beet-red face staring down at him. "The smoke coming out your ears tells me either we have a new pope, or this isn't good news."

"Just read it."

Jack glanced down. It didn't take him long to see the problem.

INTEROFFICE MEMORANDUM

To: Detectives Henderson and
       Gilmore, R/H
cc: Detectives Larson and Randazzo
From: Captain Robinson
Re: Reassignment—Child Molester
       Killings

Pursuant to our discussion, because apparently there are now three additional murders

connected to the earlier Penhall murder, the
investigation of all four should be coordinated
under the direction of the Special Investigations Division of Robbery-Homicide. Therefore, effective immediately, the Matheson,
Knight, and Jaffe cases are reassigned to you
for further investigation and handling. Please
prepare an internal transfer order reflecting
this reassignment.

Larson looked up from the memo with an expression loosely translated as "I'm not surprised."
Randazzo was nowhere near as nonchalant. She was
fuming, her hand squeezed into a tight fist as she
spit out her words. "Those assholes. They didn't
even have the courtesy to consult with us. If they
think they can just snatch this case away, they have
another thing coming. What, they're the hotshot elite
squad and we're some dim-witted country bump-
kins? Is that what this is all about? I'll tell you one
thing—"

"Are you planning on coming up for air?" he interjected quickly. "Jennifer, this is just typical depart-
mental bullshit."

"Oh, so you're willing to just walk away from this
case?" she asked, arms flailing in the air.

"No, I didn't say that." Larson knew at this point
that nothing he said would make any difference, she
was like a gun cocked to the pissed-off position.

"Then what are you saying?"

"I'm saying that this happens all the time, especially with high-profile cases. You're gonna have to
get used to it or you're gonna give yourself an ulcer.
It's the way cases are assigned. The big ones always
go downtown."

"Oh, yeah, right. Like we couldn't possibly handle
murders as complicated as this. What bullshit. What

do they think? That we're so stupid we think a serial killer is someone who murders Captain Crunch?" Randazzo fumed. She was a whirlwind of flying hand gestures and exasperated inflections, drawing the attention of a couple of other detectives who wandered over to see what all the commotion was about.

"Hey, what's up with her?" a tanned, well-built detective asked Larson, wagging his thumb toward Randazzo.

"You have to ask?" Larson responded, pointing to the reassignment memo.

The detective looked from the memo to Randazzo, then turned back to Larson. "Good thing she doesn't work in the post office. She'd probably shoot us all."

Randazzo looked unamused. "Great! Not only do I get pulled off this case, but now everyone gets a laugh at my expense. I can't believe this!"

The detective looked off into the distance, as if to ponder the great sadness of her loss. "Randazzo's first big case and it gets kicked to Robbery-Homicide. I guess this means that it's back to purse snatchings for you. Tough break." He sighed conspicuously as he turned and headed down the hall.

Randazzo turned on his shorter, slightly balding partner, who remained behind, laughing. "What are you looking at?" she snapped.

He put up his hands and backed away quickly. Randazzo turned back to her partner. "This is just great! After all the work we've done."

"Look, Jen, you're taking this way too personally. You know we can't investigate this alone. You were the one who contacted the FBI to help us out."

"That's totally different." Randazzo didn't mind asking for help, but she didn't like being told she couldn't—or wouldn't be allowed to—handle something she felt capable of doing. "Well, I can assure you of one thing, I'm not about to lose the biggest case I've ever had. How am I supposed to get ahead in this department? How am I ever gonna move up unless they let me show them what I can do? I'm not getting off this case without a fight. I don't care what it takes, but I'm not handing off this case."

Randazzo stood defiantly, demanding Larson to do something. He thought of trying to reason with her or calm her down, then quickly dismissed such a ridiculous idea. But he'd have to try something.

"Let me see what I can do. Just mellow out." He looked at her and thought better of his last comment. Mellow wasn't a word in her dictionary. "Okay, just seethe quietly until I take care of it."

"What are you going to do?" she demanded as he started walking out.

He stopped in his tracks and shrugged. "I don't know yet."

"Why don't you start by telling them that I am sick and tired of being treated like a woman?"

Larson moved toward Randazzo, as if about to share a secret. "Jennifer, I'm afraid to tell you this . . . but . . . you are a woman."

"And if they keep treating me like one, I'll own this place. Maybe the captain needs to know about the time those sensitive guys in R-H came by to fill my locker with Tampax and Midol. What about the *Penthouse* magazines my fellow detectives thought my desk just wouldn't be complete without? Why don't you ask the captain if he knows how to spell sexual harassment?"

Larson put his hands on Randazzo's shoulders, trying to calm her down. "Before we threaten a lawsuit, why don't you let me try a more diplomatic approach? Just sit quietly and don't get into any trouble while I'm gone."

Pouting, Randazzo walked over to her desk and sat down. "I won't, unless my gun goes off by accident."

But Randazzo was incapable of just sitting quietly. She grabbed the case file and opened it to Gilmore and Henderson's disjointed report on Penhall, infuriated that the captain would even consider putting them in charge of the entire investigation. Their so-called investigation of the Penhall murder did not include going back to question his neighbors, or asking his wife or her family about their whereabouts, or ever questioning anyone related to his 288 conviction, or even visiting the Oakwood Center. They had ordered only a few photographs taken and had never even spoken with the medical examiner about his findings—too quick to accept the easy answer, not willing to look any further. Their entire report summary: "Male, Caucasian, age 36, shot six times at close range in the underground parking garage at his apartment complex. Murder weapon, .22 caliber pistol. No witnesses. Nothing taken. Apparent botched robbery attempt, consistent with crime spree in vicinity." Superficial police work at best. Randazzo knew she could do better.

The simple fact of Larson's return caused Randazzo to assume that something had been accomplished. She figured—correctly—that he wouldn't have the nerve to come back empty-handed. "Okay, let me give you the good news, first. We're not off the case. In fact, the captain has, quote, 'so much confidence in us' that he wants us to continue to participate in the investigation."

"Did he have that confidence before you threatened him with a lawsuit?"

"Well . . . before . . . after, it's all about the same."

"You really did threaten him?" Randazzo gasped. "Shit. I wasn't serious."

"Listen, what I did is my business. You just concentrate on solving these killings."

"Okay." She paused, then added suspiciously, "But what do you mean by 'participate' in the investigation?"

"Well, in the interest of harmony and cooperation which, of course, are the hallmarks of our department—I think I got the quote right—we're to work closely with Henderson and Gilmore. A 'team effort,' he called it. You know, too big of an investigation for just two lead detectives. But remember, you don't have to take any shit from those guys."

Randazzo let out a heavy sigh and smiled. "You're lucky he didn't kick you off the team and just keep me."

"I told him he'd better keep me around to keep you from biting Henderson and Gilmore in the ankles," Larson joked.

Randazzo turned back to her desk, looking at the stack of papers. "Okay, I'm sure I can find a way to make their lives a living hell. There's a shitload of paperwork that has to be done. I can let them return all the confession phone calls we've been getting. I especially enjoyed the guy who said his cat did it."

"Do you know if his cat has an alibi?" he deadpanned.

"Nope. But I'll make sure Henderson and Gilmore find out. Plus, I need someone to go through those weekly logs at the Oakwood and check the names of every employee—every therapist and secretary who had any contact with the four victims, as well as any other patient they had contact with. And we need to get the names of every person who was involved in the criminal proceedings."

"That's an awful lot of work. You are cruel." Larson smiled. "Okay, would you like to give them their first assignment, or should I?"

Randazzo picked up the phone. "Oh, please. Allow me. You're just not bitchy enough."

"You know, if a guy said that, you'd blow a fuse."

As she happily punched in the numbers, she flashed an imperious smile. "Now you see how the game is played. Let's get to work."

The intercom was usually quite an annoyance to Rebecca. However, this time it brought a welcome announcement. "Detective Larson is on the line."

Rebecca felt her heart race. "Hi," she said brightly.

"Hey, cutie." Larson was thankful for the excuse to call Rebecca. What with two new victims, he knew he'd be deluged all week with work and might have no chance to call her otherwise. And he didn't want another week to go by before he could talk to her again. How fortunate for him that Rebecca was on his investigative "to do" list. "I've missed you. Sorry I haven't called sooner, this case—it keeps getting bigger."

"I heard. You've sure got your hands full!"

"That I have. Did you know these guys? The new ones."

"Jaffe and Knight? Sure. I prosecuted them both." Rebecca looked out her third-floor window to the cluster of trees outside, a few already changing color, a rarity in seasonless Southern California. It was nice knowing she and Jack shared the same general view, his office just a few miles away. "They were just like Matheson—manipulative, conniving. Three peas in the same pod. All extreme sexual abuse—Knight raped and sodomized his daughter, with Jaffe it was a niece. And not one of them did any time, of course, 'cause we can't seem to punish people for hurting members of their own families."

He could hear the contempt in her voice. "You're not still bothered by that, are you?"

"Jack, I think you already know me better than that," she answered softly.

"Well, look, let's not waste our time discussing this crap. When do I get to see you again?"

I guess now is too soon, she thought. "It doesn't sound like you're gonna have much free time," she said, not wanting to put added pressure on him, knowing that work was pressure enough.

"I don't work twenty-four hours a day, you know. I am still a government employee after all. So how 'bout this weekend?"

"I'd love to," she said happily.

"Great. Now I have something to look forward to."

"Yeah, like another one of my speeches," she joked.

"Or another one of your kisses."

Rebecca closed her eyes and felt a tingle race through her body. "Now how am I supposed to work?"

He laughed. "See you soon."

"Bye."

Larson hung up and checked Rebecca off his list of calls for today. He made calls to get the toxicology and forensic reports on the two new victims. They were both wastes of time. He wandered over to the lunch-room in search of food, lost fifty cents in the vending machine in a failed attempt at Chee-tos, found a half-eaten bag of oat bran pretzels that someone else had abandoned, then headed over to Randazzo's desk to see if she had been any more successful.

"What is it with some people?" Randazzo said to no one in particular after hanging up the phone. "Some slime abuses her daughter, and yet the mother feels sorry for the guy."

"You're talking to yourself again, Jen. The department frowns on lunatics in the ranks," he said as he approached, waving the bag of pretzels.

She grabbed the bag out of his hands. "Obviously not. They've kept you around all this time."

Larson smiled. "Sticks and stones may break my bones . . ."

"Oh, grow up."

"Boy, you're even more cranky than usual. What, did you get two periods this month?"

Randazzo shook off Larson's retreat to juvenile humor. "I just got off the phone with Knight's ex. She broke down on the phone. She actually said, 'He's the father of my child.' I wanted to say, 'He wasn't exactly a contender for father of the year, was he?' but I bit my tongue."

"You know, you're very hard to please," he mumbled through a mouthful of pretzels. "You can't have it both ways."

"Whaddya mean?"

"You tell me that just because a guy's a child molester, it doesn't give anyone the right to kill him. Yet, you get mad when the ex of one of them didn't want him dead. A little inconsistent, don't you think?"

"All right, so I'm a complicated person." She tossed the bag back to him. "Where'd you get this crap? It's like eating cardboard. That's the problem with L.A. You people have no idea what a pretzel is supposed to taste like. And why no mustard?" Randazzo went in search of a Coke to wash down the dry crumbs and Larson tagged along as she talked. "I guess I'm just frustrated that these cases aren't making sense."

"No, they make sense. Someone is picking out these guys for a reason. Our problem is, we don't know the reason. We don't know why these guys as opposed to all the other sex offenders out there. What connects these four, that's the question. When we answer that, we'll find our killer."

Randazzo stopped and looked back at Larson. "Sometimes, you have an amazing way of cutting right to the heart of the matter."

"Why, thank you," he responded, looking quite pleased.

"I've never seen anything like this. I mean, is this a serial killer or what? Even the FBI isn't so sure what we have here."

"What do you mean? What did they say?"

Randazzo dropped her quarters into the vending machine and grabbed her Coke as it rumbled out at the bottom. She popped open the tab and took a couple of desperate gulps, capping them with an appreciative "ahhh." She offered Larson some change and he bought himself a Dr. Pepper with the donation. He looked back longingly at the other machine to see if his Chee-tos had fallen yet. They hadn't.

"I've been trying to get a profile of the killer from the FBI," she said as they walked back to their desks. "The guy I spoke with at Behavioral Science, McNamara, told me that statistically, if it's a serial killer, the killer is likely to be a young, white male, with some history of mental illness, who's motivated by a perverse sexual desire that drives him to kill. The evidence that it might be a woman would make this a highly unusual case. Female serial killers are extremely rare."

"Why's that?"

"Not to bore you with the details, but it apparently comes down to how the sexes deal with their psychological problems. Most serial killers have suffered some extreme early childhood trauma. Now, women usually internalize these traumas—turn to drugs, prostitution, suicide—whereas men turn aggressive. That's why he doubted it was a woman. But then, McNamara told me not to confuse a multiple murderer with a serial killer."

Larson slid his chair over to Randazzo's desk and sat down to finish off his morning snack. "So what's the difference?"

"It seemed like in his definition, a serial killer kills because he has to—he has some impulse, some need to punish his victims, that's the key—and he won't stop on his own. He can't. They hunt down their victims—they want to manipulate, dominate, and control them. It's a rush for them. But a multiple killer kills because he wants to—for money, to settle a score, the usual motives—and will stop when he's done."

"Sounds to me like a distinction without a difference."

"No, it's a real distinction. He says it's what separates the real loons—the fantasy-driven compulsives—from your ordinary, run-of-the-mill killer. It's the difference between our killer being nuts and being calculated."

"Which does he think fits our killer?"

"Just based on the first two killings, he voted for calculated. Now, he's not so sure. He's gonna analyze the new killings and get back to me."

"So what you're saying is you wasted your time with McNamara."

Randazzo nodded toward Larson. "Well, it's not like you're doing anything."

"There's where you're wrong."

Randazzo crossed her arms in front of her. This she had to hear. "Oh, really? And what have you accomplished?"

Larson smiled smugly. "I got a date for this weekend."

Randazzo pretended to look for her phone. "Oh, well, let me go call the chief. He'll be pleased to know."

15

Jennifer checked the clock over the cashier's head for something like the hundredth time. Twelve-fifteen, twelve-seventeen, twelve-twenty, each minute indiscriminately clicking off without any regard for her feelings. It wasn't that she was mad at Ben for being late. It was that every passing minute meant a little less time for them to be together. So here she sat, at their favorite diner, waiting for their fleeting moment together before it was back to school for Ben. It gave her time to think—time to think that she still had no real answers and few questions beyond "whodunit."

After what seemed to her like an eternity, Ben plopped down across from her in the booth, his straight blond hair falling haphazardly around his unshaven face. "I know, I'm late. Sorry."

"That's okay. I already ordered for us. You look tired."

"You look beautiful," he said sweetly. Even when he was exhausted, his otherwise glassy eyes always twinkled when he looked at Jennifer. To the guys at the station, who quite begrudgingly had accepted a woman into their fraternity, she was just another cop—the highest compliment for her abilities on the job, to be sure, but not much of an acknowledgment of her more feminine attributes. Still, to him she would always be that cute little Italian girl he couldn't keep his hands off. "I have precisely thirty minutes to eat, catch up on the latest, and tell you I love you. Then it's back to my other woman."

She was caught off guard. "Excuse me?"

"You know, the one who holds those scales."

"I don't get it."

"The scales of justice. I'm sorry, I guess it wasn't as funny as I thought." Ben leaned across the table and kissed her softly on the lips. "I missed you today."

"Stop that," a voice said. "Stop that right now. This is a restaurant. People are trying to eat their food. They can't be watchin' the two of you carrying on like that."

Ben looked up to find his favorite waitress standing above him. "And how are you, Ms. Clark?" That's what her regulars called her. Not Maxine—which her employer had emblazoned on her uniform—but the more respectful designation. With nearly daily visits, Ben clearly qualified as a regular.

"I'm fine, now eat," Maxine ordered as she dropped his usual hamburger and fries in front of him. "Then go home and do that stuff. And get some sleep, boy. You look like shit."

"You tell him. He won't listen to me." Jennifer was glad to have backup.

"Ben, you gonna lose this girl if you don't watch out. Pretty little girl like that don't need no old man with bags under his eyes. You take care of yourself."

"Yes, ma'am," he said, appreciating her concern.

"Okay. Now, I'll be back with your ketchup. See if that burger takes you more than three bites today."

Ben took two rushed bites and washed it down with half an orange soda—good for his schedule, not good for his digestion. "We talked about you in class today," he said.

"You talked about me?" She was surprised and a little flattered.

"Yeah. Well, actually we talked about your case. You'd be surprised how many amateur detectives you can find in law school. So have you come up with anything yet?"

"Nothin' really. Just dead bodies." Jennifer took a bite of her salad. "I can't put it all together yet. Right now, I'm just trying to lay out all the common factors, going by the book."

"So where do you go from here?"

"The insane asylum, 'cause this case is going to drive me crazy."

Ben looked up and said thanks to Ms. Clark for the ketchup, then fretted when he found out it was a new bottle. He tried shaking, tapping, and jiggling but the ketchup refused to move. "Oh, c'mon. I know you," he said as he poked a fry into the bottle, trying to prime the pump. He smiled with satisfaction—that worked. "You're probably not that far away from blowing it open. You just need to put together what you already know and the answer will be right there. As compulsively organized as you are, you must have a shorter list of possible suspects. I'll bet you already have some idea of who the killer is."

"Maybe," Jennifer said offhandedly.

Ben smiled. "I knew it. So what's the big mystery?"

"Okay." She leaned forward. "After I put everything together and prioritized the list of possibles, well, you won't believe who came to the top of the chart."

"Who?"

Jennifer paused, grabbed a french fry off of Ben's plate and ate it slowly, five bites by Ben's count. She picked up another and held it before blurting out, "Jack's new girlfriend." Then she bit it in half.

Ben was caught off guard and struggled to send the remainder of his hamburger down the right path. "What?" he asked, astonished.

"Jack's been seeing the D.A. who prosecuted the first two guys who were killed. He interviewed her about the first two victims and they hit it off and they started going out. No big problem, until lo and behold, victims number three and four turn up, and guess who happened to have prosecuted them both? Same person. She even prosecuted that guy MacDonald who wound up dead—allegedly a suicide, but I don't think so. That's five for five."

Ben didn't hail from Missouri, but he still needed more before he was convinced. "So?" he said.

"When you look at who knew all the victims and had access to information on them and who has a motive to kill all of them, she's right there at the top of the list. You don't know about her. From what I hear, she has a real attitude about the guys she prosecutes, and she doesn't take losing very well. Each of the first four walked, pretty much. MacDonald, too. They got a few years straight probation, but that was it. She took it very badly. So you got motive. Plus, the evidence points to the killer having long blonde hair, just like the D.A. And it's only her defendants who are getting killed. That's a little too much just to be a coincidence, don't you think?"

Ben took a long sip of his soda as he shrugged. "I hate to be redundant, but 'so?' If every D.A. who lost a case gunned down the defendant—hey, that'd be pretty cool," he kidded. "Besides, there's no shortage of women with long blonde hair in Los Angeles."

"I didn't think you had time to notice," Jennifer

needled. "Thanks for all your help." She sat back in her chair, pretending to pout.

"Well, I don't know. It sounds pretty farfetched to me."

"I know you're probably right. I mean, I have a hard time seeing a D.A. turn into a killer just because she loses a few cases. But none of the other angles have panned out. Plus, I've been asking around about her and so far everyone who knows her says she is wound tighter than a clock. Maybe she became so frustrated and angry she decided to take the law into her own hands and blow some guy's head open."

Ben stopped midbite, considered his ketchup-drenched french fry, then went ahead, popping the rest in his mouth. He had decided long ago not to let Jennifer's mealtime discussions get in the way of his food. "I don't know," he shrugged. "Does she strike you as capable of something like this?"

"I haven't actually met her yet. Maybe I should ask Jack if we could all go out together, you talk to him about sports while I find out if she has an alibi for any of the killings."

"That's subtle."

"I don't know what else to do. I just have this feeling that she's involved, and I don't have much to go on except this feeling. I think we should check her out, but obviously I can't count on Jack. Unless it's to do a strip search, that is. But I feel weird investigating her. What do you think I should do?"

"I think if you investigate her, you should do it quietly."

Jennifer lifted her eyebrows. "So you don't think I'm crazy?"

Ben reached for her hand. "Not while you're the only one who brings home a paycheck."

✧ ✧ ✧

"We've got to stop meeting like this. People are beginning to talk again," Tom kidded as he stood in the office kitchen, waiting for the coffee to finish brewing. He silently cursed whoever took the last cup and had the audacity to leave without starting up a fresh batch.

"You know, I don't even want any. I just come down here out of boredom," said Rebecca.

"Me too. I've spent the whole morning behind my desk. I'm drowning in paperwork. God, I love my job—what it lacks in pay it more than makes up for in monotony. File a motion, oppose a motion, get a cup of coffee, file a motion, oppose a motion, go to the bathroom."

"You know, if you gave up the coffee, you could also give up going to the bathroom. That would simplify your day."

"Very funny. So what are you working on?" Tom asked.

Rebecca leaned on the counter and watched as the coffee started to drip into the pot. "Catching up on some unfinished business. Going through some of my old files, nothing exciting. I don't even have any trials scheduled till next month, and I'm all ready for it, so there's not much more to do."

"Your life sounds as dull as mine. You need to get out and have some fun so I can at least enjoy life vicariously." A touchy subject Tom handled gingerly.

Rebecca thought for a moment. Why not tell him? She was a grown woman, he was married, certainly she could date whomever she pleased. "Actually, I just started to see someone," she said coyly, waiting for Tom to take the bait. No reason not to have a little fun with her revelation.

"That's great," Tom said, a bit too enthusiastically. "Who's the lucky guy?"

"Funny you should ask. It's Jack. Jack Larson. You remember him. Your best man," Rebecca deadpanned.

If Rebecca wanted a reaction from Tom, she wasn't disappointed. He looked like the proverbial deer in the headlights—right after the truck ran him over. Startled and unsure what to do next, he tried to hide his well-telegraphed shock. "Really. You and Jack." A weak laugh. "Wow. I—uh—well, that's just great. Really." Tom pieced it together, a sharp stab of pain. "I gave him your number," he said with resignation.

"Thanks," Rebecca said brightly. "I'm sure glad you did. He's a great guy."

He ran his hand through his hair, not at all surprised to find much of it sticking between his fingers. "Yeah, great guy. Wow, you and Jack."

"You said that already."

"So I did." Tom suddenly grabbed the pot and filled Rebecca's cup, the last drops from the coffeemaker sizzling on the hot plate. "You know, I never would have put you two together. I thought he only went for bimbos."

"Oh, you mean the type you marry?" she snapped.

"That was uncalled for," Tom shot back.

Rebecca recoiled slightly, a little embarrassed. "You're right. Sorry."

Tom hastily filled his cup, passing on the cream and sugar to save time. He knew he better get out of there before either of them said anything else they might regret later. But it was all her fault, he decided, sneaking up on him like that. What was she expecting him to do, throw them a party? "Well, I really should get back to work. Say 'hi' to Jack for me."

"Sure will. And give my best to the missus." A little too flip, Rebecca thought. But appropriate.

Rebecca enjoyed the sight of Tom twisting in the wind. She had grown tired of his pity. Turning the tables was starting to feel real good.

Wednesday night at the Oakwood Center brought with it the usual assortment of sexual miscreants. Anita had a roomful of incest offenders, Valerie was surrounded by "queers"—as the other men at the clinic derisively referred to the gay child molesters— and David was up to his eyeballs in flashers. Anita checked her roster—three missing. These days, roll call took on a new meaning at the Oakwood. Absenteeism no longer meant that one of the men was ditching group. Now death was a plausible reason.

Anita came in tonight sporting a new hairdo, her hair cut in blunt layers around her attractive, subtly made-up face. Outfitted in a narrow red skirt with a slit up the back and matching, fitted jacket, she looked like a stewardess for a Scandinavian airline. None of this was done for the benefit of her group. With two new murders of fellow child molesters weighing on them, they didn't notice Anita's appearance anyway.

"Well, let's get started. Who wants to go first?" Anita asked, looking around the room for a volunteer. The men were uncharacteristically silent. "Doesn't anyone have anything to say?"

Most of the men looked around at each other, no one wanting to begin. They breathed a collective sigh of relief when Hal leaned forward, signaling he'd take the lead. "I heard that two more guys were killed. Have you heard anything about it?"

Anita wasn't surprised that Hal led off the

evening. He always had something to say, except when it came time to discuss why he taught his six-year-old daughter to orally copulate with him. "Well, what do you want to know?" she asked, careful always to answer a question with a question.

"I don't know, I'm just worried. I'm sure everyone is," Hal added, speaking for the group. "Obviously, someone's out there killing child molesters."

Anita nodded to herself. She had expected this would be the topic for some time—at least as long as new victims turned up. "And do you think that you're at risk?"

He bristled, thinking her question ridiculous. "What do you think?"

"It's not important what I think. What do you think?" Anita tossed it back at him with an unnerving smile. "Are you scared?"

"Only if the police don't do something soon. I don't know how long that fucking list is."

Anita noticed a number of men nodding their agreement. "My understanding is the police are doing their best to catch the killer," she offered.

The room filled with sarcastic laughter. "Yeah, like the cops are going to spend a lot of time on this case," said Carlos, a heavyset man with a thick black mustache. "I don't think so. The only reason they're going to want to catch the killer is to pin a medal on him."

"Or her," added Hal.

"That's right. It's women who get all bent out of shape about this stuff. They're the ones who can't understand our perspective. Women just don't appreciate our urges and impulses," added Carlos.

"Quite frankly, I'm not sure there is anything to appreciate about your urges. Do you?" Anita glowered. She was incensed with Carlos's automatic retreat into excuse making and minimization. She was never one to be impressed with rationalizations or easily swayed by self-pity. True, many of the men in the group had troubled childhoods. Hal had been beaten by his alcoholic stepfather, Marty was abandoned at two by his mother and raised in abusive foster homes, and Carlos had been raped by an uncle at nine. However, to her mind, that in no way entitled any of them to continue the cycle of abuse.

"I didn't mean it that way," Carlos recanted.

"Let's hope not."

"What if it's not one killer?" Marty interjected. "What if there are different killers? Maybe when they heard about the murders, with everyone talking about a serial killer, some guy's ex or whoever said, 'Hey, what a great idea. I can kill the guy and no one will suspect me.'"

"Oh, thanks. That makes me feel much better. Now all I have to wonder is whether my sister is sitting at home sharpening her knitting needles," said Drew, an ex-marine who had an unfortunate problem of liking little girls and little else, his niece included.

"Does anyone else harbor some fear that they could be next?" asked Anita.

"Yeah. Just last week my ex was giving me some crap about child support. I'm supposed to pay five hundred dollars a month for a kid the court hasn't let me see in three years. I told her to go fuck herself and the lawyer she rode in on. 'How'm I supposed to pay my bills? Don't you care about that?' I asked. And then she goes off about how I should have my dick cut off and shoved down my throat. Now I'm thinking—maybe she'll do it. Christ, like I don't already have enough to worry about," Hal complained.

"I'll tell you, I fired off my child support payment

so fast—don't want nobody to get any funny ideas," Marty added.

"Is anyone else concerned about their safety?" The irony of the situation was not lost on Anita, who stifled the urge to laugh out loud.

"Not me," said Frank, here on a makeup for an earlier missed session. "I'm just too cute to kill."

"Oh, spare me," said Hal.

Frank ignored him. "You know, one of the detectives came by the Monday group a week ago, and I can tell you, they don't know shit. They're looking in all the wrong places."

"Well, that makes me feel much better," Marty said with a halfhearted laugh.

"You know, I saw this show on TV. All these 'experts' saying how the problem is we can't be treated and that we should be kept off the streets permanently. Why wasn't Hillerman on TV protecting us, saying how therapy works?" Paul asked. A thin man who could make coffee nervous, he was one of the rare true believers in the merits of therapy, coming to the clinic for individual, group, and even family sessions.

"Is that what's bothering you, Paul? That Dr. Hillerman hasn't come to your defense?" Anita asked. "Believe me, he is working very hard to gather data to be able to show once and for all that therapy works and is a far better solution for everyone than prison. But he's not the kind of expert who will just go on TV making bold assertions without the supporting data. When the time is right, he'll lay it all out, and that should help debunk some of the misunderstandings."

"Yeah, but in the meantime, couldn't he just say that we're not all these monsters who are finally getting what they deserve? Couldn't he explain that we're in treatment to get better? I'm so sick and tired of watching on the TV all these people trying to explain the murders as understandable and expected. Like, sure, why shouldn't child molesters be killed? I mean, nobody seems the least bit bothered by the killings. Nobody mentioned that the guys had been in therapy for all these years and were getting help," said Paul, his fingers darting nervously around his face as if stroking an invisible beard.

"He's right, you know. Not one person has gone on TV and said how the guys who were killed were victims. No one seems troubled that some crazy person is killing guys for something they did years ago," said Jerome, an older man with thinning gray hair and stooped posture. He maintained a firm belief that what's past is past, including his two-year history of fondling his granddaughter.

"Guys, I do think that you are blowing this somewhat out of proportion. I know most of you think you've been treated rather unfairly—that between the courts, the probation officers, your exes, and the lawyers, you've been, if you pardon the pun, screwed. But let's be real. The world isn't 'out to get you.' It's natural for people to be talking about the killings. The killings have just brought to the surface society's hatred of child molesters. You can't be all that surprised?" Anita asked incredulously. "The public has gotten tired of reading about child molesters who pass through the system only to molest again. So seeing the tables turned, in a manner of speaking, and someone getting to child molesters before that can happen—well—that's intriguing to a lot of people. Not that it's right, necessarily, but it does tap into the public's frustration."

The men grumbled, convinced Anita wasn't seeing things through their eyes. Hal spoke up. "Aren't you supposed to be on our side? I don't want you to think I'm minimizing, but most of the guys in this room, I just don't think we did anything that horrible. Not to get killed for."

Anita raised an eyebrow. How, after all this time, could Hal continue to believe he hadn't done anything that bad? She called on her training to maintain an empathic demeanor. "I am on your side, but I think some of you are acting a little paranoid about all of this. I wonder if this isn't unearthing some deep-seated feeling in all of you that maybe you do deserve this kind of punishment? A number of you seem to think that all child molesters are in danger of being killed, and I'm not ready to concede that. Why do you feel this way?"

Hal's jaw dropped in disbelief and he looked around the room for support. Surely the other guys would see it his way. "Don't you watch the news?" he asked Anita.

"And you believe everything you hear on the news?" Anita retorted.

"I believe that four guys are dead, that's what I believe," said Hal. "That's not just a coincidence. Who are you trying to kid? There's something going on here and we're just sitting around waiting to see who's next. I've talked to a lawyer and he says you guys have a duty to protect your patients and you better tell Hillerman that he better start doing that. I don't know about the rest of you, but I'm not going to hang around here waiting for someone to call my number."

Anita wrote up a few notes about the session and then scored everyone's participation on a scale of one for snoring through the session to five for dropping to their knees begging forgiveness for their crime. Most got a three for piping up with something halfway meaningful somewhere during the two

hours—as they did each week they were there—
which was all they needed to keep their probation
officers happy. Anita finished her paperwork and
started to pack up to leave. She was startled when
Hillerman came into the conference room after it had
cleared out. He was usually there only nine to five,
leaving his minions to work after dark.

"Anita, how was your session? Were you regaled
with hours of sorrowful contrition from our clien-
tele?" Pronounced clee-untel, for maximum affecta-
tion.

Anita smiled at Hillerman's attempt at humor.
"Not tonight. All anyone wanted to talk about were
the killings."

He nodded knowingly. "Well, you can understand
why. These men are pretty egocentric to begin with,
so the fear that they might be next must occupy their
every thought. Oh, well, I'm sure you'll find a way to
use it in a therapeutic way."

Anita couldn't tell if he was being sincere, and she
was unsure how he felt about her abilities as a therapist. Unsure how he felt about her at all anymore. "I
suppose," she mumbled. She passed her hand
through her hair, hoping he'd notice the new cut. He
had complained that the long, straight look was not
flattering, and she was sure he'd appreciate the
change. But he seemed to be looking through her.

"Anything of interest come out of the session?
Anything of which I should be aware?" he asked, getting to the point of his unexpected visit.

Anita cleared her throat. "Well, one of the guys
mentioned suing you or the center, something about
all the victims being tied to the center. He said you
have to protect them."

"And who is this 'he'?" Hillerman demanded.

"Hal."

Hillerman threw his head back and laughed in an

exaggerated gesture. "Oh, Mr. Complainer. As I recall, Hal has wanted to sue us over everything from the air conditioner not working to your less-than-favorable last report on him. Anyone else say anything I should know about?"

Anita shrugged. She wasn't sure what Hillerman wanted to know and concentrated on replaying the session to see if she had anything to offer him. "No," she said finally, then quickly added, "I mean, they're clearly worried. There's no question about that. The killer's sure got their attention."

"Well, that's good. Maybe they'll become even more committed to their rehabilitation now." Hillerman turned on his heels and headed for the door.

"Would you—uh—like to go out for a cup of coffee?" Anita sputtered. "Do you have to get home right away?" She looked up at him, with a slight smile on her face. She took a couple steps toward him. "We haven't talked in a long time."

"No, sorry." He looked around the room, as if trying to find something. "I must head off. You have a lovely evening, Anita."

Anita looked hurt, but Hillerman didn't notice. He turned and walked out, leaving her standing alone in the conference room. "Thank you, Dr. Hillerman," she called after him as he left. "I will."

16

Usually, Hal had no trouble putting the group discussions out of his mind. As he saw it, his sentence only required him to attend group; it didn't require him to think about it afterward. But he couldn't get the thought out of his head that he might now be on somebody's list. Hal felt anxious as he approached each intersection, hoping for a green light so he wouldn't have to sit there waiting for something to happen. He looked around furtively, wondering. Would he even notice if someone were following him?

As he turned onto his street, Hal started to talk himself out of his panic almost as quickly as he had talked himself into it. This is ridiculous, he told himself. I am not going to be spooked by this. It's probably just a coincidence, just like some of the guys said. L.A. was a violent town, after all, and lots of people were getting killed every day over less than nothing. And, anyway, compared with some of the guys in group, he was a saint. Shit, Carlos fucked his niece in the ass so hard she needed stitches. And

Marty was going down on his daughter even before she was out of diapers. Let them worry. There's no need to change my routine, he told himself, fairly convincingly.

As he turned the key, Hal could hear the familiar panting on the other side of the door. He opened the door and was instantly pounced on by his flea-bitten mutt of a friend, short tail wagging in orgasmic frenzy. Hal grabbed the leash, a jacket for himself, and headed out for Rocky's nightly walk. It was a brisk night. That day's strong winds had left the sky so clear that even all the city lights couldn't obscure the stars. Hal tried to slow the dog's frantic pace, wanting to unwind in a leisurely stroll, but Rocky had other ideas—setting a new record for most deposits left in the shortest amount of time. They rounded the block, with Mrs. Sherman's petunias, Mrs. Weinberg's begonias, and Mrs. Williams's geraniums all being fair game. A half hour later, Hal led Rocky back to the apartment.

Rocky pulled on the leash, back toward the street. "Oh, come on, Rocky. That was a long enough walk. It's starting to get real cold. Let's go inside." He dragged the reluctant dog through the door.

Rocky apparently was the first to realize they weren't alone. He growled, bared his teeth, and jumped at the figure on the couch. The gun exploded, and Rocky let out a high-pitched cry as he fell to the ground.

"Got him on the rise."

"Oh, my God! Oh, my God!" Hal cried as he looked down at what no longer resembled his dog.

"I didn't know you were so religious, Hal. Self-centered, self-absorbed, yes. But, pious? What a surprise."

Despite the cold, Hal was immediately soaked in sweat. He dropped to his knees to hug his beloved pet.

"You know, it never ceases to amaze me how people who care so little for their fellow humans can be so enamored of stupid animals. It's just a dog, Hal. I've got a joke. What's black and white and red all over? Give up? Your dog." With that, the killer shot Rocky again. Hal jumped back as the animal slumped to the ground.

"Why are you doing this? What did I do? Why me?" he shouted, his voice choked with terror.

"'Why?' is not the question. 'How?' is. And I just can't decide. But I've got some ideas. However, first, would you be so kind as to put the masking tape over your mouth? I've laid it on the table for you."

Hal sat on the floor, staring at the tape.

"Hal, I believe I just gave you an explicit instruction. You have one second to comply and then there will be a penalty, a death penalty so to speak. Although I guess that's not much of an incentive, since you're going to get that penalty anyway. Oops, did I give away the surprise?"

Hal looked up helplessly, overwhelmed with fear, realizing for the first time that his life was about to end. Finally, his trembling hand reached out and fumbled for the tape. He started the tape and began to place it across his mouth, whimpering as he tore it off the roll.

"Good. Now we won't have to hear from you again. By the way, did you know that you were hyperventilating? You must try to relax. And really, Hal, the tears are rather unbecoming."

Hal decided his only chance was to go for the gun. It looked so small, he thought even if he was shot he still might make it. He leapt forward, aiming for the gun, and was surprised by the two quick pops and the burning sensation in his stomach. As he looked down, he saw blood pouring from the small wounds. He gasped with pain and fright and fell backward over the coffee table. His blood ran freely onto the floor, meeting the stream of Rocky's blood to form a crimson river.

"Not fast enough, Hal. Good try, though. As Lou Grant said to Mary Richards—'You've got spunk. I hate spunk.'" The killer rose slowly from the couch. Consumed with anger, the voice twisted into a sing-songy whine. "You know, Hal, I suppose I should feel very sorry about this." Another shot ripped through his cheek. "But I don't."

Hal's screams were distorted and muffled by the tape. He clasped his cheek, his hand feeling the warmth of his blood.

"Oh, who am I kidding? I do feel a little sorry for you. Just like the others, you don't seem to appreciate how amusing this all is—watching you cower and whimper and cry out in pain. You should be having the time of your life. What there is left of it, that is. Which, in all candor, really isn't much now." The killer shot again, hitting Hal in the leg. "That one was for sport."

Hal's hands clawed the air in vain, his screams replaced by a repetitive moaning, barely audible.

"You know, you and your dog really make quite a lovely picture. I've got an idea. Wait right there. Please, don't get up on my account." The killer went into the kitchen, returning with a small carving knife. The killer looked down at Hal's contorted body and smiled. "Well, you've been a wonderful host, but I've got to go. However, before I leave, I have something special for you, in honor of the season. Maybe if you have an out-of-body experience, you'll get to see it."

When Hal Riddell was found the next day, he was so covered in blood the details of the carving were lost. It was the medical examiner's assistant who first caught a glimpse of the happy face carved across Hal's chest.

✢ ✢ ✢

"This is Linda Marquez, Channel Ten news, reporting to you live from City Hall where Police Chief Peter Bellamy is about to make a statement regarding the recent string of child molester murders." Her voice was breathless with excitement, her dark eyes twinkling with glee. "Early this morning Harold James Riddell, thirty-six, of Venice, was found dead in his apartment, an apparent victim of the Child Molester Slayer. Both he and his dog had been shot to death. Like the other victims, Mr. Riddell had a felony conviction for incest and was currently on probation, having served no prison time for his offense. Okay, Chief Bellamy is approaching the microphone. Let's listen."

"Excuse me, Dr. Hillerman. You wanted to see me?" Valerie asked, oblivious to Hillerman's focused attention on the television in his office.

Hillerman kept his eyes on the TV. "Valerie, not right now. Can't you see that I'm busy?"

"Oh, I'm sorry. I saw the message you needed to talk to me and I thought—"

"After the press conference is over!" Hillerman snapped. "I want to hear this. We lost another patient last night."

Valerie walked over to the TV. "Is it about the killing? What are they saying?"

"If you'd stop talking, I'd know."

Valerie sat down quietly on the edge of a chair, watching the TV as the chief began to speak.

"Thank you for coming," Chief Bellamy began. A tall, powerfully built man, the chief silenced the room with the first sounds of his booming voice. "I'd like to make a brief statement and then we'll take questions. As you are aware, this morning the body of Harold Riddell was discovered. He is the fifth convicted child molester killed in the last two months. While we cannot conclusively state at this time that all five murders are related, we are obviously investigating that possibility. Regardless of the potential connection, however, there has been some suggestion that because the victims were all convicted child molesters the department is not devoting or should not devote its full attention to this matter. Let me state unequivocally that we are putting our maximum effort into this investigation."

"Dr. Hillerman?" Valerie interjected.

He snapped his head to look at her, his eyes as scolding as his tone of voice. "Valerie, I want to hear this. You'll just have to wait until this is over."

"Now to answer your questions, I have with me today"—Chief Bellamy looked down at his notes to make sure that he had all the names right—"the two lead detectives assigned to this investigation, Detective Jack Larson and Detective Jennifer Randazzo." Randazzo smiled at the official designation—lead detective. Bellamy continued, unaware. "They are coordinating the investigation with the FBI, Robbery-Homicide, Special Investigations, and the West L.A. and East Valley divisions. They will answer your questions to the extent they can without compromising the integrity of the ongoing investigation. Also with us is their captain, Hank Robinson, Detectives Jonas Henderson and Mark Gilmore from Robbery-Homicide, and Lieutenant David Andrews from the North Hollywood division."

The shouting began. "Detectives, why do you believe that the murders are all the work of the same killer?" As both Randazzo and Henderson moved forward, Chief Bellamy whispered "Jack" and nodded toward the microphones. Larson acknowledged the sign and positioned himself to answer the question.

He looked over apologetically to Randazzo before he began.

Larson squinted in the glare of the camera lights. "As you know, we cannot at this point divulge any specifics of the evidence found at the scenes. However, there are certain similarities between the murders, which suggest that the same person may be responsible for all five killings—dating back to the murder of Eric Penhall. The fact that each victim was a convicted child molester is, of course, a common factor that cannot be ignored." Larson was proud of himself—he had said nothing, but nevertheless sounded intelligent. Randazzo was fuming, and it showed.

"Detective, do you believe the killer to be a woman, as some have suggested, and, if so, wouldn't that be highly unusual, a female serial killer?" another voice called out.

"We are not ruling out the possibility that our killer may be a woman. But, yes, based on what we have learned, female serial killers are the exception, not the rule," Larson stated.

The group of reporters all shouted out at once and Larson pointed at random, letting them figure out who was next. "Have there been any witnesses? We've heard reports that the police have a description of the killer. Can you confirm this?" asked a young female reporter with an oversprayed auburn flip.

Larson wondered why—since the reporter seemed to know as much as he did—there was even a need for a press conference. "What you may be referring to is a description we have of an individual seen in the vicinity of the last murder. By tomorrow, we will be circulating a sketch of the person. At this time, we are not saying that this person is a suspect in the killings. It is merely someone we would like to talk to."

"Have you talked with the victims of the child molesters for their reactions? They must be pretty relieved," said a middle-aged male reporter in heavy makeup.

"We have had conversations with some of the victims, but beyond that, we cannot elaborate," answered Larson. "We'd like to honor their privacy as much as possible," he added diplomatically.

"What is the police department doing to protect other potential victims?" The reporter's question was barely audible from the back of the pack.

"Well, certainly, we do not have the resources to provide round-the-clock protection to every child molester on probation, but we can do our best to catch the killer before any more victims turn up. And that is what we are doing."

"So the streets can be safe for child molesters once again?" A woman snickered from within the throng.

Bellamy moved forward. "That is just the sort of attitude that the police department will not condone." The chief's noted temper flared, index finger pointing in the direction of the offending remark. "We are as committed to finding the killer of these men as we would be if the victims had been nuns on their way back from an orphanage," Bellamy said disingenuously. No one believed him, but it made good copy. "Next question."

"Detectives, can you confirm that the bodies were mutilated?" one of the tabloid "journalists" asked, more interested in his question than in the anticipated answer.

"Were the men sexually abused in any way?" another chimed in.

A third decided to be less vague. "Is it true their penises were cut off?" he asked, having no idea if such a rumor even existed.

"We have not officially released any of the findings about the conditions in which the bodies were found, in order to protect the investigation and any later criminal proceeding. Any rumor about the conditions in which the bodies were found is just that, for now—rumor," Larson answered.

The chief had said all he'd planned to. He'd certainly heard enough, so he stepped back in front of the microphone. "We appreciate you all coming down, and we will certainly notify you of any further developments in the investigation." With that the press conference was over. The media throng shouted their obligatory last questions, which the chief, following protocol, ignored as he and the others left the stage.

The raven-haired reporter turned swiftly back to her camera for her sign-off. "That was Police Chief Peter Bellamy and part of the police team investigating the murders of now five convicted child molesters. To review, the police have no leads in any of the murders, although they are looking for a witness seen near the site of last night's murder for questioning. In addition, the police stressed that, regardless of public opinion, they are conducting their investigation to the fullest extent possible. We will have an update on this story at four. This is Linda Marquez, Channel Ten news."

"What a bunch of idiots." Hillerman snapped off the TV and turned to face Valerie. "Now, what were you saying?" Without waiting for an answer, Hillerman continued on. "Can you believe that? It's almost ironic. Harold Riddell threatens to sue me for not protecting my patients and look what happens to him. Well, I guess he won't be filing that lawsuit now, will he?"

"No," Valerie said softly.

"I'll tell you one thing—we're well rid of him. I just

hope that the added publicity doesn't hurt us too much." Hillerman rose to pour himself another cup of coffee. "Now, Valerie, the reason I wanted to talk to you is because I am very concerned with your work performance around here. Deeply concerned." He sat back down behind his desk in his slightly elevated chair, where he could lower his head to look down at a visibly nervous Valerie. "You know, since you were Herman Kingsley's daughter, I took a chance when I hired you and I expected you to rise to the occasion. However, that has not been the case. Your work is subpar, you have been behind in your reports, your groups are disorganized, and with what happened with Matheson, your participation in the family study has been less than impressive. Much less."

Valerie's heart was pounding and she bit her lower lip nervously. "I know, Dr. Hillerman. That was a terrible mistake, but I promised it wouldn't happen again. And it hasn't."

Hillerman shook his head gravely. "I'm just not sure you're up to the job. I've tried to help you, I've been more than patient. I was willing to give you a little extra time to prove yourself, but I have seen absolutely no improvement." He sighed heavily for effect and noted to his enjoyment the little mannerisms that told him she was distressed.

"I'm sorry. I've been trying, really I have. I just need some more time. There was so much to learn and I keep getting more groups and covering other people's groups when they need the help. I guess I get overwhelmed sometimes." Valerie fiddled with a small charm hanging from a solid gold chain she wore around her neck.

"Well maybe you need to say no more often." Hillerman jabbed his finger toward Valerie, emphasizing his point. "If you can't cover a group, just say so. There's no reason for you to compromise the center merely because you don't want to hurt someone's feelings. You cannot take on more than you can handle." He leaned forward, his arms stretched out in front of him on his desk. "Valerie, I have given you far more chances than anyone else would. But this is not the time for me to have any weak links in the center's chain. I need everyone to perform at their peak. I need the probation department to be catered to—their reports sent out on time, their phone calls returned promptly, all their needs met. Without them, we are out of business. Do you understand?" He paused to let his words register. When he saw her falter, he knew he'd been understood. "I cannot tolerate anything that causes them to be unhappy. They can just pull all the patients out of here at any time and send them to Elmhurst or some other center. Do you see how important this is?"

"Yes, of course. I don't want to do anything to hurt the center. I've been working hard to get better. You'll see. If you give me another chance, you won't regret it. You'll be very proud of me." Valerie's voice became stronger. "I really like it here. You know that. You've helped me so much and I want to repay you by doing the very best I can. I really appreciate the time you've spent with me." She leaned forward and reached across the desk and squeezed Hillerman's hand. "I really think I would have been lost without you."

He looked down at her hand, smooth and supple against his dry, ruddy skin. "Valerie, I have told you and told you, you can be as good or as bad a therapist as you want to be. It is all up to you." He patted her hand. "I will give you a little more time to pull yourself together. But I must see improvement."

Valerie exhaled deeply as the relief spread across her. "Oh, thank you. I promise I won't disappoint you."

Hillerman smiled. "I'm sure you won't."

As Valerie got up and started out the door, he added, "See you after work," more as a statement than a question. Valerie paused for a moment, nodded her head, then kept walking.

Chief Bellamy stayed for a perfunctory, but necessary, visit with his detectives. "Thanks for coming for the show. Now, if there is anything else you need, more manpower—excuse me"—he laughed, looking over at Randazzo—"person power, more lab help, whatever, give me a call directly. Let's catch the killer. All right?"

"Thanks for your support, Chief," Larson said, extending his hand to Bellamy. The chief left quickly, accompanied by a phalanx of advisers and aides.

Randazzo stood watching the chief and his entourage walk away, her hands on her hips. "'Person power,' oh, save me. He practically threw a body block on me to keep me from answering any questions. What an ass."

"Jennifer—"

Randazzo cut him off. "Don't 'Jennifer' me."

"Maybe he just wanted someone with a little more experience dealing with the media. You know, someone—"

"—with a dick."

Larson chafed. "That's not what I was going to say. Anyway, Henderson has a dick and the chief didn't let him talk either."

"Fine." It came out "foin." Brooklyn came back strong when she got irked. "So I'm little Miss Oversensitive. I just want to know if all the time I'm spending bustin' my butt to solve this case is gonna end up makin' you and all the other golden boys look like heroes. Nothin' personal, pal, but I'm not workin' this hard to make you look good."

"Listen, hotshot. You solve this one and I'll personally go on TV and give you all the press you could possibly want. I'll even take out an ad in the *Times* touting your unequaled talents as a detective. Fair enough?"

"You'd better." She flipped open her notebook, the new one labeled Harold Riddell. She was about to read from her already detailed notes when she was interrupted by a tall, dark, and menacing presence—Henderson in a bad mood. An otherwise handsome man with mocha skin and intense brown eyes, Henderson's anger caused a deep inverted v-shaped crease above the bridge of his nose and forced his mouth downturned and hard.

"Nice move, Larson. I didn't know at your age you could cut and run so well," he groused as he walked over to Larson.

Larson turned to face Henderson, who stood glaring at him, his face in a scowl. Larson just shook his head—first Randazzo, now Henderson. "Not you too! Jesus, is this an investigation or media event? I'm sorry if I pissed everyone off, but it was the chief's call."

That didn't mollify Henderson. "It's a white man's world, that's what it is." He sneered. "There's no other reason you're in charge of this case, Larson. I tell you one thing, I'm not about to carry your bags on this one. No motherfucking way."

Larson was visibly annoyed. "Oh, God. Here we go again. Would you leave it alone, Henderson? It's getting real old."

"Don't want to hear the truth, do you?" Henderson poked Larson in the chest. "You know they say the cream rises to the top, but then, so does scum. You can do all the press conferences you want. You can think you're running things. But this was my case from the beginning, and it's gonna be mine in the end. Count on it." Henderson stormed off, not wanting to lower himself to arguing with a Valley cop.

Larson turned to Randazzo. "Did I mention that guy's an ass?" he asked.

"You didn't have to. Some things are obvious," she said.

"Okay, so tell me more about our eyewitness," Larson asked. To save time and not be late for the press conference, they had split up, Larson following the body to the morgue while Randazzo stayed at the scene to oversee the criminalists.

Randazzo checked her notes. "She's a nice, older woman who lives in the duplex next door. She said she was looking outside her window and thought she saw a woman entering Riddell's condo—a white female, tall, slim, with long light brown or blonde hair. But she didn't hear anything. When I went in to talk with her she had her TV on pretty loud, so it's possible she missed the gunshots. The uniforms asked around the complex and found a couple who thought they heard either shots or a car backfire at around eleven and a man who heard Riddell's dog barking also around eleven. But the elderly neighbor was the only one who claims to have seen something."

"Well, if it's detailed, the sketch oughta help," Larson offered.

"Don't get too excited. I'm not going to try to build an entire case on this eyewitness," Randazzo said, shaking her head. "She's like Mr. Magoo in drag. My grandma wore glasses like that. She always thought I was my cousin Constance. We wouldn't make it past the prelim on her ID alone." Randazzo closed her notebook and put it behind her back. "So what did you find out, hotshot?"

"You'll love the photos. He looks like chopped liver. First he was shot, then he was carved like a pumpkin."

"How festive. It's just like McNamara told me. It's textbook, for heaven's sake. Once the killer starts, he can't stop. There'll be more and more till we catch him. And he'll need more gore each time. Except that it still looks like our he's a she."

"So where to now?"

"Well, obviously, we need to go back to the Oakwood, and then maybe we should, or maybe you might want to, you know . . ." Randazzo hesitated. "Check out who prosecuted him. Twenty bucks says it was Fielding."

Larson missed the reluctance in Randazzo's voice. "The way it's been going, I'd bet you're right," he said offhandedly.

"Doesn't that strike you as odd, Jack? That she prosecuted each of the five?"

He looked at her, confused. "No, why should it? That's her job."

Randazzo wanted to say something, to grab him by the shoulders and shake him awake. But she had decided to keep her concerns to herself until she had something concrete, so she did the hardest thing for her. She said nothing.

17

Although Randazzo had little more than a hunch to go on, she did have some free time to go along with her nagging curiosity. A dangerous combination for someone who needed all questions to be answered. So she used Larson's dentist appointment to delve into Rebecca's background. Ralph Simpson was only too happy to indulge her suspicions, artfully hinting at what Randazzo was already thinking, leaving her more convinced than ever that what she started with might turn out to be much more than just a hunch.

"Well, you've really been a big help, Mr. Simpson." Randazzo snapped her notebook shut and put her pen in her purse. "Thanks for all the information."

"You know, I certainly wouldn't want to do or say anything to hurt Rebecca, Detective." Ralph's usually shifty eyes went wide with innocent concern. He put his hand to his chest for added effect. "But I feel it's my duty as an officer of the court to tell you what I know. Thinking back to when I first met Rebecca, even then I could tell there was something strange about her—" He leaned back and clasped his hands behind his head, ready for another story.

"That's okay, Mr. Simpson. I think I have enough for now. Again, thanks for all your help," Randazzo said, cutting him off as she rose from her seat and extended her hand. She had gotten what she needed and had been trying for the past five minutes to get out of his office. Randazzo was beginning to feel uncomfortable, as if she were going behind Jack's back just by being there. If she got back to the office before Jack, she wouldn't have to make up a story about where she was.

Ralph rose to his feet—his shirt partially untucked and his tie just a little short—and shook her hand firmly, like old pals. "I'll call you if I think of anything else you should know."

Randazzo was pretty sure she'd hear from him again. "Thanks."

As Randazzo hurried out the door and into the hallway, she practically crashed into Rebecca. "Sorry," she said quickly, before looking up.

"Narrow halls," Rebecca noted with a smile.

"Oh, Detective Randazzo, one more thing," Ralph called out the door. He stopped in his tracks when he saw Rebecca. The three of them looked at each other. "That's okay, I'll call you," he said and quickly withdrew into his office, shutting the door behind him.

Rebecca noticed Ralph's odd behavior, his apparent unwillingness to talk in front of her and quick retreat, but decided to ignore him, a habit she wished everyone would develop. She instead focused on Randazzo. "You must be Jack's partner."

"Yes. Yes, I am," Randazzo answered, her curiosity only fleeting as she quickly figured out who she'd run over.

Rebecca extended her hand. "Hi. Rebecca Fielding. Jack and I have been, uh, well, we've talked about the child molester killings you're working on." She smiled brightly, pleased to be meeting Jack's partner.

Randazzo studied Rebecca for a moment, the tall, WASP goddess type that had been the bane of her high school years. She had outgrown taking an instant dislike to her based solely on Rebecca's cursed good looks, but her suspicions caused a definite aloofness. Her face remained blank. "Yes, I've heard a lot about you."

"All good I hope." Rebecca smiled.

Randazzo didn't return the smile. She furrowed her brow and narrowed her dark eyes. Her cover blown, Randazzo figured she had nothing to lose. "Well, one thing I've heard is that you greatly disliked several men who have now turned up dead," she said, her voice unnaturally light in contrast to her words.

"Just a coincidence, I suppose," Rebecca said, looking off back toward Ralph's door. She lingered a beat before locking her eyes back on Randazzo.

Randazzo met her gaze directly and spoke without hesitation. "You know, I don't mean this to sound rude, but my dad was a cop for thirty years and one thing he always said to me is that there's no such thing as a coincidence."

Her forthright comment caught Rebecca off guard. Rebecca tilted her head, as if assessing Randazzo, and crossed her arms in front of her—not really sure what to make of her comment. "What is it you're saying?"

Randazzo looked up and down the hallway and saw a number of Rebecca's co-workers milling about. This was not a conversation to hold in public and she had probably said too much already. "Why don't we talk in your office?"

Ralph, who had been standing by his door, straining to overhear the conversation, cracked it open wider to find out what was going on. He was greatly disappointed to find the women walking away, frustrated that he'd now have to guess at the rest.

Rebecca led her down two doors to her office, wondering and yet knowing what Randazzo meant. She let her in and shut the door behind her slowly, the sound punctuating the tension in the air. Rebecca sat behind her desk and motioned to Randazzo to take a seat as well. She switched off a small stereo she had behind her desk, and the room became noticeably silent as the two women settled into place. "Now, what's this all about?" Rebecca asked finally.

Randazzo was uncustomarily at a loss for words. This scene was uncomfortable and tricky. If her hunch was wrong, then this conversation would no doubt come back to haunt her in a big way, courtesy of her partner. But if she were right, then she'd be giving an advantage to the killer, letting her know the police were close. It could blow the case. And yet she had to say something.

"I've been investigating these killings for some time," she began, "and I know that if I figure out the motive—why these men in particular were chosen—I'll find the killer. So I look at who knew all of these men and who would have a motive to want them all dead." As she spoke, she held her notebook on her lap self-consciously, knowing inside were notes of accusations and rumors about Rebecca—support for what she had hoped for Jack's sake was an insupportable theory.

Rebecca leaned back in her chair and rested her chin on one hand. She wanted to force Randazzo to spell it out. "What does that have to do with me?"

she asked, wondering but afraid to find out if Randazzo was here merely doing Jack's bidding.

Randazzo looked around Rebecca's stark office, noting the bare walls and unadorned furniture. Am I reading too much into the lack of decoration here or is this woman a little too absorbed in her work? she thought. She sat forward. "As I look at each victim, I keep coming back to one thing. One common trait all these men shared is that they were all prosecuted by you and you couldn't get jail time for any of them. And you hated each of them for that." Randazzo left out that Rebecca also vaguely matched the artist's rendering of the suspect. She scanned Rebecca's face for a reaction but saw none. If anything, Rebecca looked more amused than irate at what she was hearing.

"And you think I would kill them because of that?" Rebecca laughed. "That's ridiculous."

Randazzo considered her for a moment—cool, relaxed, even lighthearted. Was this the posture of an innocent woman or of a calculated killer? Randazzo couldn't yet read her, but was immediately struck by the fact that Rebecca didn't deny involvement in the murders. Taken literally, Rebecca only said that her theory was ridiculous, not that it was untrue. "Well then how would you explain it?"

Rebecca shrugged. "I don't know that I have to." She spoke evenly, without nervous mannerisms—no averting her eyes, no fiddling with her pen, no clearing her throat. She just sat with her hands clasped in front of her, implacable.

Randazzo sighed. "Well, something doesn't seem right." She looked Rebecca squarely in the eyes, trying to find the answer there, yet seeing nothing—not the anger of an unjust accusation nor the fear of detection—but cold indifference over the deaths. "You really hated those guys, didn't you?"

Rebecca's face dropped its pleasant expression and her body noticeably stiffened. "What does that have to do with killing them? Do I have to love child molesters to avoid being a suspect? If I were you, I'd be a lot more suspicious about people who claim not to hate these scum." Rebecca sat quietly for a moment, then something seemed to click and her face softened. "This is because of Ralph, isn't it? You spend a few minutes with Ralph and think you have the inside scoop. But you don't know me. I'm as shocked as anyone over what's happened." She smiled a little self-consciously. "Not exactly upset, mind you. But very surprised."

"Don't get me wrong. I'm not accusing you of anything." Randazzo could have kicked herself—both of them knew that's precisely what she was doing there, and her efforts to deny it only made it more obvious. She was irritated with herself for not heeding Ben's admonition of a quiet investigation. "Look, we seemed to get off on a bad foot. I'm sorry. I probably sounded a little harsh. I'm just trying to put together a very confusing puzzle and I don't know where you fit in."

"I don't fit in at all."

Randazzo paused, looking at Rebecca and hoping for Jack's sake she was right. "I better be going." She got up and put her purse on her shoulder, then sighed. "I'll tell you one thing, I'll sure be happier when this case is over."

"Me, too."

"Well," she added weakly, "thanks for your time." Randazzo rushed out of her office, wondering what to make of the visit and how to explain it to Jack.

Ralph had been hanging out by his door, dying to find out what was going on in Rebecca's office. He pulled back into his office when Rebecca's door opened, then watched as Randazzo left, noticing her awkward good-bye and hurried gait. He waited until she was out of sight before making himself at home in one of Rebecca's guest chairs—even though that would hardly describe his status in her office. "Well, well, you seem to have become public enemy number one. Did she read you your rights? I sure hope you didn't talk to her without a lawyer, Becky. You should know better than that."

Rebecca ran her hands through her hair, pulling it back off her face. She looked in her drawer for a scrunchie to tie it back. Right now her hair was as much an irritation as Ralph. "Ralph, is being an imbecile your only pleasure in life? It's like you're an idiot savant, but without the special gift."

Ralph ignored the dig. "Becky, do you realize that if murder figured into your conviction rate, you'd be tops in the office right now? I bet all your old defendants are shaking in their pedophilic boots," Ralph said with a hearty laugh. He had to laugh at his own jokes, because Rebecca clearly was not going to.

She continued searching in her drawer, but found only useless paper clips and a few sunflower seeds and slammed it shut. She looked back up at Ralph. "Isn't there some Three Stooges film festival you should run off to somewhere? Or is that too cerebral for you?"

"Oh, ouch. You sure told me." He laughed as he gestured, as if to fend off Rebecca. "I'd better back off. I sure don't want to get you riled. No telling what you'll do."

Even after Randazzo's visit, Rebecca still couldn't muster the energy to take Ralph seriously. She dug through her purse as she spoke. "Tell me, have you ever considered becoming the poster child for retroactive abortions?"

"Yikes, sounds like I'm interrupting something," Jack said with a smile as wide as a river. Rebecca's relief was palpable as she looked up to find him standing in her doorway. Ralph recognized him from the press conference and instantly felt a little confused. Why was the other detective on the case there and acting so friendly with Rebecca so soon on the heels of his partner's clearly investigative visit? Had he been set up in his meeting with Randazzo? Was that why Rebecca seemed so nonplussed by her visit?

"No, of course not. Ralph was just leaving," Rebecca intoned deliberately toward Ralph, who picked up on the not-so-subtle boot and slinked out of the office, baffled and in search of an explanation.

"Sorry for not calling first," Jack said as he took a chair, "but I was in the neighborhood and I just took a chance you might be in."

"Are you here to pick up your partner?" Rebecca asked, figuring there was no reason to beat around the bush.

"No. Why? Is she here?" Jack looked back toward the door.

"She was. She just left. Rather suddenly, if you ask me."

"What was she doing here?" Jack asked, obviously puzzled.

Rebecca was pleased that Jack didn't seem to know what was going on. While his shock could be an act, ten years watching witnesses lie convincingly on the stand gave her a good feel for the truth, and Jack's reaction struck her as genuine. "I think she came here to find out if I was the killer."

Jack's jaw dropped. "Huh?"

"It's all part of her coincidence theory."

Jack seemed to be caught totally off guard. His eyes went wide and he struggled for something to say, but he could think of nothing but, "What?" He was unaccustomed to unpleasant surprises from his partner and didn't know how to react. He wanted an explanation from Randazzo and he wanted it now, but he knew that an answer would have to wait. He was rocked by the knowledge that his partner could do such a thing—accusing Rebecca of something so horrible—behind his back, and yet he couldn't stop wondering what would make her do that.

Rebecca noted the stunned look on Jack's face. "I take it that you didn't know she was coming by."

Jack's head was swimming. He was at least glad that Rebecca seemed to appreciate that he had nothing to do with Randazzo's visit, but that still didn't address his bigger problem. Why would Randazzo come here and not tell him first? He shook his head. "No, she never mentioned it. You two talked?"

"Yep. After she got an earful from Ralph—the guy who just left—she asked to talk to me. She told me that since I prosecuted each of those guys—unsuccessfully she was quick to point out—I was the logical suspect."

"She said that to you?" Jack exclaimed. "What the hell is she talking about?"

Rebecca shrugged it off, seemingly unfazed. "It's no big deal." Jack studied Rebecca's face and saw no signs that belied her words. "She was just being thorough, you know, doing her job, covering all the bases. I understand."

Jack was amazed by Rebecca's equanimity. If it were him he wouldn't take being called a killer quite so lightly. "You're being awfully nice about this."

Rebecca smiled. "Hey, I took it as a compliment that she thought I killed them."

Not the answer he wanted. Jack rubbed his forehead. "What?"

"Nothing. Sorry." Rebecca looked apologetic. "Listen, I don't think we should make too much about it. Really. C'mon, let's talk about something else. Okay?"

"Yeah, sure," Jack said slowly, unable to switch gears as fast as Rebecca.

"I saw you on TV," Rebecca said lightly.

Jack refocused his mind on the press conference. "What did you think?" he asked halfheartedly.

Rebecca looked at Jack with a warm smile, then leaned forward. "I thought you were the best-looking guy there."

"Even better looking than the anchor from Channel Six?"

Rebecca sat back as if to think. "Oh—good point," she said, laughing.

"Gee, thanks," Jack said, feigning injury to his ego. The humor seemed to lighten the tension created by Randazzo's unannounced visit. Although he wondered how Rebecca could not think that she was being suckered into the old good cop/bad cop routine. Still, Rebecca appeared so nonchalant about the whole thing.

"I was surprised to hear you say at the press conference that you have an artist's sketch. What's that all about?" she asked.

Jack started to relax again, putting Randazzo's visit out of his mind, for now. "Well, we've got a lead on a possible witness or suspect, we're not sure which."

"Really?"

"Yeah, someone saw a woman near the scene of Riddell's murder. The sketch should hopefully be all over the news shortly. Maybe something will come of it. I hope so. The chief is pushing hard for a quick resolution. He needs some good PR."

"A witness? Wow, that's great. Who's the witness?"

"Some little old lady who lived near the guy."

"What did she see? You think she's any good?" Rebecca asked.

Jack shrugged. "We're not sure. Eyewitnesses aren't always all they're cracked up to be, as you know. Especially not ours, from what my partner tells me. So I'm not that optimistic. I still have this feeling that the investigation is going nowhere fast. But, maybe you can help. Do you have a few minutes to tell me about Riddell?"

Rebecca looked surprised. "You mean you're not here because you missed me terribly?" she said coyly.

"Ahh . . . yeah . . . that was it," Jack said quickly, flashing a sly smile. "It's true, you know. I really do miss you. I can't stop thinking about you."

Maybe it was his imagination, but Rebecca's cheeks seemed to turn pinker. "Me too," she said softly.

"How 'bout you let me buy you lunch?" he asked.

"You treated the last two times. It's my turn. Let me take you out."

"It's a deal." They both stood up and Rebecca came out from behind her desk, next to Jack. Jack put his arm around her as they started out the door. Jack leaned over and whispered in Rebecca's ear, "Oops, I guess I shouldn't do that while we're both on duty." He dropped his arm and continued out the door, with Rebecca at his side. "So let's just pretend like we're holding hands."

Rebecca took Jack to a cozy Thai restaurant a few miles from work. Linen tablecloths and inflated luncheon prices kept the chances of running into any of their co-workers down to a minimum. The drive was too short for them to find a song they liked on the radio, even the usually reliable KROQ playing only a string of commercials for ski weekends, eighteen-and-over clubs, and the far-off Acoustic Christmas. They chatted about nothing in particular and enjoyed just being together.

As the waiter took their menus, Jack said, "Why don't we get the police work out of the way first?" instantly realizing he'd said that before. Already they had an established routine, an odd mixture of work and play. "What did you think when you heard about Riddell? I mean, another victim so soon. Pretty amazing, don't you think?"

"That's one way to describe it."

"So what about Riddell should I know?"

"What can I tell you about Hal?" Rebecca asked with a heavy sigh. "Not a lot out of the ordinary, except he was very good at crying on cue. At the arraignment, at the prelim, at hearings, whenever he thought it might help."

"It must have worked. He didn't do any time, right?"

Rebecca took a long sip of ice water, careful to avoid the thin lemon slice that floated on top. "Not a day. Hal was well coached. He said he was sorry for his 'mistake' and the judge—as usual—bought it hook, line, and sinker. A mistake! Another lovely euphemism." She seemed disgusted. "I tried to tell the court that a mistake is putting the wrong kind of gas in your car or giving someone the wrong change, not having sex with your daughter. But the judge wasn't interested. He fell for one of my all-time favorite bullshit arguments—'How can I take care of my family if I'm in prison?'" Rebecca gulped some more water, then sighed. "The judges like to fall for that one. 'We'd only be punishing the family further to lock him up,' they say. Yeah, right. And who cares about the message it sends to the victim?" Rebecca looked down and saw that her hands were clenched. "I'm sorry. Didn't take me long to make a speech, did it? I can't believe I haven't scared you away yet."

Jack looked at Rebecca curiously. "Why, do you want to?"

"No," Rebecca said too quickly, her voice tinged with nervous laughter. "It's just that most of the time we're discussing my least favorite topic, my work. And I know how I must sound."

Jack smiled warmly at Rebecca. "What you sound most like is someone in need of a break."

"My sister said the same thing to me. She said I should take a sabbatical."

"So why don't you?"

The waiter brought over the drinks, and Rebecca took the opportunity to slowly sip her Thai tea as she considered Jack's question. "I don't know," she said as she put her glass back down. "I guess I'm afraid to. You know, no one who ever breaks out of jail goes back voluntarily. If I get too much distance from my job, I might never go back."

"So? You've spent a decade there, that's enough time for anybody. That's more than you get for manslaughter."

Rebecca looked at Jack incredulously. "This from a man who's already passed almost twenty years with the same employer."

"But I like my job."

"And you're saying I don't?"

"No. You're saying you don't."

Rebecca said nothing, realizing just how right Jack was, yet still unwilling to give in and admit it. "I guess I wasn't paying attention," she joked, a subtle diversionary tactic.

Jack saw a somberness in Rebecca and reached across the table, taking her hand, gently touching her smooth skin. Her arm tingled at the touch, as if electricity passed between them. Rebecca lost herself in Jack's eyes, forgetting everything—work, Tom, the killings—everything except how nobody had ever made her feel this alive.

"If you don't stop, I'm going to have to call a cop."

"I am a cop," Jack said, using his free hand to flash his badge.

"Let me see that," Rebecca said as she grabbed it out of his hand. She tapped it with her finger. "Feels real." She handed the badge back to him. "Okay, I'd like to file a complaint then."

Jack put his badge away and pulled his small notebook and a pen out of his breast pocket, poised to write it down. "What for, ma'am?" he drawled.

"I'm falling for a guy who's going to break my heart."

"What if I get him to promise not to?"

Rebecca looked at the notebook. "Can I get that in writing?"

Jack quickly scribbled "I promise" on a piece of paper, tore it out and handed it to Rebecca. "Will this do?"

18

As soon as Larson walked into the station, he realized he was being watched. He sensed by the barely stifled laughs that he was the butt of some joke that he didn't understand. When he rounded the corner and headed toward his desk, he saw the punch line, but still didn't get it. There he saw a woman with long blonde hair sitting at his desk, her back toward him. He walked over to her and she rose slowly from her chair, displaying a curvaceous figure in a skin-tight lime green dress. She turned toward him and extended her hand coyly. "I hope you don't mind my coming by unannounced," she said in a breathy, slightly husky voice. "I just had to see you again."

He stared into her overly made-up face, her skin hidden under thick pancake makeup. "I'm sorry, do I know you?"

"How soon they forget," she said flirtatiously, flipping her hair back over one shoulder. "It hasn't been that long, has it, Detective? It was memorable for me." She giggled and batted obviously fake lashes under thick, dark brows. "Oh, enough teasing." The woman's voice dropped a couple octaves. "It's me, Detective Larson. Frank LaPaca. You know, from Oakwood."

That explained the hairy knuckles. "Oh, sure. I just didn't recognize you with the *La Cage* getup."

"Now, now. Let's not be insensitive. It's the nineties, after all. You know, I was a little nervous coming by and I always feel more comfortable this way. Do you like it?" Frank asked, turning from side to side so Larson could see the entire outfit.

Larson's attention, however, was drawn to the half-dozen detectives standing behind Frank, gesticulating feverishly like preening beauty queens. He was not amused. "Yeah, you look great. Just like Bea Arthur." He motioned for LaPaca to sit back down, hoping in vain that he'd be less noticeable seated.

Frank sat down, posing and fiddling with himself until he found the right position. "You know, that wasn't a very nice thing you said about me, Detective," he said at last. "If you don't say something nice, I won't tell you why I'm here. You want to know, don't you?"

"I'm dying to know."

"I know who the killer is." Frank sang it like a nursery school taunt. "I figured it out."

Larson rolled his eyes. "I can't wait to hear this."

"Say 'please.'"

Larson was tempted to arrest Frank for being annoying, but he couldn't think of a penal code section for that offense. "I don't have time for games. I've got a lot of work to do," he said dismissively. He turned toward his desk and started straightening the papers into neat, if still disorganized, stacks.

Frank leaned forward, placing his hand on Jack's desk. "It's Hillerman." He sat back and waited for a reaction but was disappointed by Larson's blank expression. He pressed on. "Can you believe it? Our esteemed leader, the good doctor. He's the one."

"Really," Larson said flatly.

Frank flipped his hand down at the wrist in an exaggerated move. "Okay, I can see you don't believe me. When you hear what I have to say, you will."

Larson leaned back, crossed his legs, then crossed his arms—a more skeptical body posture would have required the aid of a chiropractor. "All right, let me hear it."

Frank broke into a broad grin. He had his audience, reluctant or not. "Well, I've been around that place for a long time. I know where all the bodies are buried, as the saying goes. I knew all the men who've been killed and I can tell you one thing, they were all going to make the Oakwood look bad. Very bad."

"So?"

"You don't get it?" Frank looked at Larson with wide eyes. "Hillerman's bread and butter is in convincing people that his center works. Or else why continue sending people there, right? This isn't like the old days where the public didn't give a damn. Now they're watching him, so he can't go dumping every Tom, Dick, and Harry back on the street. Follow?"

"I guess."

"You see, the public has finally wised up and figured out that Hillerman can't deliver what he promises." Frank wiggled in his chair and finally struck a school-marm pose—his legs tightly crossed, his hands in his lap. He pursed his lips, straightened his back, and continued. "You just can't convince a guy who likes six-year-old girls to like thirty-year-old women. It just can't be done. You like what you like."

"And what do you like, Frank?" Larson could hear the sarcastic tone in his voice, but he hadn't heard anything yet that gave him any reason to take Frank seriously.

"Oh, me." Frank relaxed his posture, leaning back, arms spread out in an overly friendly gesture. "I like everybody."

"I see," Larson said slowly. He looked around the station, wondering where his partner was and whether she'd miss the show.

Frank recrossed his legs and smoothed out his skirt, using the delay to milk the moment. "Look, it's simple. The Oakwood is a farce and Hillerman knows it. But he doesn't want anyone on the outside to know. If some of the guys who give him trouble end up dead, they sure can't go out and get arrested again. You see, the guys who were killed were ticking time bombs. Hillerman just snuffed out their fuses before they could explode all over him." Frank's eyes brimmed with excitement.

"It's an interesting theory."

"It's no theory, sweetheart. Believe me, you simply never know about a man till you walk a mile in his pumps." Frank wiggled his stiletto-heeled lemon yellow shoes in the air. "I've spent a lot of time trying to figure this out and it all points to Hillerman."

Larson couldn't believe he was engaging in a dialogue with a reject from the *Jerry Springer* show dressed like a can of Sprite, but you never know where you might find answers, he figured. "All right, let's assume what you're saying is true. Then how does that explain Bradley Knight? He wasn't at Oakwood. Why would Hillerman want him killed?"

"What do you mean he wasn't at Oakwood?"

"He transferred to another center."

"Oh." Frank looked flustered, upset with himself for being caught off guard and without even a snappy retort. "I knew he was unhappy—he'd talked about leaving—but I didn't know he'd actually gone."

"Yup." Larson eyed Frank curiously. "So tell me something. How do you know all these guys? You weren't all in the same group."

"I don't limit myself to just one group. I like to spread myself around—no reason to give just one set of guys the chance to be near me. And anyway, when you've gone there as long as I have, you'd go out of your mind just sitting, listening to the same dozen guys week after week," Frank said, rolling his eyes and shaking his head.

"I guess so."

Frank stood up and pulled down on his skirt. "God, how I hate static cling. Hard to make a graceful exit. Well, Detective. That's enough for now. The chortling in the background is getting distracting. You can tell your friends it is impolite to tease a lady like that." He bent down, revealing some curious cleavage, and scribbled on Larson's calendar. "Let me leave you my number. If you have any questions, you can call me anytime," he said in a fairly accurate Mae West. "I'll keep my ears open."

Larson rose slowly, unclear on the etiquette. "Thanks, uh, Frank. You've been a lot of help." He looked behind Frank and saw that a few hairs from his wig clung to the back of the chair.

"Glad to be of service. And, if you feel more comfortable, you can call me Amber." He spread his arms out. "Frank's a little butch for this outfit, don't you think?"

Frank sashayed out of the room, hips swinging, head thrown back, chest out. Larson had to hand it to him—he sure knew how to make an exit. Frank passed Randazzo on the way out and called out "Hi, Detective" to her, but was met with a blank stare.

"Who, or should I say what, was that?" Randazzo

asked Larson, cocking her head back toward the door.

Larson moved over to the chair and picked up the hairs with a tissue paper, then slipped them in a sandwich bag. "That was Frank LaPaca, one of the satisfied customers of the Oakwood Center."

Randazzo took a seat at her desk and opened up her lunch, a submarine sandwich about as long as she was. "I can see they're making a lot of progress with him. So why was it here?" Randazzo asked, emphasizing the "it." She said it lightheartedly but noticed he was not laughing.

Larson rolled his chair over to Randazzo's desk. "I have a better question," he said angrily, taking her by surprise. "What were you doing at Rebecca's office?" Larson's face was uncharacteristically hard.

Randazzo stopped midbite. "I don't think I like the tone of your voice. Do you want to try again?" She took too big a bite and swallowed hard.

Larson fumed. As he saw it, Randazzo had a lot to explain and shouldn't waste her time complaining about his tone of voice. "You go over there behind my back and you want me to ask pretty please? I don't think so."

"Time out. I was investigating the murders. What do you think I was doing? I bumped into Rebecca, literally, and we talked for a couple of minutes. What's the big deal?"

"Why don't you tell me?" he said, his tone frosty.

"Okay, Jack." Randazzo dropped her sandwich. "You want me to say it? Fine. I thought it was a little much that all five victims just happened to be prosecuted, unsuccessfully I might add, by your girlfriend. That's quite an amazing coincidence, one you'd see if you weren't so blinded by her. Now, I didn't think I should close my eyes to the facts just because it might be a little uncomfortable for you. But I didn't want to discuss it with you, 'cause I know your feelings. So I looked into it, asked a few questions, and that's it. Okay?"

"No, it's not okay," he said curtly. "But what's done is done. Just be a little more sensitive in the future," he added, assuming it was a dead issue.

"So tell me, why was the drag queen here? What's that all about?" Randazzo picked up her sandwich and tried again.

Larson's face relaxed as the conversation turned back to neutral territory. "That's a good question. I'm not entirely sure. He came in telling me how he knows who the killer is and guess who he names? Hillerman."

"Hillerman?" Randazzo mumbled, her mouth full.

"Kinda hard to believe, huh? Hillerman's a lot of things—pompous and obnoxious immediately come to mind—but can you imagine him doing something as untidy as stabbing someone to death?"

"Maybe he hires out the dirty work," she said with a shrug. "So why do you think this guy wants to hand us Hillerman?"

"Who knows?" Larson paused. "Maybe he hates Hillerman and is trying to get him in trouble for some reason. Or he likes being the center of attention—which I think is a safe bet in his case—and so he wants to get in on the action, you know, feel like he's part of the investigation. Or maybe he's the killer. Let's have the lab check these," Larson said, lifting the plastic bag holding a half-dozen blond hairs. "It was sure nice of him to leave some evidence for testing."

"Are you going to check Rebecca's as well?" Randazzo asked abruptly.

He frowned. "I thought we had dropped that. Don't you think you've done enough damage for now?"

"You dropped it. It's still open as far as I'm concerned." Randazzo did not see the stress in Larson's eyes. "You want some?" She offered him half the sandwich. Even though it looked good, Larson shook her off—he didn't feel like doing something as friendly as sharing food.

"Why are you still talking about Rebecca? You just saw some guy in drag, with blonde hair, who knew all the victims, walk out of here and yet all you want to talk about is Rebecca? Hello . . . earth to Jennifer."

Randazzo swallowed her bite and took a gulp of Coke. "Jack, just because some freak comes in here with his nightclub act, I'm not going to ignore the fact that Rebecca is still the leading common denominator among our victims. There's just no one else with as great a connection and as much reason for wanting to kill them. What would Tinkerbell's reason be?"

"I don't know. That's what I've got to find out. But listen. It makes sense. He comes in to point us toward Hillerman. Now, I admit it's farfetched, although he made a fairly plausible argument—that Hillerman killed these guys because they were going to make the center look bad." Randazzo's face turned sour. She found that theory as ridiculous as Frank's outfit. Larson couldn't argue with her, so he pressed on. "But what I'm thinking is maybe he came by to get closer to the investigation so he could tease us, toy with us, you know, for the thrill of it. It's like the next step beyond keeping newspaper clippings on your killings, actually 'helping' the police. It opens up a whole new prospect."

Randazzo remained unconvinced. "That's fine. I'm not ignoring you, but you seem to be ignoring me. I'm trying to tell you that you better not let your relationship with Rebecca keep you from seeing the connections. Don't ignore what's right under your nose, okay? And I agree, we should check out Frank as well. Maybe he is the killer and his ego's gonna get him caught. I'm not saying don't follow up on him. But we should also follow up on Rebecca. We're supposed to investigate all leads, not just the ones that make us feel good."

Larson shifted in his chair, his frustration bubbling to the surface. He was confused by Randazzo's sudden preoccupation with Rebecca. There didn't seem to be anything there to him, yet Randazzo wasn't letting go. He wondered whether she knew more than she was letting on to. "I don't get this focus on Rebecca. You were the one who kicked me in the butt to call her for a second date, unless you've conveniently forgotten. And why would she be seeing me if she were the killer?"

"Maybe for the same thrill that you think Frank is getting out of coming to you."

"She's not like Frank. And she'd never kill someone. She's not that kind of person."

"Oh, well, that changes everything," Randazzo said sarcastically.

"I can't believe you really think that Rebecca is a hardworking D.A. by day, psychotic killer by night. Get real. You don't know her like I do."

"And maybe you don't know her as well as you think you do," Randazzo said, as gently as she could. "All I'm saying is that she fits the profile and that can't be ignored. We just don't have much else to go on other than the fact that the killer is probably a woman, who knew the victims, and wanted to see them punished . . . that sounds like Fielding to me. And she kinda looks like our artist's sketch. Or hadn't you noticed? It's sitting right there on top of your desk."

Larson refused to look over at it. "So why haven't you had Rebecca's place searched if you think it's her? Why not put a wire on me? Maybe over appetizers I can get her to confess." He felt himself getting madder and stopped himself. "Look, I know you want to make this bust, but don't take down good people with you."

"I've talked with another D.A. at her office, Ralph Simpson. He has quite a lot to say about Rebecca and her crusade against child molesters. He doesn't seem to be so sure she leaves her work at the office. He said he's been very suspicious about her for some time now. And he's not the only one, apparently. He gave me the name of a half-dozen others who he says will confirm what he told me."

Larson couldn't believe what he was hearing. He was torn between wanting to know more and not wanting to know anything. "Do you see how destructive this is? Investigating Rebecca is wrong, it's simply wrong. It's a waste of time and what's worse, it could harm a perfectly wonderful woman who has devoted her life to helping others. How can you not see that? All this snooping around, asking questions—you think it's going to go unnoticed?"

Randazzo put down her sandwich and ripped open her bag of Ruffles. "I think your judgment is being affected by your penis, as usual. So let me continue investigating her. I'm not personally involved. But you really should stay away from her. If she's the killer, it's going to look just great that the lead homicide detective was dating her."

He looked away, shaking his head. "No. This is asinine. But if it'll make you happy, I'll get her alibis for the killings. That should put this to rest. But I'm not going to pass on a chance with her just because you're feeling frustrated that you haven't caught the killer yet. You've already settled down with Mr. Right. Don't interfere with my love life and I won't interfere with yours."

Randazzo crunched a mouthful of chips. "All right. Just don't let your little head do all your thinking for you."

"Let's drop the subject."

"Fine," she said.

But Larson didn't hear her. His mind was elsewhere. On Rebecca. And how all the promise of their relationship was being crushed by Randazzo's wild theories. He rolled back to his desk and took a slurp of warm Coke. He had to find another answer—one that didn't point to Rebecca.

19

"Why are we doing this again?" Randazzo asked Larson as she pulled into the parking lot at the Oakwood, by now a familiar place to her. She maneuvered her car along the cracked pavement to one of the parking spaces designated by faded yellow lines, ignoring the suggestion that only "compact" cars take the space. She turned off the ignition and waited for the car to notice, while it sputtered to an end sounding as if it were in the throes of a death rattle. She opened her door, then turned to Larson. "You know, I'm starting to spend more time here than their clients. And I think it's doing me about as much good as it does them."

"C'mon, it'll be fun. Don't you want to meet the killer?" he said with a smile.

Randazzo looked over at him, astonished. She knew he wanted to deflect attention away from Rebecca, but she couldn't believe he would take it this far. "You really believe what Frank said about Hillerman?"

"No." Larson scoffed at the very idea, then—

hedging—he added, "Well, not really. But, since you've decided to investigate farfetched theories, why not Hillerman?"

Randazzo said nothing. She knew Larson's style was to stew for weeks on something, letting his anger occasionally bubble to the surface indirectly. But until she resolved her suspicions about Rebecca, she decided to ignore his digs, or there would be no way they could stay civil to each other. And neither of them wanted it to come to that. So she just got out of the car and slammed her door shut a little harder than she needed to, feeling about as frustrated with herself as she could. The only thing that would make today perfect would be for Ben to tell her "I told you so." But then, maybe she'd get lucky and Hillerman would just confess and she and Larson could get back to normal.

Randazzo walked briskly to the building, sprinting up the stairs to the Oakwood's offices, taking the steps two at a time. Larson lagged behind a few steps. "You okay, there, Gramps? Need some oxygen?" Randazzo teased. She hoped the levity would help ease the tension.

"What's the big hurry? It's not like they're going anywhere." As he panted up to the top, Larson figured he better spend a little less time in the health club Jacuzzi and a lot more time on the StairMaster. Apparently warm bubbling water had little cardiovascular benefit.

"I just want to get this over with. This has waste of time written all over it."

"Now, now. You never know when you'll find the one kernel that leads you to the cob," Larson said.

"Did you just make that up?"

"Yeah, you like it?"

"No."

The Oakwood had apparently responded to its

newfound notoriety with a fresh coat of paint and new furniture, Hillerman perhaps hoping a cosmetic makeover would improve public perception during the Oakwood's fifteen minutes of fame. Randazzo and Larson were quickly ushered back to Hillerman's office, as Elena had been instructed not to let them linger in the waiting room. Given who Oakwood's patients were, there was some irony in the fact that Hillerman seemed most troubled by the presence of detectives in the clinic's anteroom.

Hillerman was standing in front of his desk, with Valerie and another woman the detectives didn't recognize. "Dr. Hillerman," Randazzo said matter-of-factly as she extended her hand.

"Detectives," Dr. Hillerman responded, oozing charm. "I'd like to say that it's good to see you, but under the circumstances I'm sure you will understand. You remember Ms. Kingsley"—Valerie bowed her head in time with the greeting—"and this is Anita O'Toole. She is another of our therapists." Anita extended her hand for a firm shake, giving Larson a little longer grasp as she smiled coyly. Larson noted that Hillerman seemed to favor hiring young, attractive therapists.

Randazzo noticed as well, but something else drew her attention. "You know, I was wondering about something," she began, before taking her seat. "Who maintains the patient files here?"

Hillerman stopped on his way to his chair, turning around to face Randazzo. "Well, we don't have a formal system," he said, a bit defensively. "All the files are kept in the file cabinet in the secretarial area at the front of the office for easy access. In fact, you just walked right past them." He pointed back down the hall.

Randazzo looked back over her shoulder. "I thought so. That's why I asked. I was wondering, with the files sitting out in the open like that, how do you control who looks at them?"

"I'm not sure I need to," Hillerman said, his irritation already showing. "It's never been a problem."

"That you know of," Randazzo added.

Hillerman glared at her. "What are you suggesting, Detective?"

"Nothing, Dr. Hillerman. I'm just wondering whether someone from the outside could somehow gain access to the files?"

"I sincerely doubt it. Of course, I suppose it is possible. Indeed, anything is, as they say. But the offices are locked up at night. And I'm sure we'd notice someone snooping around the files during the day." He sat down in his chair and motioned for the others to take their seats. As everyone crammed together in front of him, Hillerman held court behind his desk.

"You're probably right," Randazzo said. "I was just concerned about security. So I gather that means you haven't had any problems recently where files were tampered with or misplaced?" She pulled out her notepad and started writing intently.

Since he figured he hadn't said anything of substance, Hillerman wondered what Randazzo could have found so interesting that she had to write it down. He tilted his head down and tried to get a peek. "Frankly, Detectives, if I were to venture a guess, I would say that you likely have better things to do with your time than worry about our filing system." Hillerman's sarcasm was not at all veiled. Valerie and Anita had been on the receiving end of it often enough, but even when it was focused on someone else, they still found it difficult to listen to. But they needn't have worried about Randazzo.

"Dr. Hillerman, we have five dead men. I'm sure you'll agree that we wouldn't be doing our job if we didn't look at everything." Randazzo did not like being told what to do, even if Hillerman might be right. "Just to be on the safe side, though, maybe you should take greater precautions with your files." She had made her point, so she could now move on. She jotted down some more notes, and Hillerman leaned forward to get a glimpse at what she was writing. He was finding her incessant scribbling unnerving, but he couldn't make out a word. Randazzo looked up, saw Hillerman staring at her, and smiled as she moved her hand to cover her notes. "Why don't we talk about Mr. Riddell? Who was his therapist here?"

"That would be me," said Anita, waving slightly. "At least for the last six months. I took over his group from Valerie when she moved to take over the errant NAMBLA members." Anita saw Randazzo's and Larson's blank expressions. She had forgotten that not everyone traveled in the same circles. "You know, men who prefer boys. And not to take to Little League, if you catch my drift." She smiled and raised her eyebrows.

If nothing else, Larson's glossary of paraphilic phrases was continuing to expand. "And how long had you been his therapist?" Larson asked Valerie.

"About a year and a half before that," she replied. "And before me, Dr. Rubin was his therapist."

"Dr. Rubin from Elmhurst?" asked Randazzo.

"Yes, that's right," said Hillerman. "You are familiar with her?"

"Yes, we are. One of the other victims, Bradley Knight, was last treated at her facility."

"I know. It's nice to see that you noticed that as well. Maybe you can tell the news media—they seemed to have missed that little tidbit. I'm tired of the Oakwood becoming synonymous with murdered child molesters. Thank heavens for Mr. Knight,"

Hillerman said, trying to sound lighthearted, but instead appearing terribly insensitive.

"I suppose that's one way to look at his murder," Larson said, noting how appreciative Hillerman seemed to be about Knight's murder.

Hillerman read the disapproval on Larson's face. "I'm sorry, Detectives. I suppose that didn't sound very good. I'm sure you can understand, this has been a difficult time for me."

Randazzo ignored Hillerman, keeping her focus on Valerie and Anita instead. She did not want to give Hillerman another opportunity to monopolize the conversation, knowing he had nothing useful to offer—at least not intentionally. "We're interested in whatever you can tell us about Mr. Riddell that might shed light on his murder. Maybe you can tell us how he was doing here."

"Not great," Anita began. She caught Hillerman's harsh glare out of the corner of her eye and quickly realized she needed to clarify. While she did not want to be caught lying to the police about something that could be checked out so easily, she also knew that she'd have to deal with Hillerman long after the police had left. So she looked to find a fair middle ground. "What I meant is while he wasn't doing great, he was improving. Overall, his participation in group was fine. In fact, sometimes it was hard to shut him up. I think he thought the more he talked, the better we'd think he was doing." Randazzo was pleasantly surprised with Anita's candor in spite of Hillerman's presence but wondered what she'd say with him out of the room.

"What did he do to get sent here?" Larson asked reluctantly, knowing he needed the information but still not wanting to hear it.

"He had molested his daughter from the time she was six until she was ten. It started with touching her genitals and having her touch his, then ended up with full-blown intercourse. I guess playing tea party with her was too old-fashioned." Anita's cynical tone appealed to Larson, who hated the sugar coating that Hillerman and Valerie usually gave to everything. Randazzo also noticed the difference in approach and took an instant liking to Anita, who seemed under no illusions about who she was treating. "Anyway, the girl's pediatrician noticed the scarring. At first Riddell said the girl had done it to herself, then he said his wife had done it to set him up." Anita shook her head. "He never did admit that he'd done it."

"What a piece of work," Larson said, disgusted and unable to keep it to himself.

"Now, Detective," Hillerman chided, "we do not judge our clients by what they did before they came here."

I do, Larson thought to himself, not so willing to start with a clean slate. What's wrong with making people take responsibility for their actions? he wondered.

Randazzo shifted the conversation back on track, turning to Kingsley. "Ms. Kingsley, did you share Ms. O'Toole's opinion of Mr. Riddell?"

Feeling a little uncomfortable with her colleague's candor and recklessness, Valerie glanced over at Anita. She felt her loyalty to Hillerman and the Oakwood was paramount and that there was nothing wrong with slanting facts in a light favorable to both. She wondered whether Anita was trying to make the center look bad to get back at Hillerman for ending their relationship. But she didn't want to get in the middle of their problems any more than she already was. So she stayed on the fence. "Uh . . . yeah . . . sure. I guess he wasn't progressing as much as we had hoped." She looked over at Hillerman. "I mean, we were just starting to make some progress, but he died before we were through with him."

"Doesn't it get frustrating?" Randazzo asked, more out of personal than professional curiosity. "I mean, after so many years, the best you can say was that he was starting to show progress. How did you feel about the likelihood of him leaving here pretty much the same as when he had arrived? And not just him, but the others too, from what we've heard."

Valerie appeared flustered. She seemed to be taking these questions as a personal attack, Randazzo noticed. As Valerie struggled, Hillerman stepped in, unwilling to risk a slipup again. "I think it is a mistake to assume these men were unchanged by their time here. Just the exposure to our philosophical teachings, and some of the behavioral exercises we employ, enlightens them, gives them a new understanding of their behavior and how it affects others. Some men are defensive and do not wish to let down their guard. They may appear unchanged and hostile, but they do not leave unaffected by their participation in group. In that way, I would say all are success stories."

Larson was tired of hearing the same old public relations bullshit. He was not as tolerant as his partner. "What can you tell me about Frank LaPaca?" he asked, desperate to wrestle the floor back from Hillerman.

Hillerman seemed taken aback. "Frank?"

"Yeah, he was in Matheson's Monday night group, right?" Larson said.

"Frank's in every group," said Anita with a little laugh. "He can't get enough of this place. He fancies himself our resident expert." She rolled her eyes and smiled, making it clear that she found Frank trying at best.

"How'd he get along with the guys who've been killed?" Larson asked.

Hillerman sat forward. "Is Frank a suspect?" he asked.

"Well, we're exploring many things," Larson said. A nice way of saying, "It's none of your damn business, just answer my question."

"Look, Detectives, if one of our patients here is a suspect, I believe we have a right to know. The safety of our patients is of the utmost concern," said Hillerman. Too bad I couldn't get that on tape, he thought. Stan would be proud.

"Dr. Hillerman, we don't know anything at this point." Except that Frank thinks you committed the murders, Larson thought to himself. "We're just trying to get some background information on Mr. LaPaca. We saw his name in the same groups as the murdered men, so we thought we'd check him out." Larson figured he'd better come up with a reason he'd mentioned Frank before Hillerman wondered what was going on. Just in case Frank had anything useful to say, no reason to let on he was giving information to the police.

Anita leaned forward and spoke up to get the conversation back on track. "Frank doesn't really get along all that well with the others. He has a tendency to irritate people—he's so over the top, so flamboyant. I think he does it on purpose—it's his way of keeping from connecting with the other men in group. Plus, he tries to take on the role of a co-therapist. It's also part of the reason I think he likes to go from group to group. It's all part of some plan to keep him from being 'one of them' and he can playact like he's one of us instead."

"But do you sense that he has any grudges against any of the other group members or that he had anything against any of the victims?" Larson asked.

Anita furrowed her brow, considering the question. "I really don't know," she said finally. "Because of some of Frank's predilections—his sexual preference and his dabbling in cross-dressing—he gets into it with some of the more homophobic guys. But he dishes out as much as he takes. I think he likes baiting the other guys and getting into it with them. Valerie, do you remember any problem with Frank in any of your groups?"

Valerie had been looking absentmindedly at the clouds forming outside the window and was pulled back by Anita's question. "What?"

"Frank. Did he get along in your groups or was there friction?"

Valerie relaxed, seemingly amused by the absurd question. "Frank? He lives for friction. I think he loves the verbal bickering. He goes out of his way to push other people's buttons, to stir up something. I think it's a defense mechanism though, his way of dealing with their resentment. He keeps himself separate that way. I think that's why he avoids the gay groups. It's as if he doesn't want to fit in. He wants to stay apart from the rest of the group members." Randazzo took note of the first straight answer she'd gotten from Valerie in Hillerman's presence. Apparently criticizing Frank was sanctioned by the boss.

"But have you sensed any kind of hostility between him and anyone in any of the groups?" Larson pressed.

"Nothing out of the ordinary for Frank," Anita said. "Like Valerie said, Frank goes out of his way to be a bit of a pest. But he's very evenhanded about it. He's an equal opportunity annoyer." Anita looked around the room, but no one was laughing.

"But, as his therapists, do you believe he could make the leap from irritant to murderer?"

Anita and Valerie exchanged puzzled glances while Hillerman cleared his throat deliberately. "You know, Detectives, I've wondered about Frank for some time now. I never imagined he could do this, and yet, now that you mention it, it gives me pause. This is truly very distressing to have to consider the possibility." Hillerman ran the idea around his head as he rubbed his chin. "I hope it's not true. But, we can truly never know all the vagaries of the human mind, now, can we?"

As they headed to the parking lot, Randazzo tossed the keys to Larson. "You drive, for a change. I wanna finish my notes. How many s's in asshole?"

Larson laughed. "I can see you and Hillerman are not going out for drinks when this case ends."

"Why can't that guy just answer a question? Better yet, why can't he just let the people who're asked the question answer it? I mean, it's okay for them to run groups by themselves, but they can't talk to us without him butting in? If he was as interested in helping us as he is in protecting his reputation, as if he had one, we'd have this case solved by now."

"I wouldn't say that. I doubt Hillerman has anything interesting to say. If he has, he sure hasn't shared it with us yet. But I would like to get the therapists alone without him censoring them."

Randazzo regretted not getting more out of Valerie the one time she had her alone, when Larson was meeting the Monday group. She knew that Hillerman would make sure that never happened again. "Fat chance," she said. "I bet he's keeping them on a short leash now. By the way, not to change the subject, but do you remember Velma Martinez?"

"Matheson's probation officer? Sure. Why?"

"Well, she called me today. I forgot to mention it. She told me that another child molester out on probation, Henry MacDonald, had died suspiciously a few months ago. The death was labeled a suicide, but she thought we might want to check it out. I pulled up his file. The coroner was pretty certain about suicide—gunshot to the head, powder burns on his hand. No note, but no proof anyone else was there." Randazzo thought for a moment. "Not that whoever investigated would have been suspicious enough to look for anything. There were no murders at the time. Hmmm."

"So what do you think?" Larson asked, looking for a bit of that usually keen Randazzo insight. The same insight he thought was so off when it came to Rebecca.

"Sounds like a simple case of suicide to me, except for the fact that he was an incest offender who received no jail time and was approaching the end of his probation . . ."

". . . and was being treated at the Oakwood Center?"

Randazzo nodded. "You got it. I think it's worthy of another investigation."

"Go to it. You have my blessings."

"I wasn't sure you'd say that."

Larson looked baffled until he figured out what she meant. "Why?" he asked anyway, to hear it from her.

"Because he also has one other common fact."

He couldn't believe Randazzo's stubbornness. She refused to let go, no matter what he said. "Don't start up with that crap again. I've heard it, and I'm not impressed," Larson snapped, cutting off the conversation. Randazzo said nothing, which was fine with him. Time would prove him right about Rebecca. Larson was sure of that.

20

Jack drove the short distance between his Marina del Rey apartment and Rebecca's Santa Monica condominium. Hitting nothing but red lights along Lincoln Boulevard helped turn a five-minute trip into a half-hour excursion, unfortunately giving him ample time to think about Randazzo's continuous insinuations. How could she expect him to even consider the possibility that this beautiful, intelligent, warm, accomplished woman had flipped out and become a raving homicidal avenger? He was sorry he'd ever taught Randazzo that she'd never get burned overestimating her fellow man's ability to do evil. She'd obviously taken the lesson to an absurd extreme this time, jumping on every piece of evidence that so much as hinted that Rebecca was the killer.

He parked in the visitors section of Rebecca's underground garage, wishing that he were more than that. Rebecca's condo was on the top floor, with a side view of the ocean, as the realtor had called it, which meant that if you stepped out onto the balcony and craned your head around the corner of the building, you'd get a peek at the water. But the condos with the direct views were way out of her price range. As it was, Rebecca could afford to buy her condo only after the Los Angeles phase of the nation's recession demolished the real estate market. Triumph out of tragedy.

Jack's finger had no sooner left the buzzer when the lobby door snapped open. He walked past the pool area, noting for future reference the cozy Jacuzzi under the lights. He took the elevator to Rebecca's floor and walked down the hall, where she was already waiting with the door opened. He looked at Rebecca, the lighting from inside creating a halo effect around her exquisite face, and instantly forgot Randazzo's warnings. Rebecca greeted him with a soft kiss on the cheek that melted his defenses, leaving his heart unprotected and highly vulnerable.

Rebecca invited him inside. She had the CD player on softly and the living room was scented with fresh cut roses. Jack looked around at the cherry-wood furniture, English country prints, and floral chintz fabrics. The accessories were sparse but precise, just a few well-selected pieces. "This is nice," he said, impressed. The room was filled with a coziness usually reserved for a country cottage and not for a modern condominium. Jack liked the warm feel of the room and felt it represented the softer side of Rebecca—the side she hid behind her hard, professional exterior.

"Well, thank you," Rebecca beamed. "Here, let me show you the rest of the place."

"Wow, did you do all this yourself?" he asked as the tour began.

"You think I could afford a decorator on my salary?" she joked as she led him by the hand.

As they headed down the hall, Rebecca showed

him her bedroom, decorated in matching blue and yellow Laura Ashley prints from the quilt and bedding to the walls and window treatments. A room Jack—a self-respecting red-blooded male—would never have stepped into, save for the opportunity to be there with Rebecca. He had to force himself not to stare too long at Rebecca's bed. Maybe later, he thought.

"Can I get you a glass of wine?" Rebecca offered as they worked their way back to the kitchen.

Jack suddenly felt like a jerk for not remembering to bring any. He didn't know whether to apologize or just continue looking awkward. He decided to ignore his faux pas, hoping that Rebecca would too. "That's perfect, thanks," he said as they returned to the living room. He took off his brown blazer and draped it over the back of a chair. White button-down shirt, worn blue jeans, and cowboy boots completed his off-duty uniform. "You sure have a beautiful place. Doesn't look like a lawyer lives here."

Rebecca looked incredulous. "What, you expected a house full of pit bulls and aquariums filled with piranhas?"

"I was thinking sharks, not piranhas," he joked. Rebecca pretended to glower. "I guess that means I shouldn't tell you the new lawyer joke I heard?" he asked with a smile.

"Not unless you want to hear how many cops it takes to change a light bulb," she kidded. She handed Jack his glass, and then looked around the room. "Actually, though, I know what you mean. I threw out all my Daumier prints last year along with most of my Nordstrom suits." Rebecca let out a little laugh, thinking back to what a walking stereotype she had been. "I may as well have had lawyer tattooed on my forehead. It was like that's all I knew how to be."

"I think I know how you feel. When you spend all your time doing something, it tends to take over your life. I can't help but see the world from a cop's perspective. It's not just what I do, it's who I am. It's hard to separate the two," Larson said as he settled back on her sofa. Rebecca sat facing him on the other side of the couch.

Rebecca could hardly believe she had found someone who not only listened to her, but really seemed to understand what she was trying to say. She sat forward as her words rushed together. "Exactly. It ends up slanting your perception of the world. I know in my case, I tend to see the world through the eyes of a prosecutor. I assume that people are always lying to me."

Jack couldn't help but flash on Randazzo—what would she think if she heard Rebecca? "I think you need that break we talked about. You know, all work and no play—"

"I know, I know. Look, I do have other interests, you know."

"Yeah, right. Like what?"

Like you, she thought as she looked into his eyes. She kept her thought to herself. Instead Rebecca scrunched up her face as if struggling for an answer. "Hmmm. Other interests?" She paused and looked up, perplexed. "Give me a minute, I'll think of some."

"See?" Jack said, laughing.

"Okay, I got one. Cooking. I love to cook. I find chopping vegetables to be very therapeutic."

"I'm not surprised."

"And I've taken up Tae Kwon Do."

"You sure have some violent hobbies," Jack kidded.

"Yeah. So don't mess with me," Rebecca teased. "Anyway, not everything I do is violent. I volunteer sometimes at the children's hospital. My sister's a pediatrician and I guess I was feeling envious of her ability to help kids. So I go, read stories, blow up balloons, hand out stuffed animals. It's not much, but it feels pretty good."

Jack felt a little overwhelmed—all this from a woman who was notorious for being a workaholic. "I don't know what to say. The most ambitious thing I've done all year is clean out my closet. I found an autographed baseball signed by the 1988 Dodgers which I was sure I'd lost. It's as close to God as I've been in years," he said with a laugh.

"Well, if you're anything like Tom, baseball may be your substitute for religion."

Jack thought back to when he and Tom would hang out at the ballpark. "When it comes to baseball, we do share a certain obsessive interest. A girlfriend of mine once started talking during baseball highlights—I doubt her body will ever be found," he quipped. Then, turning serious once again, he added, "But I'm nothing like Tom if he's the kind of guy to let someone like you get away."

Rebecca looked away suddenly. "I said the wrong thing?" Jack asked.

"No, that's okay," she said softly.

"I'm sorry." He could have kicked himself. "I never want to get in the middle of what went on between you and Tom. It's just that since I've had the chance to get to know you, I'm really at a loss for why he ended up with Claire instead of you. The guy must be out of his mind."

Rebecca agreed with the diagnosis, and yet she didn't want Tom to take all the heat, as usual. "Don't blame Tom. It was a long time ago, and I was every bit as much to blame for our breakup as he was. It's just that since he found someone else and I hadn't, he tends to look like the bad guy. I guess I liked it better that way. But I wasn't ready to make a go of a serious relationship at the time."

Jack looked at her quizzically. Rebecca wanted to explain more and yet felt uncomfortable opening up, even with someone as trustworthy as Jack.

"I'm being vague. I'm sorry." Rebecca rubbed the back of her neck, feeling the tension immediately hit. "Suffice to say I had a lot of personal issues to deal with that I just swept under the rug. I'm sure I must have driven Tom crazy, because as much as part of me wanted him, I did everything in my power to push him away." Rebecca paused, nervous about revealing so much, and yet wanting to let Jack in. She rolled her head around to unleash some of the stress. Then she continued, hesitantly, still afraid she'd say too much and scare him away. "I was sending mixed messages, you know, why won't you commit, why won't you leave me alone. I guess one day he just decided he'd had enough. He declared himself the winner, and left."

Jack knew from experience never to second-guess other relationships, but he couldn't shake the belief that Tom was nuts for letting her get away. "Why couldn't he try to understand you—to understand what was going on with you?"

"I didn't understand it myself until a year and a half of therapy opened my eyes. By then, it was too late," Rebecca said with resignation. Then, as if banishing the negativity, she shook her head. "Now, my sister would say that though it may be too late for Tom and me, it's not too late for me to find Mr. Right. I'm just not sure I agree with her."

"You know, I think your sister has keen insight. In fact, you may not have to look too far to find him, if you're looking." Jack grinned and Rebecca melted into his dimples.

"Oh, really? Do you happen to know someone

who is available and who gives great neck massages?"

Jack motioned to Rebecca. "Come over here." She moved closer to Jack, sitting with her back to him. He gently stroked her long hair and then tossed it over one shoulder to begin massaging her neck.

"Ooh," Rebecca sighed, "that's good. I could get used to this."

"Thank you, ma'am. Glad to be of service. Too much taking on the problems of the world. Those are some pretty sore shoulders." Jack kneaded her back—his thumbs pressing in between her shoulder blades with slow, rhythmic circular motions. He worked like an expert, his hands hitting all the right spots, helping take the stress out of her body.

"Mmmm. Has anyone ever told you you're too good to be true? What's the catch?"

"I guess I am," Larson joked.

"Cute."

"And that too," Jack agreed. "But don't fool yourself. You're the real catch. I'm a lucky guy." He leaned forward and kissed her softly on the back of her neck, sending a shiver down her spine. "Ticklish?" he asked.

"No. It just feels very good."

Jack continued to massage Rebecca, his warm hands relaxing her shoulders and calming her nerves. He moved his head into the small curve of her neck, taking in the hint of lilac from her floral perfume. When he could stand it no longer, Jack slowly turned Rebecca around, cupped her head in his hands and kissed her gently on her slightly trembling lips. Rebecca stiffened at first, her hands clutching Jack's shoulders, her body rigid, her breathing shallow. Then, all at once, her body turned supple and yielding as she surrendered to Jack's touch.

"For someone who pretends to be so tough, you're really just a sweet little girl, aren't you?" Jack whispered as he moved his mouth from Rebecca's and began nibbling her neck. "You just gotta stop taking work so seriously and let that little girl out to have some fun," he said between bites.

As he started to kiss her again, Rebecca pulled away, her face turned hard. Flustered, she pantomimed a check of her watch, her eyes elsewhere. "We're late. Let me find my keys and we can walk over to the restaurant."

"Oh . . . okay," Jack said as he rose from the couch, confused.

"I just don't want to lose our reservation. We should get going," she stated matter-of-factly. As Rebecca searched in her purse for her keys, Larson was sure he caught a glimpse of steel. It was fleeting, a small, barrel-shaped glimmer, but he knew what he saw. Why does she have a gun, he wondered. She should know better. He made a mental note to check to see if it was registered. Then he made a separate note to call himself a prick for so quickly switching to cop mode.

"I found them," she chimed, her voice artificially bright. "I'm ready if you are."

The date was over by eleven, when Rebecca suggested that it was late and Jack needn't walk her to her door. He obliged. Jack knew the evening had been a disaster, but without a little black box to play back what had happened, he was clueless. How could something so good have turned so bad so fast? he wondered. But he was in no position to answer any complicated questions, having drunk his way through dinner. So he passed out on his bed and hoped that when his mind cleared, the answer would come into focus.

Rebecca walked into her condo, tossed her purse on the chair, stepped out of her shoes, and lay down on her bed. She picked up the phone and dialed Tom. There was something wrong about this, turning to Tom tonight of all nights, but Rebecca didn't know where else to turn. Arctic reception from the missus or no, she needed to talk to him, and it couldn't wait till tomorrow. Rebecca got lucky; Tom picked up on the first ring. "Hi. It's me. I need to talk to you." Tom heard the forced effort to sound calm, but the word "need" had a desperate sound to it.

He looked over at Claire. She didn't return the glance. She probably already knew it was Rebecca and was preparing her verbal darts for when he hung up. "What's wrong?"—this time, he silently added.

"Well," she paused, nervously. "Jack and I went out tonight."

"You two are really becoming quite an item," Tom stated without hiding his surprise. Claire glared at him. Tom took the portable receiver and left the bedroom for the den.

"Not after tonight. Jack said something that got me upset. It was stupid really, it was an innocent comment. I just overreacted. It pushed some buttons in me and I just turned off. By the end of the evening I couldn't wait for the date to end. I didn't even let him walk me back to my place. I don't think it mattered. He was pretty drunk by then. It seemed the more aloof I got, the more drinks he ordered. I guess we both pulled away."

"Hunh," Tom grunted. "Well, getting close is not your strong suit."

"And why do you think that is?" she snapped. "I learned that some people don't want to get too close to the real me. It causes them to behave strangely, like running off to marry the first woman they find." Rebecca couldn't stop the rush of words from this old hurt, which had never healed. And Tom's words from so long ago still echoed in her mind: "I need my space." Being dumped with a withered cliché was bad enough, but finding out through an announcement in the office newsletter that a month later Mr. Space had run off to Acapulco with someone he'd just met was more than Rebecca could take. So she shut down and kept her feelings inside, boiling over only in the occasional snide one-liners. Yet her anger had never been fully expressed.

"You know, you really have your nerve," Tom shot back. He hated getting whipsawed by her. "You call up asking me for advice and then start berating me. Why don't you try to get your head together before you cause any more damage?"

"I'm sorry, I'm sorry." Rebecca started crying. "Don't hang up. You're right. I did it to Jack and now I'm doing it to you. It's like I can't stop pushing everyone I care about away. Tom, I don't know how you've stuck in there all these years. You must be a saint."

Tom paused. He hated when Rebecca would take the blame for everything. It wasn't right and it made her more resentful when she calmed down. But psychological analysis wasn't what Rebecca needed right now, so he kept his observations to himself and tried to lighten the conversation. "My mother would be so happy. Twelve years of Catholic school apparently didn't go to waste. Saint Thomas. Wait, I think somebody beat me to it."

She managed a weak chuckle through the tears.

"Rebecca," he said, adopting a big brother tone. "You need to call Jack and tell him the truth. Don't worry, he'll understand."

"I hope so."

Tom found solace in trying to help Rebecca. It also made him feel magnanimous—and it helped ease his guilt over hurting Rebecca so badly. "I know you didn't call asking for my blessings for you and Jack. But, since you sainted me and all that, I guess a benediction might be in order. Jack's a great guy. Hell, he saved my life. I think he might be good for you." Better for you than I was, Tom thought, but not as good as I'd be if I ever had another chance. He quickly ended that thought. He knew Rebecca would never give him another chance, even if he had the nerve to divorce Claire and bring shame to the entire Baldwin clan. He looked toward the bedroom, seeing the light from the TV flicker, but no sign of Claire. And yet he was sure she was listening.

"Maybe," Rebecca added, feeling less confident than her voice sounded. She looked over at the clock radio on her nightstand. "Well, it's getting pretty late. Do you have time for a less emotional question?"

"Sure." I'm in enough trouble already, he thought. What's a little more ammunition for Claire? "Shoot."

"My phone's been ringing off the hook, all the local channels want me to comment on the killings. I wanted to stay out of the media circus, but they keep pestering me. One reporter suggested that if I give her an exclusive, then the other stations will stop bugging me. She seemed nice enough and said we could run through the questions ahead of time. What do you think?"

He took off his glasses and rubbed the bridge of his nose, then slipped them back on. "You're asking me if I think you can trust a reporter?"

"No, I'm just trying to figure out the best way to handle this. Campbell thinks I'm making the office look bad by not going on TV to denounce the murders. He mentioned that my assignment is up for reconsideration and that I should think about that."

First love advice, now career advice. I should be getting paid for this, Tom thought. "If you have to go on TV to keep the brass happy, then maybe that exclusive deal is the best way to go. But watch what you say. You know how you get when you get started on the subject."

Rebecca smiled to herself. She knew precisely what he meant. "I'll try to keep it short and sweet—'Child molesters are bad, but killing them's not the answer.' I only hope I can say that with a straight face."

Tom could hear the change in her voice and he commended himself on a job well done. "You'll be terrific. Aren't all great attorneys great actors?"

"Does that mean you think I'm a great attorney?"

"You already know the answer to that. Stop fishing for compliments. If you believed in yourself you wouldn't care about my opinion. Or anyone else's for that matter."

"All right. Enough with the pep talk. You made your point. See you at the office."

"See you on the news."

After Tom hung up, he sat in the darkened den, thinking. He wasn't happy with Claire, and he knew she wasn't any happier with him. Maybe fifty years ago people stayed together in lousy marriages, and some still did for the sake of the children. But there was nothing keeping him in the marriage other than stubbornness, inertia, and the fact that he was a former altar boy who wanted to believe in till death us do part. He wondered if death of the relationship counted? He decided to sleep in the den. He turned on the TV quietly. In the morning he could pretend he fell asleep watching—not that he chose to stay away.

21

Waking up hung over was far from a new experience for Larson, but the throbbing in his head and the stiffness in his body convinced him that even he was getting too old for this. Next time he wanted to drown his sorrows, he might consider a pool instead. He doubted he could maneuver his way to the bathroom, let alone manage a trip down to the station. He hoped this would be a quiet day.

As he rubbed his face, trying to kick start his circulatory system, his thoughts turned to last night, the confusing events swirling around in his head, searching for a rational place to land. The evening had started out so great, maybe too great. He remembered kissing Rebecca, and then just like that she seemed to turn off, as if someone had flicked the wrong switch. Larson wasn't sure if it was something he said or something he did, or both. All he knew was it was the first promising relationship he'd had in a long time, and now it was, in all likelihood, in the toilet.

Larson wandered into his kitchen in a vain attempt to rehydrate his body—although it was probably too late for water to do him any good, since his headache was already in overdrive. A handful of aspirin and a hot shower were definitely in order. But first, he needed to sit and rest. Apparently, while he was sleeping, someone had greatly lengthened the walk to the kitchen.

The aspirin downed, he stood propped against the wall of his shower, eyes closed, the water just this side of too hot pounding his back. Usually fifteen minutes of hot water and steam were enough to overcome the effects of pickling his body. However, he was well beyond that—and no closer to restoration—when he realized that the phone seemed to be ringing incessantly. Larson ran out of the shower and grabbed the phone before the next ring could explode in his still-pulsating head. "Yeah?" he managed.

"Yeah, what?" Randazzo blurted out, exasperated. "Do you know it's ten o'clock!"

"No, but thanks for letting me know. I'll look forward to your call at eleven."

Randazzo was not in the mood for humor. "What is going on? Why aren't you here yet?"

"Jesus, what crawled up your ass and died? Isn't it a little early for you to be so testy?"

"What crawled up my ass?" she asked incredulously. "We got dead guys coming out of our ears and you're dragging your butt."

"I'm sorry. I had a late night with Rebecca," he said automatically, before he realized he had said precisely the wrong thing at the wrong time.

"I figured," Randazzo said, furious. She could feel herself squeezing the receiver as her efforts to remain calm were rapidly failing. "Look, maybe you don't care about your career anymore, but I care about mine. There are dozens of other detectives, not the least of which are our R-H friends, who would like nothing more than to push us aside and take credit for the collar. If we don't keep up, we're going to lose out in a big way. Don't you understand?"

Larson carried the phone back to the bathroom to grab a towel. His carpet was soaked, he was freezing, and his head was still throbbing, yet he had the feeling that this might be the high point of his day. "I know, I know," he said earnestly.

"I don't think you do. I'm not going to let an opportunity like this one slip away. If you're not up for it, I'll get a new partner." She hated giving him an ultimatum and wasn't even sure she could follow up on it, but she saw no other option.

Jack felt like he had just been slapped in the face. A punishment he needed, and apparently deserved. "You're right. I'm sorry," he said, wondering how he always ended up in messes like this. "I wasn't thinking about you. I have a lot on my mind."

"Like getting Ms. Fielding to wiggle her tiny little butt for you? Well, what's it gonna be, Jack, her or me? I'm your partner. You used to think that meant something."

That quickly answered the question whether Larson could feel any worse today. He rubbed his forehead, feeling the pressure of her words. She sure knew how to get him where it hurt. "Okay, enough. Can you just let it go? I said you're right. I'll be shaved in no time and I'll see you at the station before you know it. I won't let you down again, I promise." Besides, he thought, after last night, solving these killings seemed to be easier than figuring out Rebecca. Unless, of course, solving the killings meant figuring Rebecca out.

Larson walked to his desk to find a pile of wadded-up paper on his chair and his partner barely stifling a smile. Apparently in his absence she had found a new way to play paper basketball. He put the stack on his desk, planning on firing them back if necessary.

Randazzo called over to him. "So tell me, Romeo. Did you find out if your girlfriend had an alibi for any of the murders?"

This was precisely what he did not want to talk about. He grabbed a scrunched-up piece of paper and fired it at Randazzo's desk, getting the bounce off the side to land the paper in her trash can. "It didn't come up, and she's not my girlfriend," he growled. "I told you, if you want to investigate her, go ahead. It's your time you're wasting. You haven't turned up anything yet, so go ahead with your crusade against Rebecca," Larson said with due conviction, belying the fact that he was defending someone who had just cast him aside.

Randazzo rolled her chair over to his desk. "As a matter of fact, I did investigate a little more. And you're not gonna like what I turned up."

"What are you talking about?" he said in measured tones. He got up suddenly and headed toward the coffeemaker. Whatever she had to say to him, he figured it was better to hear it with some caffeine in his system.

Randazzo followed behind, a little apprehensive. "Now don't get mad when I tell you this."

Larson always rankled when told what not to do. The easiest way to get him mad was to tell him not to get mad, and Randazzo knew it. "When you tell me what?" he snapped.

"Well, I've been asking around the D.A.'s office and around the courthouse . . ."

Larson stopped walking and turned around. "And?" he interrupted, his eyes narrowing.

Randazzo swallowed hard. "I discovered that Rebecca has hired a private investigator in the past—on her own—to investigate some of her old defendants, including Matheson. She was called on the carpet for it—it almost cost her the head of the department.

Ralph Simpson's been gunning for her for a while, and he's been a busy little beaver compiling evidence of her obsessive interest in her cases. He's got phone records showing calls to the defendants' homes and work. He told me there have been complaints about her following these men and snooping around asking questions about them." Randazzo looked up at Larson, her eyes filled with compassion. "She's got a problem, Jack."

Larson wanted none of her pity. He turned on his heels and continued down the hall, with Randazzo still following. "No, you have the problem. How do you know Simpson's not just jealous of her? Maybe he wants her job and he's using this character assassination to try to get her removed. Even the most elementary police work would have showed you that he has a motive to make up stories about Rebecca."

"That was uncalled for," Randazzo interrupted.

Larson didn't feel much like apologizing. He reached the coffeemaker and poured himself a cup, then leaned back against the counter, facing Randazzo. "While you've been checking up on Rebecca, I've done some checking around on my own. Would you like to hear about your informant? Ralph Simpson, bottom third of his class, small problem with gambling, bigger problem with a wife who spends more than he makes. Dearly wanted the thirty-thou-a-year promotion that Rebecca got. He'd love nothing more than to serve her up as some psycho nut so he could waltz into that job." Larson took a sip and looked around for the customary box of donuts. As usual, his late arrival meant nothing was left but a maple and a coconut. He picked up the maple and took a bite. "You know, you really ought to consider the source before you give too much weight to the information you get."

Randazzo noticed some other detectives walk into

the kitchen and didn't want this broadcast for everyone to hear. She waited for them to leave, then leaned in toward Larson, speaking with a stage whisper. "I am considering the source. He's in there, in the office, able to observe what she's up to. And a lot of what he said, you've confirmed. You're the one who told me that she was a little intense about this stuff. All I'm saying is you're not seeing just how intense she might really be."

Larson paced in the small kitchen like a caged tiger. "I think you're just a little too quick to accept anything that points to Rebecca and ignore everything that points in another direction."

"Like what?"

Larson stopped pacing and looked at Randazzo, anxious to give his alternative theory. "Like what about LaPaca, or even Hillerman? Maybe Hillerman and Rubin are killing each other's patients?" he said.

"Now why would they do that, Sherlock?"

"I don't know. Maybe because they're taking a lovers' spat to a new level. Maybe they're trying to put each other out of business. Did you ever think of that? Don't you find it odd that the Oakwood is being so secretive with us? That's where you should be focusing your attention. Don't you wonder why they're not turning over all of their files? Every time I ask Gilmore where their reports are, he just shrugs and says they're not giving us anything. Maybe they have something to hide. Maybe it's one of the blonde therapists they have there, which is just about the only kind of therapist Hillerman seems to hire. You could get pretty tired sitting, listening to all that crap week after week. Maybe one of them decided to thin out their patient list."

"Maybe, Jack, maybe." Randazzo motioned for Larson to join her at the small table over by the sink. "But, just listen to me for a minute." She reached forward and touched him on the shoulder. She didn't want to fight, but she was afraid that what she was about to say would send him through the roof. "I also did some other checking up on her and I found out that she was molested by her father when she was a little girl. She thinks it's this big secret, but apparently everybody in the office knows. Think about it. It makes sense. She spends her life trying to put away molesters so she can get even for what happened to her. But what happens? They don't do any time. The system is stacked against her, so one day she snaps. She probably can't stop herself. But we're gonna have to stop her."

Larson remained quiet for some time, surprising Randazzo. She was waiting for him to explode, to yell at her, get in her face about checking up on Rebecca. Instead, he seemed lost in thought and, oddly, mildly relieved. "You know something? It would make sense. Last night. I couldn't figure out what had happened. We seemed to be getting along great, then all of a sudden, I'm the kiss of death. I replayed the evening in my mind and it didn't make sense until something you just said." Larson seemed to fade away. "There I was, going on about what a little girl she is—how was I supposed to know? Why didn't she tell me?"

Randazzo looked at Larson, confused. Was he coming around? Was he finally seeing the obvious? "Okay, so you see what I'm saying?" she asked slowly.

"What?" he answered, startled back into the conversation. "No, no. I was just trying to piece together something that happened last night. You don't think I'm buying into your bullshit theory about Rebecca?" He scoffed. "You've just made me realize what an idiot I was. I've gotta call her and apologize. I accidentally put my big foot right in my big mouth." He smiled with relief.

Randazzo started rubbing her temples furiously.

She never had headaches until this case, but now she kept running out of Tylenol. She tried to speak softly, evenly, repressing all emotion. "Jack, I think you should ask for a reassignment. You and I are on two totally different wavelengths here. You're sitting here worrying about your love life while I'm trying to explain that your girlfriend could be a cold-blooded killer. What the hell is going on here? Wait. Don't answer," she implored. "I don't want to lose this case. I've worked too hard. But I think you've lost whatever objectivity you ever had. She's the best suspect we've got and I'm gonna nail her before she kills anyone else. I don't care that the victims are all child molesters. I don't care if she thinks she's doing God's work and I don't care if she's just a poor, pitiful, psycho case. It's my job to catch the killer, and I'm gonna do that with or without you."

Randazzo got up suddenly and walked out of the room. This time she meant it, and Larson knew it. But at this point, he wasn't sure he cared about the case. All he knew was that for the first time in a long time he cared about someone besides himself. That had to be worth more than losing a partner, right? "Oh, hell. What have I done?" he muttered to the empty room.

Rebecca popped her head into Tom's office, greeting him with a little wave and an offer of a handful of M&M's. Tom was happy to see Rebecca looking rested and happy—a far cry from the woman he'd talked to last night. He worried about her, a habit he long ago tried to shake. He wondered wearily if he'd ever pass the mantle along to someone else who would become her guardian angel, a job with too much responsibility and not enough reward.

Rebecca handed him the candies, a thank-you

present. "I know I said it last night, but thanks for being there. I don't know what I'd do without you."

Great, put more pressure on me, he thought. "You know I'll always be here for you," he said. She looked up at him and smiled. He wondered why Claire couldn't make him feel that needed, that important.

"Well, I cleared it with the brass. I'm going to be interviewed on the news the day after tomorrow. Ten o'clock, Channel Ten. It's going to be a call-in. Maybe you can phone in with a nice softball question. Now that I agreed to it, I'm petrified."

Tom's secretary walked in with his morning mail and he thumbed through it as he spoke. "I'm sure you'll do great. You don't need my help." He dropped the stack of letters into his to-do basket. "By the way, did you give any thought to how you're going to deal with Jack?"

Rebecca looked out the window, counting the broken windows in the empty building across the street, courtesy of the last big earthquake, and found herself angry that no one cared enough to repair the damage but left it standing as a hollow monument to the disaster. She thought how easily her relationship with Jack could stand like that building unless she cared enough to fix it. "I'm gonna have to be honest with him. It's going to be scary, but I've got to take the chance one of these days or I'll end up miserable my whole life, and I really don't want that."

"Good luck. Jack won't let you down," Tom said convincingly. He hoped he was right. And yet part of him—the part he didn't want to see—was afraid of Rebecca finding true love. If she no longer needed him, what would he have left? A loveless marriage and a miserable, going-nowhere career. It was as if all he had was his role as Rebecca's safety net—and he wasn't prepared to lose it.

22

L arson, get your ass up here. You got a delivery," the beefy desk sergeant barked into the intercom.

"What the hell?" Jack blurted out as he walked out to the front and saw a huge bouquet of flowers waiting for him at the front desk.

"It's so cute, I could puke," grumbled the sarge as a red-faced Larson retreated with his haul.

At first, he had an unsettling thought that it might be from Frank, but then he read the card, relieved— "Can we try again? Dinner, my place, Saturday night? Soft music, good food, an explanation. Rebecca." It was an offer he couldn't refuse. He called Rebecca at the office and told her voice mail that he'd be delighted. When he hung up, he thought, did I really say "delighted"? I must be in love. I've lost my mind.

Valerie had paced her five-by-five cubicle and rehearsed her lines. Now, standing in his doorway, she was as ready as she would ever be. "Dr. Hillerman, I was wondering if we could have a talk."

Hillerman didn't look up from his computer. It wasn't that he was doing work of any importance; it was just that he didn't feel like being polite. "It's really not a good time. Can't it wait?"

"If I don't say what I have to say right now, I'm not sure when I'll ever be able to." Valerie came in and closed the door. "You know, you've been so good to me and I really appreciate all you've done for me. I don't want you to think I'm being ungrateful or anything. And I want you to know that I love working here and hope that I can stay here for a long time. So I don't want anything I say to detract from that."

Bored, Hillerman turned away from the computer and looked up at her. "Valerie, perhaps you might get to the point?"

Valerie felt a dryness in her mouth and looked down at her clasped hands. "I think that maybe we should stop seeing each other."

Hillerman broke into a broad smile. "You're breaking up with me?" He laughed, astonished by her boldness.

She closed her eyes, took a deep breath, and pressed on despite Hillerman's unexpected reaction. "This is really hard for me to do because I think so highly of you and I've been so flattered by the attention. But I think it would be best if our relationship went back to the way it was. I want to continue to work here and learn from you. I really do. I enjoy what I do and that's what I'd like to concentrate on. I worry that my work has suffered because of our relationship."

Hillerman couldn't drop the amused expression from his face, incapable of taking her words seriously. "I'm not sure what to say. I thought you enjoyed your time with me."

Valerie blushed and her resolve began to falter as she realized that rehearsing alone was no preparation for facing Hillerman. If only she didn't have to face him, if only she didn't have to look into his eyes. "It's not that. I mean, you've been wonderful. It's just that . . ." Valerie paused, searching for the right words, not really sure they existed. "I'm afraid you're going to leave me some day and I think if we just call it off now, that won't happen and we can go back to how it was. I want to stay here. I don't want to have to leave like Dr. Rubin did."

The mention of Rubin's name caused Hillerman's face to drop its bemused grin. He looked back at his screen and clacked on the keys noisily. "That was before your time," he said firmly as he continued typing, "and I think it would be better if you stayed out of matters that do not concern you. Her leaving had nothing to do with that. I think we should all be professional about this and keep our personal life separate from business. If one no longer works, there's no reason to end the other. They are two totally different matters. But right now, they both seem to be working just fine for us." Hillerman stopped his typing and turned back toward Valerie, who remained standing, still too uncomfortable to take a seat. "Is it the age difference? Is that what is really bothering you?"

"No, no, not at all. I feel very comfortable with you." She looked away as he searched her face.

"But?"

"But I'm not sure that we should be doing what we're doing. I just thought that maybe we should stop that part of our relationship and just stick with business. I mean, it's been really great and all, but I guess I don't want anybody to get hurt."

Hillerman had grown tired of looking up and gestured for Valerie to take a chair. She obliged. "No one has to get hurt," he said. "How can anyone get hurt when it feels so good, so right. We're two intelligent people who want to please each other. There's nothing wrong with that at all. If we decide to stop, that can be a decision we both make and agree upon."

"What about Anita? I didn't get the feeling that's what happened with her. I got the feeling she was upset when you two stopped seeing each other."

He looked at her coldly. "That was Anita. We're talking about you now."

Valerie seemed to visibly shrink, becoming smaller as each of her arguments failed. "I don't know what else to say," she said with a weak shrug. "I'll have to think about what you said."

Hillerman sat back in his chair, suddenly looking relaxed and satisfied. He found mind games quite enjoyable—so long as he won. "You know, it's a good thing that we're having this talk. If at any point either of us wants to stop seeing each other, we can talk about it like mature people. There's no reason for us to stop now just because you're worried about the future. Why deprive me of pleasure today simply because you fear that there might be pain tomorrow? Enjoy, live life. You're far too young to be worrying about the future. Now I know you can't mean that you really don't still want me?" He pouted playfully.

Valerie smiled weakly. "No, no. Of course. That's not what I was saying."

He looked at her with boredom in his eyes, his tone dismissive. "Well, when you do know what you mean, why don't you come back and let me know. Next time you should consider thinking before you speak." Hillerman turned back to the computer and started to tap the keys rapidly.

Valerie stood and started to say something, then turned suddenly and ran out of his office. Anita saw her run down the hall and thought she saw tears. She wasn't surprised.

✢ ✢ ✢

As he was dressing for his date, Larson realized what an excellent job he had done not thinking about what Randazzo had been telling him all week. It was a gift, to be able to so totally put disturbing information out of his mind. He couldn't help but feel guilty, like he was cheating on his wife or something—going out with Rebecca behind Randazzo's back. He didn't much like being forced to choose between two women he cared about, but he hadn't yet figured out how he could keep Randazzo as a partner and Rebecca as something more. Not unless he could convince Randazzo she was dead wrong about Rebecca. He should have brought a lie detector to tonight's date. He could just imagine it. "Rebecca? Can I ask you a few questions before dinner? Would you mind if I just hooked you up to this little machine?"

The sound of Jack's footsteps coming up the corridor sent a rush of excitement mixed with fear through Rebecca, like the first day of school. Wanting to turn back, repelled by fear, and yet propelled forward by hope and anticipation, she took a deep breath, then opened the door. Here we go.

Jack smiled, not sure what to say. He started simply. "Well, you scooped me on the flowers. So, I brought you these instead." He handed her a small package—flat, square shaped, wrapped with a large pink bow. Rebecca took the package and let Jack in, shutting the door behind him. She quickly opened up the present to find two CDs. "You said these were some of your favorites but that you never get around to buying them." Rebecca scanned the selections— Natalie Merchant and Gin Blossoms. A bouquet of music, she thought, even better than flowers. This man has been paying attention.

"Excellent choices. You always did know how to make a good impression," she said warmly.

"I try."

She walked over to her CD player and loaded the CDs, setting the volume low, while he took off his jacket and settled on the couch.

"Can I get you a drink?" she offered.

"No, not right now. Come, sit down. Let's talk. About the other night. I think I owe you an apology."

"It's not you who should be apologizing." Rebecca tentatively moved toward him, his seeming composure heightening her schoolgirl nervousness. She knew she had to say what was on her mind, to take the risk now before she lost her nerve. She sat facing him, looking small and delicate, swallowed up by the overstuffed love seat. "Jack, I—uh—I need to explain about that. There's a lot you don't know about me."

He knew enough to know when not to speak and let the pause linger, allowing Rebecca to choose her time.

"This is not going to be easy," she said, stating the obvious. "The other night, I know you must have wondered what the hell was going on. And, I wanted to explain. There's never—there hasn't been anyone since Tom. No one that I've gotten close to. I don't get close that easily, it's hard—trusting someone enough to let them know you is hard. I guess when I felt we were getting that close, I just panicked. I started doubting myself and doubting you. I didn't know what to do, and withdrawing seemed like the best choice at the time. But I don't think it's a decision I can live with. I think if I don't try, well, I'll always wonder, what if?"

Jack held her gaze securely but silently. He wanted to tell her that he knew, that he understood, and that it was all right, but he felt that it was important for her to continue.

"I wasn't completely open with you the other night. About why Tom and I broke up. It's a very difficult subject for me, it's not something I've been willing to face." She looked down at her hands, afraid to see any doubt in his eyes. "You see, for a long time, I was convinced that I was damaged goods, because I know that's how Tom saw me. Or at least that's how I felt." Rebecca slowed herself down, feeling herself spinning out of control. A deep breath helped calm her. "I didn't give you the entire answer before when you asked me why I prosecuted sex offenders. I stay in the sexual abuse division not just for the kids. I stay there for me, too. I guess it's my way of trying to fight back. The way I couldn't when I was younger. My father . . . I was sexually abused when I was a child." Her voice stayed strong, her eyes stayed level. She looked for a sign of retreat, a subtle revulsion, but saw acceptance instead. She took strength from his unspoken support. "From the time I was eight until I left home at sixteen, it was . . . All I had was school, it was the only place I felt safe. It paid off. I got straight A's and got into Stanford and out of the house. But I guess I never really left it behind me. I kept it a secret from Tom, from everyone. I was ashamed. . . ." Rebecca quickly brushed away a small tear, a remnant of old hurts she wanted to bury once and for all. "It was so hard to get close to him and open up. It took years. And when I finally trusted Tom enough to open up and tell him what had happened to me, I could see something in him change. I felt that his feelings for me changed. Maybe I was wrong, but I don't think I misread him. He couldn't handle it. I don't know why. But he drew away from me. It was never the same. I was devastated. I blamed myself for a long time." She bit her lip as she worked to hold back more tears.

"What a jerk," was all Jack could manage through his anger.

Rebecca shook her head. "I don't want you to be mad at Tom. I don't want you to do anything at all. I just wanted to tell you what was going on the other night. When you kissed me, I could feel myself starting to let go. But then you made that comment about my being a little girl and I know you meant it in a nice way, but it just brought it all back. It hit real close to home. I just reacted instinctively. Suddenly I felt as if things were happening to me beyond my control. I just needed to get back in control, so I turned off. That's what I learned to do as a little girl, just turn off." Rebecca sighed and closed her eyes, worn out by the truth and yet resolved that she wasn't going to be a prisoner of it any longer. "But I don't want to turn off. I really do care for you, I want us to be closer. I was afraid if you knew me . . . I just didn't know if I could trust you, to tell you the truth." She paused and swallowed hard. "The other night, I wasn't sure who you were anymore. And I wasn't sure you'd still care about me if you knew who I was."

Jack wished Rebecca could see inside him, to know that his heart was hers for the taking. He had fallen hard and fast for her, and—to Randazzo's great disappointment—there wasn't much Rebecca could do to change his opinion. But how could he convince her? "I was such an idiot. I don't want to lose you over such a stupid comment. I care about you more than I've cared about anybody in a long time. I thought we had a chance and I don't want to do anything to spoil that."

Rebecca put her hand up to brush his hair back off his forehead. "Jack, you didn't spoil it. But I almost let my fear do just that." She smiled, a crooked nervous smile that he melted into. "But no more. I'm being as open as I can be. I'm scared of relationships. I've never been in one that worked and I've never even seen one that worked. But I know I'll never be in one that works if it's based on keeping secrets. This is me, this is who I am. No hiding, no games, no secrets."

Jack, who never was at a loss for the right move to make, was suddenly immobilized. "Rebecca, I don't know what to do. I want to hold you and have you not pull away. I want you to know you can trust me. You tell me that this is the real you. Well, I like what I see. I like this person. I'm not Tom—you haven't scared me away. The real me is someone who's not going to run away from the real you. I'm here for the long haul, if you want me."

"I do." She wiped away a stray tear.

"I like the sound of that," Jack said as he wrapped her up in his arms, pulling her tight against his chest. They sat holding each other for what seemed like an eternity, rocking gently in time with the music. Jack noted with irony the song they were listening to— "Found Out About You." He flashed on Randazzo then shook his head, as if he could somehow rid himself of her. She didn't belong here, not tonight.

They stayed like that for what seemed like a lifetime, Rebecca releasing years of bottled-up fears and doubts, feeling emotionally exhausted and yet renewed at the same time. Finally, the soft rumbling of Jack's empty stomach broke the mood and left them laughing out loud.

"I can take a hint. I guess I should feed you." She smiled and let out a deep sigh, freed of the tension that had been bottled up inside. "Go sit at the table. Tonight, I serve."

"Would it be too chauvinistic of me to say that I like the sound of that, too?"

"Yes," Rebecca said with a hearty laugh. But she

didn't care, tonight she liked being old-fashioned. She retreated into her kitchen to finish readying dinner. She heated the oil to fry the crab cakes she'd made earlier in the day, sliced lemons for garnish, and checked the remoulade sauce, upping the red pepper just a notch for an extra kick. Rebecca couldn't remember enjoying putting a meal together more. She had puttered around all afternoon nervously anticipating her talk with Jack. Now that it was over and he was still here, she felt relieved and hopeful, and yet not fully rid of a nagging doubt that things weren't supposed to work out for her. Still she was willing, for now, not to give into that doubt, to trust that this might be different. That Jack was different.

Jack went over to the table, already set with fruit-and-berry-trimmed stoneware, and decided he'd feel silly just sitting there waiting for his food. He popped his head into the kitchen to see if he could help but was quickly shooed away. So he hung out in the living room, checking out Rebecca's small and decidedly narrowly focused CD collection and her larger and far more eclectic array of books as his nose was teased by the aroma emanating from the kitchen.

When Jack could stand it no longer, Rebecca called out "Dinner's ready," and he scrambled to take his place at the table. She emerged from the kitchen feeling lighter, the great burden of her shame and doubt lifted from her shoulders. She had to check to see if her feet were still touching the floor. She felt as if she were Alice, beyond her own personal looking glass, seeing the world as she never had before, as a safe place, a loving place, with promise for happiness stretching out before her. She couldn't wait to share this new world with Jack.

Jack's heart swelled as he saw Rebecca absolutely glowing, her face flushed and her smile a mile wide, coming into the dining room, a huge platter of crab cakes in her hands. He decided to take her lead, put the intensity of the discussion behind them and just relax. "That looks incredible," he said.

"Me, or the food?" Rebecca said with a smile, as she went back into the kitchen for a bottle of chilled Pinot Noir.

"Both," he called out. Jack picked up the serving spoon and dug out a large serving of crab cakes, piling them high on his plate. "Heart-to-hearts give me a healthy appetite."

Rebecca sat back down, uncorked the wine, and poured two glasses, handing one to Jack. "Apparently."

"To a wonderful dinner," Jack toasted.

Rebecca lifted her glass. "You haven't even tried it yet."

"Just sitting here with you makes this wonderful. If the food is good too, that's just an added bonus." Rebecca looked down and felt her cheeks grow warm again.

Jack took a bite and nearly passed out. "Mmmm. Why did we ever go out? This is fabulous," he exclaimed. "Better than the ones I had when I went to New Orleans."

"Thanks," she said brightly.

"Some people tout their cooking skills and then when you take a bite it's pretty gruesome."

"Well, glad to know it's not gruesome," Rebecca said with a laugh. She took a bite, happy to be sharing a simple pleasure with Jack, but her mind turned to his work, as it always did. "So, speaking of gruesome, anything new on the case?"

Her question caught him by surprise, causing the food to catch in his throat. A quick gulp of wine helped it down. Anything new? Besides my partner still suspecting you, not much, he thought. "No, just a lot of waiting and wondering. There hasn't been a killing in two weeks, I think the killer's due."

"That reminds me. Did I tell you I'm going to be interviewed on TV next Tuesday? Thanks to your case, I'm suddenly in demand as the resident expert on the prosecution of child molesters. So I get a few minutes to make a speech and field some callers' questions. It should be fun."

Jack could just imagine what Randazzo would make of this. "You're going on TV to talk about the killings?"

"Not exactly the killings. Mostly I'll be talking about sentencing issues. My goal is to use the killings as a springboard to discuss how inadequately the system punishes child molesters, especially incest offenders. Listen, this is the chance I've been waiting for."

"Are you sure it's such a good idea?" He wondered how much ammunition this would give Randazzo for her theory.

Rebecca stopped midbite, a little puzzled. "Why?"

"Well, I don't know." He fumbled for something to say. "Just be careful. You know how people can twist what you say around or misunderstand the point you're trying to make."

She laughed off his concern. "Don't worry. It'll be fun. Just remember to call and tell me how cute I looked."

"I thought you only worried about truth and justice?"

"And how my hair looks. It's a genetic flaw, those two X chromosomes."

He laughed. "I'm sure you'll look beautiful, as always."

"Flattery will get you anywhere."

✤ ✤ ✤

After dinner, Jack considered going for the Kahlúa cheesecake. But, as much as he wanted dessert, there was something he wanted more. He got up and took Rebecca by the hand, walking toward the living room couch.

Rebecca had other ideas. She led Jack down the hall toward her bedroom, looking back at his slightly dubious face.

He pulled back slightly. "I'm not rushing you," he stressed, fearing she was acting out of obligation. Rebecca put her hand to his mouth. "Don't be silly. I think I may be rushing you," she said. "Now, of course, if you don't want—" she said playfully.

"No, no. I do want," Jack interrupted. "I've wanted to ever since I first saw you."

She laughed softly as she walked on ahead of him, down the hall, then turned around and beckoned him with her upturned palm. Jack dropped his head along with his resolve and went willingly wherever Rebecca wanted to take him.

23

Rebecca thought about what she could accomplish tonight. She finally had the audience she longed for and the chance to get her message out. Knowing that helped to ease her nerves as the red light on the camera blinked on and the news anchor began to promote Rebecca's segment.

"This is Clint Nolan. Good evening and welcome to the award-winning Channel 10 News at Ten." The handsome, young anchor dropped the smile to assume his serious pose. "Tonight, the child molester murders again top our news. Tonight's live viewer call-in segment will feature Rebecca Fielding, the head of the sexual abuse unit of the Van Nuys district attorney's office and the district attorney who prosecuted each of the recently murdered child molesters. She will talk with us about the legal system and its handling of child molestation cases."

Rebecca looked straight into the camera without expression—smiling into the camera seemed inappropriate following that introduction.

"Okay, we're clear," the director announced, allowing

Rebecca to exhale and slump in momentary repose. "We'll give you a two-minute warning. Just relax and take it easy."

"Okay, sure. Thanks."

Ralph Simpson flipped to another channel. He knew he'd turn back. As pissed off as he was that Rebecca was, once again, the anointed expert and he was, once again, a nobody watching her run the show from afar, he knew he couldn't resist the temptation to watch. There was always the chance she'd make a fool of herself. Maybe she'd panic, eyes frozen ahead as the anchor kept calling her name. Or she could let loose on one of her famous tirades and look like a nut in front of the whole city. The call-in number registered in his head. Sometimes it's difficult to resist having a little fun.

Not far from Ralph's condo, the Oakwood was still abuzz with activity, the last groups for the night midway through their allotted time. Valerie was finishing up this month's reports while the TV quietly hummed in the background. Hillerman came up from behind and put his hands on her shoulders. "The faster you type, the sooner we can get on with the evening."

"But I have so much work to do. I'll probably be up typing all night."

Hillerman dropped his hands to his side. "And what am I supposed to do? You really must learn to organize your time better. If you shut off that TV you'd probably get your work done faster. I'm so tired of listening to this drivel and I really don't want to hear what that bitch has to say about our patients. Isn't there any real news?"

"I'm sorry. I thought you were interested in this, too."

"Now what would give you that idea?" Hillerman

turned to walk out. "Let's just forget tonight. I'll see you tomorrow."

"Three, two . . ." The director pointed a finger at the anchor who sat and nodded a silent greeting to his audience. "We'll be taking your calls for our in-studio guest, Rebecca Fielding, a ten-year veteran of the district attorney's office prosecuting child molesters. Here is Linda Marquez with her exclusive interview."

"Ms. Fielding, thank you for joining us tonight. The recent killings of five convicted child molesters on probation have spawned a country-wide debate on the appropriate punishment of child molesters. You've been prosecuting child molesters for almost ten years. I guess first and foremost on everyone's mind is: what is the typical sentence that first-time offenders receive and is it unusual that these men receive no jail time?"

Rebecca was thankful that the first question was such a slow pitch. "By statute, first-time offenders may get up to eight years in jail, plus additional enhancement time if their offense was committed under certain circumstances. But in reality, unless the victim was a stranger to the molester or the molester had multiple victims, most get one year or less for the first offense. Indeed many, especially incest offenders, do no time at all and are simply put on probation."

"That's unbelievable," the interviewer said, looking surprised. While this reaction was for show, when she had first heard this statistic an hour ago, she had been genuinely surprised, as had most of the crew.

"Unfortunately, it's true," Rebecca continued. "While society seems to uniformly abhor what child molesters do, there is a surprising lack of public demand to increase the penalties or to ensure they are enforced as written in the law. Right now, judges have an incredible amount of flexibility—what they call judicial discretion—which permits them to give sentences far more lenient than you would imagine. Judges have virtually no accountability for the sentences they hand down, and legislators typically are not held to answer for the laws that they do not pass. So, until the public demands that the legislature abolish the discretion judges are given in sentencing child molesters, we will continue to have inconsistent and insubstantial sentences." Rebecca was feeling comfortable now, emboldened by her rare opportunity to give her opinion to an audience far larger than the occasional co-worker or two hanging out by the coffeemaker.

"But judges aren't the whole problem, are they?" Well-rehearsed, the reporter read her line smoothly, giving Rebecca the segue she needed to her next point.

Rebecca took a deep breath. She knew she had to watch her words carefully, since she appeared in front of many of those judges on a regular basis. "No, of course not. There are a number of other reasons. First is the way the law is written. Jail time should be a requirement and not an option. Second, in the case of incest, the families themselves surprisingly do not push for a severe sentence. These families convince themselves that the molestation was a one-time occurrence and believe that if the perpetrator promises not to offend again, there is no reason to take him out of his home, put him in jail, have him lose his job, and have the family lose his income. The sad reality is that many families view having a bread-winning father to be their first priority and not necessarily the psychological well-being of the child. Another reason families don't push for severe sentences is that these men are not seen as threats to society. They are our fathers, uncles, grandfathers, neighbors. They molest children who they know, using persuasion or threats rather than actual violence. So I think that families believe, albeit incorrectly, that now that the offense has come to light, it won't happen again."

"So are you saying that incest offenders are treated differently from other child molesters?"

Rebecca smiled. She was getting it. "Precisely. It's similar to the problem in domestic violence cases. If a man punches a co-worker, he'll do some time. If he punches his wife, he gets probation. For some bizarre reason, violence and abuse within the family are not treated as harshly by the courts as violence and abuse outside the family. That is particularly unfair to children, who are stuck in horrible situations and unable to get out. While we can debate whether battered wives are partially at fault for staying with their abusive husbands, there is absolutely no question that incested children are totally blameless."

The reporter took the cue from her director. "Well, our lines are already lit up, so why don't we take one of the calls? This is Howard from Los Angeles, go ahead."

"Yeah," he began in an exaggerated New York accent, "since you prosecuted all the men who've been killed, have you participated in the investigation? Do you have any idea who might be the killer?"

Rebecca's nerves kept her from detecting Ralph's rather poor attempt to disguise his voice. "Answering your second question first, obviously I don't know who the killer is. I've spoken with the police detectives who are investigating the killings," and a little more, thought Rebecca, "so to that extent I guess you could say I'm participating in the investigation. But, as a district attorney in the sexual abuse unit, I work exclusively in the prosecution of sex offenders and do not as part of my job work homicide cases unless they're tied to a sex crime."

"Can I ask another question?"

"Well, we have a lot of other callers—" Marquez tried indirectly to move on.

The caller missed the subtlety. "Why do you think it is that only the men you prosecuted have been killed?"

Rebecca momentarily looked flustered. She'd thought about how to answer that question as each murder added to the scorecard, and still she had no ready response. "I have no idea," was all she could manage.

"Our next caller is Roberta from El Monte. Go ahead."

"Hello. I was wondering what your guest thinks about the reporting laws that require the police to notify residents when a child molester moves into the neighborhood. Do you think it will result in more violence against the child molesters?"

"No, I don't believe it will. While I'm aware of a few incidents where neighbors reacted with violence when they discovered that a child molester lived nearby, I think by and large notification is an excellent idea—as is the registry that lets the public call a number to find out if a person has a record of child molestation. Both procedures help to give parents the information they need to protect their children, and keeping children safe is more important than keeping criminals from being inconvenienced. It's not that child molesters should be denied access to housing, necessarily, but parents should be aware of who these people are and where they live so that they can keep their children away from them. These laws ensure that parents won't unknowingly hire a convicted child molester to baby-sit or do work around the house. I think these laws provide excellent safeguards and should be upheld and enforced." Linda started to turn toward the camera to take another call, but Rebecca gently interrupted. "But I want to stress that by far the greatest threat to children is from people they know, love, and trust, not from strangers. That's the sad truth about sexual abuse."

Linda nodded solemnly. "Okay, we have a call from Stacy in Pomona."

"Hi. How do we get rid of the judges that let the child molesters off so easy?"

Rebecca stifled a smile. She thought of suggesting the caller gather a posse to run them out of town, but knew she needed a more diplomatic answer. "I would suggest reviewing the record of the judges to see what type of sentences they hand out compared with what sentences the law provided for. I think those statistics should be made available so that when we have elections, we can make an informed choice about our judges. But also, bear in mind that judges have only as much discretion as the law permits. An obvious solution to that problem would be to pass laws enacting strict, mandatory sentencing guidelines that take the discretion away from the judges. But as we learned with the three strikes law, the courts don't take too kindly to their discretion being removed."

"Okay, we have Debbie from Van Nuys."

"Aren't you ignoring the fact that many child molesters are sick and in need of mental help?" The voice was barely a whisper. Soft, childlike.

"No, but I am saying that focusing only on the child molester's so-called illness sends the wrong message. It's a way of taking the blame off the perpetrator— using what may be a partial explanation for his crime as an excuse for his criminal behavior. It's all part of the nonresponsibility trend in psychology where everyone is a victim and no one is responsible for their actions. We've moved away from personal responsibility to a place where if someone can articulate a reason for why he or she behaved in a par-ticular way, they free themselves of the responsibility for their behavior. So, alcoholics who become violent aren't responsible because their alcoholism excuses their behavior. Poor people aren't responsible for stealing, dealing drugs, or killing—their poverty excuses their behavior. And with child molesters, many say their own history of abuse excuses their behavior. I say this kind of thinking is damaging to society. It takes the obligation off of each of us to rise above our particular baggage. Taken to its logical extreme, this nonresponsibility movement could lead to the abolition of the criminal justice system. I mean, why punish anyone? People just can't help who and what they are, right?"

The interviewer stared blankly at Rebecca. This philosophical discourse was not part of the script. The director apparently had the same reaction as he gestured furiously for her to take the next call.

"Dan from Venice, you have a follow-up question?"

"Yes. I take it that you don't believe therapy works for child molesters and that it's better to just lock them up?"

"Personally, I don't believe that therapy is the answer. I support long mandatory sentences both for whatever deterrent effect they may provide and, most importantly, to keep the offender from having the opportunity to reoffend."

"I see," Marquez said, not knowing how else to respond. "Next we have Glenn from Tujunga."

"Hello. I belong to a group you may have heard of, VOCAL—Victims of Child Abuse Laws. I was arrested, jailed, I lost my job, my house, my good name, all because my vindictive ex-wife dreamed up some bullshit charges against me . . ." The news director cringed and used the three-second delay to bleep the caller's profanity. "She claimed I molested my baby daughter. And even though she had no proof, there was no physical evidence of any kind, no witnesses, nothing, I lost everything." Glenn's voice resonated with anger across the line. "What are you doing to prevent men from being victimized by false accusations? What are you doing to protect our rights?" he demanded.

After all she had experienced, Rebecca didn't have much room in her mind for the concept of a wrongly accused parent and found it hard to be sympathetic to his plight. "In my capacity as a prosecutor, all I can do is try to ensure that the cases I bring to trial are real cases. The difficulty is that most molestation occurs in private, so there are no witnesses other than the perpetrator and the victim, and there often is no physical evidence whatsoever. If we don't proceed with cases solely on the basis of victim testimony, then guilty men won't be prosecuted. I do realize that a very small fraction of women, and some men, may use the claim of child molestation to gain leverage in a divorce or custody battle, for example, and that a few false accusations are made. I regret that and would hope that the prosecutors would do their best to ferret out erroneous accusations."

"Well, that didn't happen in my case," the caller challenged. "My attorney forced me to accept a plea bargain, said if I didn't and went to trial and lost, I'd be put away for ten years. He told me that if it was my word against my wife's, she'd win. And I'm not the only one that this has happened to. There are thousands of guys out there who've been falsely accused and convicted or forced to accept a plea bargain when they didn't do anything."

"Sir," said Rebecca, clearly irritated, "I think you exaggerate how many false accusations get to court. It's far more common for a guilty perpetrator to get off with a very light sentence because either the victim is unwilling to testify, the evidence is weak, or the courts are overcrowded. You know, plea bargains started out as a necessary evil and I think since then they've become more evil than necessary. Ultimately, the only answer lies in our jury system. If twelve impartial citizens believe beyond a reasonable doubt in the guilt of the accused, then that's as good a safeguard as we have in this country. So if you were really innocent, you should have gone to trial and not pleaded guilty."

The reporter cringed. Rarely had she seen a caller dressed down like that. "Let's move on to Sue in Gardena," said Marquez at the behest of the voice in her ear urging her to move along.

"What do you say to the people who applaud the recent murders of these convicted child molesters as vigilante justice?"

Rebecca measured her words carefully, lest her answer send her boss into convulsions. "I can understand the frustration of some people who may feel that vigilante justice is better than no justice at all. We see news reports of child molesters who go free, or who are released after serving short prison terms, and quite understandably we're angry."

"So you condone the actions of the killer or killers of these child molesters?" the reporter asked, aghast.

Think before you answer, Rebecca warned herself. "Understanding frustration is not the same as condoning it."

"Thank you, Rebecca Fielding, and thank you .to the callers. We'll be back."

The screen flashed as they went to a commercial.

Jimmy Hempstead sat stone drunk in his recliner watching the TV, seething, his eyes burning a hole in the middle of Rebecca's head. Before she had finished, he decided he'd heard enough. Someone should shut that fucking cunt up once and for all, he thought. Only "the fucking cunt" was audible over his private mumbling.

"What?" said Mary, his dull-eyed girlfriend, as she dutifully brought him the last of his nightly six-pack.

"Nothing. I'm going for a drive." He took the can of beer, grabbed his keys, and charged for the door. "Don't wait up."

"Jimmy. Wait. You're in no condition to drive." She ran after him, shouting. He hopped into his dented Blazer, gave her the bird, and was down the driveway and onto the street.

Channel 10 was only a few blocks from his house, in a seedy Hollywood-adjacent neighborhood. He didn't have a plan, wasn't sure what he'd do or say when he saw her. He was propelled by alcohol, and reason was the first casualty of his intoxication.

"That wasn't too bad. I told you the screener wouldn't give you any nut cases." Linda spoke while one of the stagehands disconnected Rebecca's microphone.

"There were actually some good questions. I was surprised how fast the time went. But I couldn't believe how nervous I was."

"Live TV will do that to you. But you were great, just great." The reporter dropped her voice a notch and leaned in. "Just between you and me, how do you really feel about the murders? It's got to be just a little satisfying for you."

Rebecca smiled. "One thing I've learned is to disregard the phrase 'just between you and me.' I think I'll stick with the answer I gave on camera. You know, though, I do find it amazing how many people seem to be happy about the killings. I'd hate to be a child molester in this city right now."

"Yeah, they might as well walk around with a bull's-eye on their foreheads."

Rebecca smiled, shook her hand, and thanked her for her professionalism. She felt she'd made a good choice trusting the reporter and felt she'd gotten a rare chance to share her beliefs with a fairly wide audience. She walked out, her keys in her hand, eager to go home and call up Jack for his instant review. She didn't notice she was being watched.

Jimmy caught a glimpse of Rebecca leaving the studio and followed her with his eyes as she headed for her car in the parking lot. He trailed her down La Brea to the Santa Monica freeway. Traffic was light and he had no trouble following her—she didn't dodge in and out of traffic, didn't speed, and didn't run the yellow lights. Shit, he thought, and Mary said I was too drunk to drive. This is a piece of cake. He popped open the beer can and then slid it into one of those phony soda pop can holders. What beer? Just drinking a soda, officer.

"Where the hell are you going, little missy?" he wondered aloud as Rebecca got off the freeway at Lincoln and headed for the supermarket. "I thought you were gonna take me home." She parked under a lamp. For safety. Nice try. Jimmy pulled over to the side, got out with the engine still running, and grabbed Rebecca from behind as soon as she lost the protection of light.

"Well, that was a fine fucking speech you gave,"

he sneered as he put his hand over her mouth. Rebecca tried to scream but the sounds were muffled by his beefy hand. She struggled against him, kicking her legs and twisting her body, and tried to pull free, but he had a hundred pounds on her. "Well, Miss Big Shot, do you feel so high and mighty now?" He smirked. Rebecca fought him, trying to squirm out of his grasp, trying to scream, trying to draw attention. But no help came. She couldn't see anyone around. Rebecca couldn't think. She just felt the aching pain as he wrestled her back to his truck. He opened the rear door and then threw her in the back. She fell back and he leaned in, looming over her, smelling of beer and sweat. He hauled back and slapped her hard in the face. "That was to get your attention. Now, you make any trouble and I'll kill you. But first, I'm gonna make you feel good, real good."

He jumped into the driver's seat and Rebecca felt the truck lurch forward. She reached to unlock the doors, to dive out of the truck to safety, but in the dark and in her panic she couldn't find the handle. She looked up to see his eyes in the rear-view mirror. "Just sit there and don't try nothing stupid. You ain't goin' nowhere." Rebecca felt trapped. She could feel her heart pounding in her throat. Her whole body was shaking. She couldn't breathe. She couldn't think. It was happening too fast. Her mind raced. "Gonna fuck you up, real good. Yes, ma'am," he snarled. He grabbed the can and threw back a slug of beer then broke into a frightening, malevolent laugh.

She clutched her purse, squeezing it tightly, as if it were all she had in the world. And then she knew what to do. She pulled out her gun, raised it to the back of his head. Jimmy looked back over his shoulder and found himself looking straight into a deceptively small .22 caliber handgun. Rebecca squeezed the trigger and shot, once, twice. His face seemed to explode then completely disappear as Rebecca heard the loud, sharp sound of stray bullets shattering the windshield.

The truck slammed into a light pole. Rebecca was thrown backward by the impact, the gun flying out of her hand. She bolted out of the truck, and without hesitating ran across the parking lot to her car. She fumbled for her keys, jumped in, and sped out of the lot, leaving a couple feet of tire tracks and a few confused bystanders behind.

Rebecca drove without thinking, her car almost psychically trained on her condo. She tried to piece together what had happened but bewildering thoughts crowded her mind. She couldn't sort them out. Who was he? Why did he grab me? He'd mentioned the speech. He'd seen me on TV, Rebecca thought. He was angry. He was going to kill me. But he didn't get the chance. There were witnesses. Many of them. And they saw me. When Rebecca got home, she collapsed on her bed, sobbing, until, exhausted, she fell into a deep sleep.

There was no hope that last night was all a terrible dream. The dried blood on the front of her clothes was just the most obvious testimony to the events of last night. Then there were the pictures flashing in her mind, mostly of exploding glass and blood splattering inside the truck. Rebecca sat on the edge of her bed, as frightened as she was mad at herself for allowing this to happen.

The ringing of the telephone startled her. She picked it up automatically. "Hello?" Her voice was shaky.

"I don't know what's going on and right now I don't want to know. All I can tell you is that I just learned that the Santa Monica police are coming to arrest you for murder. They should be there any minute. I wanted to save you the embarrassment. I know you won't run. I think it'd be best if you surrender yourself at the nearest station. Try the one on Fourth Street. Once you get there have them call me and I'll come down to meet you." He paused. "We never spoke, okay?"

"Okay, Jack." Her voiced cracked as she started to cry. "Thank you."

She stood holding the dead receiver, staring ahead at her reflection in the bedroom mirror. In such a few short minutes, her life had been turned inside out. She tried to stir herself to action. A voice in her head barked out instructions, but to no avail. Put down the phone, get your keys, get out of there. Run. Instead, she remained frozen, as if her stillness could stop time. Her paralysis was broken by a pounding on the door. She dropped the phone and went into the living room.

"I'm coming," she called, an obvious resignation in her voice. As she reached the door, she looked through the peephole to see a solid chin and thick neck above a blue uniform. She took a deep breath and opened the door.

"Rebecca Fielding?"

"Yes."

"You are under arrest for the murder of James Hempstead." The officer handed Rebecca a stapled document, which she instantly recognized as an arrest warrant. How strange to see her name there, as the suspect.

The moment became even more surreal as the familiar routine continued. "Ms. Fielding, you have the right to remain silent. If you give up that right—"

"I know, I know." She could quote from the original *Miranda* decision, she didn't need some rookie telling her what she already knew. But more than that, she didn't need any more proof that she was in trouble—terrible trouble.

"Excuse me, Ms. Fielding. But I have to read you your rights." He completed the verbatim recitation without further interruption as Rebecca closed her eyes and tried to push away the fear.

Rebecca was keenly aware of the sensations—the metal pulled tight against her wrists, her arms strained awkwardly behind her, her heart beating deep within her chest. She tried to regulate her breathing, concentrating on each breath, in and out, slowing the repetitions. When she felt ready, she spoke, her voice weak and halting. "May I call my attorney from here?"

The arresting officers looked uncomfortable at the suggestion that they deviate from the book. But knowing that their arrestee was a district attorney, they assumed that bending the rules would be allowed. "Sure."

Rebecca was unprepared for them to grant her request. She had no "attorney" in mind. She knew a few defense attorneys that she regarded highly. She knew far more whom she wouldn't trust with her car. But even those she thought honorable, she couldn't envision trusting with her life. There was only one attorney she wanted to call. He'd let her down once before, but he wouldn't do it again, she hoped. Unfortunately, he also happened to be a D.A.

"Give me the number," the policeman directed, and she gave him Tom Baldwin's home number. He held the phone to Rebecca's ear.

"Tom? It's Rebecca. I don't have long to talk. I'm being arrested and . . . wait, just listen, I'll explain everything to you later. They're taking me to—" She looked to the young officer for an answer. "Santa Monica station," he replied. "To the Santa Monica station for booking. Please meet me there. Okay?"

Tom, his head swimming in confusion, muttered,

"Okay," a simple word that meant the world to Rebecca.

She passed by nearly every occupant in the large condominium complex as she was escorted—in cuffs—to the patrol car. She was too stunned and shaken to feel embarrassed by the scene. Rebecca sat low in the back of the patrol car, feeling small and weak, like a child waiting in fearful anticipation for the promised punishment. She looked out the window at a world that seemed foreign to her now. When she was a little girl, she could conjure up a fantastic castle with high ivy-covered walls where she, the princess, could play safely inside, surrounded by an infinite moat that no evil could cross. She closed her eyes and tried to imagine herself back in the castle, but the walls turned to bars and the moat became a raging sea threatening to crash through and drown her.

24

Fingerprinting, first the right hand, next the left, slowly, each finger lifted, rolled in ink, and then rolled again on paper. When Rebecca had registered to take the bar exam, she'd been fingerprinted too. It was exciting then, another step toward a goal, not a sobering slap in the face identifying her as an accused criminal. Next the mug shot, one picture, head on, "look straight, please," flash. "Step this way, please." The pat down, a simple search for weapons or contraband. Quick, impersonal, expertly performed by a square-shouldered female officer. The clothes, now evidence. "Please put this on." No privacy now. Then the wait in a cramped, fetid holding cell. Rebecca tried to occupy as small a space in the cell as possible, avoiding eye contact with everyone and nervously awaiting Tom's arrival.

Rebecca struggled to stay calm, not to let her mind race off, not to let fear take root. Yet her pounding heart was an ever-present reminder of the real panic inside. She replayed last night over in her head, trying vainly to make sense of the confusing blur of images. She could still feel his hand over her mouth, his hot breath in her ear, and the sting of his hand against her cheek. She could still hear the sound of her gun exploding over and over, splattering blood everywhere, and the sound of her own voice screaming.

Rebecca was startled by the sound of the metal bars sliding open, signaling her time to leave the cell. She was led into the conference room by two large, female sheriff's deputies, who marched her wordlessly to a table for her meeting. Tom was already seated and waiting for her, looking confused and worried. The sight of Rebecca, shaken and haggard, disquieted him. In less than twelve hours she had aged a decade. He hoped his face wouldn't betray his shock at her appearance.

Rebecca sat down across from Tom and stretched her hands out to him, desperate for contact. He grasped her icy hands and stared into her panicked eyes. He knew she needed him to be strong for her, but was he up to the task? he wondered.

"What happened?" he asked with equal measures of compassion, fear, and bewilderment.

"All I can tell you now is that I've been arrested for murder. I'm not guilty. I didn't do anything wrong." She hesitated, fearful of the answer to her next question. "Tom, I need you to be my lawyer."

"Wait." He put his hand up. "Slow down. I don't even know what's going on."

"I want to tell you the whole story, but I can't unless you're my lawyer. Otherwise, it won't be privileged. You know that. So, will you do it?" Rebecca bit her lower lip, her heart pounding in her chest. She was afraid of Tom's answer, afraid what she'd do if he said no.

"I can't just represent you like that. I'm a D.A., for god's sake. I'm on the wrong side."

"But I don't have anyone else to turn to. I need you, Tom."

He ran his hand through his hair, trying to think, feeling totally off-kilter. He looked at the door. "I can't just quit like this. I've got to talk this over with Claire. I don't even know if I can represent you. I need time to think about this. Maybe you can get advice from someone else right now and in a few days—"

Rebecca leaned forward, looking squarely at Tom, forcing him to make eye contact. "I don't have a few days. I need you now, Tom. Please," she begged him, her voice trembling as she forced the word out.

"Rebecca, how can I make such a major decision on the spur of the moment?" Tom's eyes pleaded with her for understanding. "You've got to give me some time."

"Tom, I can't. You've got to decide right now, because if you're not going to represent me, I've got to stop talking to you. Look, if it's money you're worried about, I'll pay you. You and Claire won't starve. I'll sign over my condo, you can have my car and anything else I have. Whatever you need. I have a lot saved up and I'll borrow money from Elizabeth if you need more." She sounded desperate. Her eyes stayed fixed on Tom, tears welling.

"Oh, shit. Don't look at me like that." Tom felt backed into a decision he didn't want to make. He'd spent half his life avoiding making hard choices, not wanting to face the consequences of a wrong choice. The last big decision he'd made was to break it off with Rebecca and turn around and marry Claire, and he'd lived miserably with that mistake for years. And now she was pleading with him—no, demanding him—to make a life-altering decision in an instant. What did she expect of him? he wondered.

"Please, I'm begging you. I don't want to go

through this alone. You've got to help me. For old times' sake?" She laughed weakly, her eyes fearful, her words imploring. Tom felt the tug. Don't let her down. Not this time.

He ran his hand through his hair, then grabbed a handful and tugged, as if to make sure he was fully aware of this moment. Claire had been looking for a way out and this would sure give it to her, he thought. Funny, she'd always said he should leave the D.A.'s office and go make some real money. He just didn't think she had in mind him leaving it all behind to go defend Rebecca.

Tom sat quietly for several minutes, thinking, twisting his wedding ring absentmindedly. Finally, he looked directly at Rebecca, and with a determination that had eluded him for so long, spoke. "Okay. You've got yourself a lawyer." The words were almost a surprise to him. A welcome one. "But before you say anything, let me go to the phone and quit. I don't want to blow my first case by having a conflict of interest." Then, quietly, he added, "I guess I should also tell Claire."

"Thank you," Rebecca whispered. Tom smiled faintly—a poor excuse for a hug, but all that the surroundings would permit. He then rose from his seat, leaving Rebecca behind to wait. She felt relieved, as if all her problems had been erased with his decision to help her. From experience, she had learned to try to appreciate the small comforts that came her way. She tried not to think about the nightmare she was facing.

Tom returned several minutes later, heartened to notice that at least Rebecca appeared stronger. "Well, it's done. I called Campbell and gave him the news. The law offices of Thomas Baldwin are officially open for business. And you're my first and only client."

"What'd he say?"

"Not much. Something about how either I have a fool for a client or you have a fool for a lawyer. Forget about it. Now"—Tom paused to switch into his lawyer mode, which was what Rebecca needed most now—"tell me what's going on."

She began replaying the events of last night, her words spilling out. She hoped that in the telling, somehow it would all make some sense. As Rebecca spoke, Tom took notes and asked questions to fill in the gaps. "What exactly did this man say to you?"

"I don't remember now. It was something about my being on TV. Something like, 'nice speech you gave.' I know it doesn't sound threatening. But it was the way he said it. He sounded very angry and very drunk. He smelled like stale beer and he slurred his words."

"Did he have a gun?"

"I'm not sure. I guess he did, but I never saw one. He grabbed me from behind. He was so much bigger than me, there was nothing I could do. It all happened so fast, I didn't know what was going on. I just knew that he wanted to hurt me."

"Why?"

"I don't know. Something I said must have upset him and he was coming to teach me a lesson."

Tom held his hand up to stop her as he scribbled furiously. "Okay, let's focus on that for a minute. Did you feel like he was going to kill you?"

"I guess," she answered wearily. "What else was he going to do?"

"Well, you have to tell me. I can't make up an answer for you."

"I'm not asking you to make up something for me," Rebecca stated indignantly. "He grabbed me, slapped me, dragged me to his car, and was driving away with me in the backseat. What do you think he was going to do? Give me a lift home?" Her sarcasm was laden with grief and Tom realized he was upsetting his first client when he was supposed to be helping her. On-the-job training was never supposed to be like this, he lamented.

"I'm sorry. I'm not used to being on this side."

"This isn't exactly old hat for me either," she said evenly.

Tom took in a deep breath then blew it out loudly, rubbing his face with his hands. "Look, can I just make a blanket 'I'm sorry' to cover the rest of this discussion?" he offered. "Otherwise we're never going to get through it. I don't know the right thing to say, but I do know the right questions to ask, so just let me do that."

Rebecca knew he was right, and yet she also knew she needed to talk. "Okay, but I don't want to be prepped for a deposition. I just want to tell you what really happened. Just let me tell you about last night, 'cause right now it's not making much sense to me either."

"Okay, fine. Just remember, though, if you confess to me, I can't lie for you. Whatever you tell me today, you're stuck with it, understand?"

"I don't care. I didn't do anything wrong," Rebecca said, her voice stronger, almost indignant. "The guy kidnapped me and I fought back."

"Why were you carrying a gun in your purse?" Tom asked suddenly, too impatient for an answer to that nagging question to let her just tell her story. "A concealed weapon, for god's sake. It's illegal. It's not going to look good."

"I was worried about my safety," Rebecca said, her jaw tight.

"But why didn't you get it through channels? Why not petition for a permit?"

Rebecca shrugged him off. "I didn't get around to it."

Tom sighed. She wasn't going to make this easy. "How long have you had this gun?"

"I bought it about six months ago."

Six months, he jotted down, circling the words. Even with her workaholism that delay would be tough to explain. Tom noticed to his dismay that quite a few items were now circled on his notes. He continued gathering details. "Was there a struggle when he grabbed you? Do you have any bruises?"

"I'm not sure. I know he grabbed me hard." Rebecca pushed up her sleeves. Two small bluish marks were on the outside of her left forearm.

"Let me get a picture of that. That's great." Finally an item got underlined on his notes. He flipped the page of his legal pad. "Did you take a shower or bath after you came home last night?"

"No, I just passed out on the bed. I was just waking up, trying to sort out what happened, when the police arrived."

"Where are the clothes you were wearing last night?"

"They took them when I was booked. I was covered in blood. They're probably processing them for evidence."

"Maybe they're torn. We could sure use evidence of a struggle, proof that he grabbed you against your will. Let me think, what else could prove an abduction?" His mind raced. He tried to picture the struggle. Would she have scratched him or kicked him? He'd need pictures of the deceased for signs that she had fought him. "We should have your fingernails checked. I don't want to miss anything," he said anxiously. "You said he slapped you—where?"

"On my face." Rebecca automatically reached up to touch her cheek.

Tom frowned—he couldn't see any marks. "Maybe

the bruises will show up later." What else? He racked his brain.

"Tom," she said quietly. He looked up expectantly and saw desperation in her eyes. "You've got to get me out of here."

"I know." He gently squeezed her hand. "You haven't talked to the police yet, have you?"

"No, you're the first person I've told this to."

"So they don't know the whole story about last night?"

"No. I told you, I wanted to talk to you first."

Tom looked back at the door. "Hunh. Well, that explains their attitude."

Rebecca looked hopeful. "Maybe if I tell them everything . . ."

"Now you know better than that."

"I know. I know. But once they realize I was only acting in self-defense, that should change things, don't you think?"

Tom sighed and shook his head. "Yeah, maybe, but I would be crazy to let you do that. All my years of experience tell me an accused should never make a statement." He stopped, realizing for the first time that the person he was lecturing knew as much about the law as he did, maybe more. "Listen, I'm dead set against it, but you know the risks. If you think it will help, I'm willing to trust your instincts."

"It may be the only way. If I can just explain to them what happened, they'll see that this isn't a murder case. That I had no choice. That I didn't do anything wrong," Rebecca said slowly but emphatically. Tom could see how much she wanted to be believed and couldn't help but wonder if this was somehow related to her old issues. The ones he'd so studiously avoided in the past.

"Do you think you're up for it? You've obviously

been through a lot in the last few hours. I don't want you doing this if you're not thinking straight."

Rebecca looked around the cold gray walls of the conference room. "I'm more up to that than sitting in jail. Frankly, I'm not sure I could survive jail."

"Okay, I'll go set it up. I'll see if we can't get something out of it. But you have to promise me one thing. If at any point I say stop, you stop. All right?"

She nodded. "All right."

He got up to leave and she grabbed him by the arm. "Tom, I'm scared."

He patted her hand. "It'll be okay. You just hang in there." He hoped he sounded reassuring.

Rebecca got up and circled the table as she waited for his return. She tried not to think about anything, concentrating on the pattern of the phony tile squares on the floor, so that her mind wouldn't turn to the scariest "what if"—what if the police didn't believe her? When he returned, Rebecca thought she saw the glint of a smile.

"Okay. It's a done deal. You talk and they won't fight us on bail, for now, anyhow."

"Really? I'll be able to go home?" She sounded surprised and greatly relieved to have her wish granted.

"Now, I don't want you to get too excited. The vultures are circling. But this at least buys us a little time." Tom was quickly learning the ropes of being a defense attorney. Right now it meant getting his client whatever concessions he could from the police and keeping her hopes up.

25

After dropping Rebecca off at her place, Tom went back to the office to clean out his desk, reassign his cases, and exchange awkward good-byes with co-workers who would now become his opponents. It was such a surprisingly easy farewell that Tom couldn't help but wonder just how selfless his decision to represent Rebecca was.

He was more uncertain about what his return home would offer. Tom was a little surprised to find it empty. Leave it to Claire to choose this moment not to make a scene, he thought with tired amusement. As he walked into the kitchen, he noticed the note on the refrigerator. In hastily scrawled pencil it read: "Tom, I'm spending the week at my parents'. I've already spoken to an attorney and he says we can do a 'no fault' divorce. Sounds quick and painless, although I'd quarrel with the name. Please be out of the house by Sunday. Leave me your new address. Let's get this over with quickly. I'm sure you'll agree—it's what you've wanted for some time, after all. Claire."

It was a sad commentary on the marriage that Tom

felt only relief that it would be over quickly. He felt
more loss over cutting ties with the D.A.'s office. And
yet both decisions came too quickly, as if Rebecca
had provided him with the excuse he had wanted for
years. Having ended the two longest relationships he
had in one afternoon, Tom felt surprisingly unbur-
dened. He had no responsibility, no commitment
other than to help Rebecca through this mess.

As the night wore on, Rebecca sat in her living room
absentmindedly flipping channels on the TV, needing the noise to make her feel less alone. A mistake.
Her face stared back at her from a small box in the
upper corner of the screen as the talking head news
anchor broke the story. ". . . arrested early this morning on suspicion of murder in the killing last night of
a convicted child molester." She quickly shut off the
TV, hoping that with it the memory of the last day
could be shut off as well.

She sat in the darkened room and wondered if she
was the top story in the Bay Area too. Although she
had briefly filled Elizabeth in earlier, she worried that
her sister would be sitting up there fearing the worst,
so she decided to call her and allay her fears. As she
dialed, Rebecca was struck by the fact that she was
more worried about Elizabeth than herself. Old
habits die hard. "Hi, it's me."

"Oh, Rebecca. I was so worried when you didn't call
back." Elizabeth's palpable concern quickly bridged the
miles between them. "What's happening? Where are
you?"

Rebecca heard the panic in Elizabeth's voice and
tried to keep her voice modulated and her words cir-
cumscribed. "Home, for now. I'm sorry I didn't call
back sooner."

Elizabeth's words poured out in a flood of pent-up

emotion. A day of waiting and wondering had taken its toll. "You call to tell me you killed some guy who tried to abduct you and you're being arrested and then I don't hear from you again! I was worried to death. What's going on? Do you need me to fly down? I can get someone to handle my patients while I'm gone. I can leave any time."

Rebecca tucked her feet up under her as she curled into the corner of the sofa in the hope that she could find some comfort there. She reached up and turned on the lamp next to her, not needing the dark to accentuate her fear. "Why don't you wait? This might be over quickly, or it could go on for months," she said, trying to sound detached and professional. "I'll have a better idea of what's ahead after they complete their investigation, and that could last a few days or even longer. Don't mess up your work schedule yet. I may need a rich relative and I can't risk you losing money."

"Oh, Bec. I'm sorry, I wasn't even thinking. Do you need money? I mean for, you know . . ." She struggled not to say the wrong thing.

"Bail?" Rebecca said.

Elizabeth winced at the word. "Well, that, or an attorney. You're not going to represent yourself, are you?"

"No, of course not. I hired Tom." She said it offhandedly and then remembered Elizabeth's last comment on the subject of Tom—"if you want to remain friends with that creep, that's your problem." She had, up until now, diligently avoided mentioning his name.

"Tom Baldwin?" Elizabeth asked, her voice a mix of shock and rage.

Rebecca got up and walked into the kitchen. If there was going to be a fight, she at least needed a Coke to nurse. "Yeah," she said, a little chagrined.

"You're kidding? You're putting your future in his hands? As I recall, the last time you tried that, you got six years. Maybe this time he'll get you life."

Rebecca opened the can and gulped loudly into the phone. She didn't want to have this discussion. "Elizabeth, I know you don't want to hear this, but he really has been a good friend over the years. He was just a lousy boyfriend. Trust me, I know what I'm doing," she pleaded.

"Not where he's concerned, Rebecca," Elizabeth scolded. "I'm sorry, but your track record with him stinks. He's burned you before and you shouldn't give him the chance to do that again. This is much too important. I never understood how you could stay friends with a man who would take the best years of your life, string you along, and then dump you with not so much as an apology. You are a glutton for punishment. I can't believe you did this!"

"This is really not what I need to hear right now," Rebecca said, her voice cracking. "I need your support. I made a decision and, like it or not, this is how it has to be. You're not helping me by arguing about it."

"Fine," she snapped. Then, realizing Rebecca was right, Elizabeth's voice softened. "I'm not going to get into a fight with you about this. I just hope you're right. Look, if you need anything, money or whatever, let me know. Remember, I'm here for you."

Rebecca walked back to the couch, sitting down with her legs spread out across the cushions, and sighed, comforted by Elizabeth's words. "Thank you. That's what I needed to hear."

"So how are you holding up?" Elizabeth closed her eyes and shook her head. "I'm sorry, that's a stupid question. I just don't know what to say."

"No, it's okay. I'm doing fine, really."

"Why were you carrying a gun?" Elizabeth suddenly blurted out.

"Why is that everyone's favorite question?" Rebecca felt herself becoming defensive. "For protection, why else?" she retorted, her voice tinged with indignation at the question. "Don't you carry something—mace, pepper spray, anything?"

"No. I guess I should. I didn't think you were allowed to carry a gun."

"Well, I didn't think it was fair that the criminals could and I couldn't. I didn't want to be that vulnerable. It probably saved my life." Rebecca flipped the TV back on, switching to MTV, hoping for a soothing video. She wasn't disappointed. She saw Michael Stipe staring back at her telling her that even if it was the end of the world, he was apparently not too upset about it. She smiled at the message.

"I guess so," Elizabeth said. "So you are all right, aren't you? You weren't just trying to keep me from worrying?"

"I'm fine. Just a couple bruises," Rebecca said, shrugging it off, not wanting to burden Elizabeth with the terror she'd felt last night.

"Thank God. You must have been scared out of your mind."

"It all happened so fast."

"It seems so weird, you know? On the news they said he'd been a convicted child molester and that you'd prosecuted him. Like all those other guys who were killed. That's so strange, don't you think?"

Rebecca shrugged as she fumbled for an answer to Elizabeth's question. "It's not that strange. I've pissed off a lot of child molesters in my time. It's not all that surprising one came after me. It's part of the job."

"I guess. It just struck me as, I don't know, just strange. The timing, that is." Elizabeth trod carefully, keeping her doubts to herself and giving Rebecca what she needed—unconditional support. "Well, anyway, if you need anything, anything at all, just let me know. You can call me anytime, you got it?"

"I got it. You don't know how much I needed to hear that. I'm feeling pretty alone right now."

"You're not alone. I'm always there for you."

"I know."

After Elizabeth hung up the phone, doubts and questions nagged at her. The bizarre nature of all this overwhelmed her. Her sister, the defender of justice, representative of the people, was an accused criminal. She had been—no, she still was—so proud of her sister, following her conscience to right wrongs. Still, she had always questioned why Rebecca chose this line of work. Didn't it get to her, hearing the same stories over and over? Didn't it just bring back all those horrible memories? Did Rebecca see herself in the eyes of the little girls, telling frightening, horrific stories of how Daddy brutalized them? Why not just let the past lie? Why bring it back up over and over? Rebecca never had an answer that suited Elizabeth. Sure, there might be some small satisfaction from getting a conviction or sparing some child, Elizabeth thought, but by and large it seemed to be so frustrating for Rebecca. Maybe it had gotten to her, maybe . . .

The sound of the buzzer startled Rebecca. "Tom?" she asked with some trepidation. Earlier, when she had arrived home, a half dozen reporters were there waiting for her in the lobby, thrusting microphones in her face and asking her about the shooting. Apparently, the local media thought a district attorney arrested for killing anyone was newsworthy enough, even without having all of the facts in yet. She had hurried by them without a word, but worried this was one of them trying to get some comment before the evening news.

Instead, the voice on the end of the intercom turned out to be a familiar one.

"No. It's Jack. Can I see you?"

She stood there for a moment, her body resting against the wall, trying to summon what little remained in her depleted reservoir of strength. She wasn't ready to see Jack, not now, not the way things were. And yet, she needed him. She needed to find out if he was still there for her, all the while fearing that he couldn't be. With her voice faltering, Rebecca answered, "Yes," and buzzed him in.

She waited for him to knock then slowly opened the door. Jack stood looking at her for just a fleeting moment before pulling her to him and squeezing her tightly in his arms. The gesture unleashed a flood of tears in her. They stood, Jack holding her close as her waves of sobs swelled and then ebbed.

When Rebecca could find her voice, she looked up at him and started to speak. "I was afraid I'd never see you again. I thought you'd think . . ." She couldn't continue; she dropped her head as the tears returned.

Jack tilted her head up to his and smiled through his weary eyes. "My faith in you is one thing you don't have to worry about. Didn't you know? I'm a great judge of character. No one can fool me," he added, trying to lift her spirits. "I'm a cop, remember?"

Rebecca returned the smile. "How could I forget?" Taking him by the hand, she led him into the living room. Halfway there she stopped and looked up at him, her eyes full of concern—for Jack, not for her. "Wait, can't you get in trouble for being here?"

He deflected the question. "What happened to innocent until proven guilty?"

"I think that went out with Reaganomics. Now I think it's guilty if the media says so."

Jack grabbed Rebecca's other hand and held them both tightly, looking earnestly into her eyes, wanting her to believe him. "I heard all about your statement. It's the clearest case of self-defense I've ever seen."

"You think so?" Rebecca reacted as if Jack had said the tumor was benign. Her entire body seemed to relax, and she felt lighter than she had all day. Perhaps this would blow over quickly and become no more than an unfortunate memory that would fade over time. They walked back, hand in hand, to the living room and sat down on the couch. Rebecca's face turned grim once more as her hopefulness turned back to doubt. "I didn't get the feeling that Detective Henderson saw it that way. He sure acted like I was a criminal."

Jack knew Rebecca was reading Henderson correctly, but he also knew that ultimately it was the D.A. and not the investigating detective who made the final call about filing the case. "Don't worry about Henderson, he's got this bug up his ass about the child molester murders, some bullshit jealousy. I guess he thinks Jennifer and I pushed him and Gilmore out of the lead position or something. Playing hardball with you may be his way of getting even. What about the D.A.? What'd he say?"

"She, actually." Rebecca shrugged. "I couldn't get a read on her. She just sat there during the statement, let Henderson ask all the questions, and she just stared at me with this cynical look stuck on her face. I imagine it's the same look I have when I hear false claims of innocence." The lack of acceptance from her brethren clearly weighed on Rebecca. "I wish I understood her reaction. I've never even met her before. You'd have thought she'd see my side of it. I mean, what would she have done in my shoes?"

"She would have done the same thing. If she was smart enough to carry a gun, like you." Jack drew

Rebecca to him, her head resting on his chest. He gently stroked her hair, suddenly aware of how precious their time together was. "You know, when I first saw you had a gun, I was a little surprised. Now, I thank God you had it."

Rebecca pulled her head back and looked up at him. "You knew?"

He looked down at her, surprised. "Of course. You have a habit of ransacking your purse anytime you're looking for something."

Rebecca laughed nervously. "Oh, guess I wasn't as discreet as I thought."

Jack gave her a quick squeeze, wanting her to know how he felt, yet eternally tongue-tied when it came to speaking from the heart. "I wish you had called me when all this happened. Maybe there was something I could have done." His voice caught as a rare feeling of powerlessness came over him. "I just wish I'd been there." He paused, wanting to ask her about it, yet wanting her to choose when she was ready. "If you want to talk about it," he offered, "if you think it might help."

Rebecca closed her eyes as the memory of the events flooded back. "It all happened so fast, I didn't know what was going on. I just wanted to get away so bad—that's all I could think about. When I got home, I just shut the door behind me, hoping it was all a bad dream. But it was worse. I can't stop thinking about it. I keep replaying it over in my mind, wondering, why? What did he want?" Rebecca looked up at Jack, her eyes asking him to help her find the answers. "What could I have done differently?" Her questions hung in the air as Rebecca dropped her head back down in resignation.

Jack saw the tears welling and wanted to make them go away. "You did what you had to do to survive and that's all that matters. You're here with me and some creep who tried to kidnap you is dead. What's wrong with that? Nothing," he said firmly.

They sat there together, holding each other, as they had done a lifetime ago. "It won't do any good thinking about what you could have done differently. What's done is done," he said.

"I guess you're right. It's just . . ." Rebecca looked up at Jack and hesitated. "I killed someone. I did that. I can't forget that. No matter whether there was a good reason, everyone will look at me and know I was capable of taking another person's life. That will never go away. I'll have to live with that the rest of my life."

Jack wanted to shake her, to snap her out of her self-blame. He knew she did what she had to do, it was only her decency that made her question her decision. And yet he realized that he was one of those people who had thought her incapable of killing another person, and now he knew that to be wrong. But this was different, he told himself, then turned his attention to convincing Rebecca. "But at least you still have a life. If you didn't do what you did, you'd probably be dead now."

She heard his words, but couldn't accept them. "You don't know that for a fact," she said, her voice barely audible. "And neither do I. I can never be absolutely sure I did the right thing."

"Well, I'm sure."

Rebecca was drained and yet still managed a jaded laugh. "It's almost funny. If I had seen him grab a child, I would gladly have shot him. But because all I saved was myself, I'm not sure I had the right to do what I did," she said softly.

"You did the right thing. You're here with me and that's all that matters."

"You don't know how much it means to me to hear that right now." She leaned her head on his chest. "Just hold me and let me pretend everything's going to be all right."

Jack hugged her and kissed the top of her head. "You don't have to pretend. It will be. I promise."

As she sat there in Jack's arms, the adrenaline started to drain from her body, unmasking the exhaustion she felt from her ordeal. Within minutes she was asleep. Jack quietly carried her into her bedroom and tucked her in, then returned to the living room and worried himself to sleep on the couch.

26

Diane Covington sat at her desk, writing up her preliminary evaluation and recommendation in the Fielding matter. Something about Rebecca made her feel uneasy, but none of her suspicions had added up to much so far. She didn't understand why a D.A., who could very easily register a handgun, would have a loaded, unregistered one in her purse. She didn't understand how an athletic, young woman could be kidnapped by a drunk, unarmed man in a public parking lot without drawing any attention. And she didn't understand why the same woman would show virtually no physical signs of a struggle. Her instincts told her there was more to Rebecca than this incident, but so far she couldn't prove anything more than one count of manslaughter. At least, not yet.

Her secretary interrupted her concentration, telling her that a witness in the child molester murders was on the phone. When she heard who it was, she thought of blowing her off but decided to take the call. "Diane Covington."

"Miss Covington, this is Mildred Walker." Her thin

voice quivered on the phone, like a radio set between two stations. "Do you remember me?"

"Yes, of course I remember you." How could I forget, Covington thought to herself. You were a big disappointment, you old bag. Mrs. Walker was the neighbor of Harold Riddell who had seen a woman outside of his apartment shortly before he was murdered and had provided the police with the information for the artist's sketch. Covington had met the elderly woman the day before when she was brought in to look at a photo lineup to see if she could identify Rebecca as the woman she saw. But Mrs. Walker was unable to make a positive identification, saying only "I'm just not sure" when pressed. Covington had smiled understandingly, thanked her for her time, and waved a pleasant good-bye, then cursed the woman all the way back to her office. "What can I do for you, Mrs. Walker?"

"I just saw something on TV I thought I should tell you about."

"And what was that?" Covington started checking her report for typos.

"I saw the woman I'd seen before the murder. The one outside Mr. Riddell's apartment."

Covington put the report down. "Where did you see her?"

"I was watching the morning news and they showed this girl, they said she'd shot someone and was being questioned about that. I wrote down her name. Oh, where is that? Here it is, I found it. Rebecca Fielding. Does that help?"

Covington stifled a sarcastic "No, what D.A. wants an eyewitness I.D.?" and struggled to maintain a sugary demeanor, speaking slowly and softly. This was potentially too big to blow by being cantankerous. "Now, Mrs. Walker, when you came in to look at the pictures that we showed you, one of them was Ms.

Fielding. But you weren't able to identify her." No matter how long I pointed at her picture, Covington thought. "What changed?"

Mrs. Walker picked up the remote and turned the sound down on her TV. That did little to help the noise level, since the set in her bedroom was still blaring away while the radio blasted from the kitchen. "You know, I had a hunch at the time, but it's so hard to tell when you're just looking at a picture, and I didn't want to say anything if I wasn't absolutely sure. On TV they showed her moving around. They had a closeup on her face, too. That's when I was sure it was the young lady I'd seen before."

Pretty good. A witness who rehabilitates herself, Covington thought happily. Too bad this conversation wasn't taped. Covington hastily scribbled notes to document Mrs. Walker's words, although she knew that her notes would be of little value if the woman was unable to deliver on the witness stand, so she took a breath and tested her witness. "Now you're absolutely sure she's the woman you saw outside Mr. Riddell's apartment the night of his murder?"

"As sure as I can be."

"And you'd be willing to swear to that under oath, in court?"

Ms. Walker hesitated for a moment and Covington's heart stopped, waiting for her answer. "I suppose so," she said finally. "I've never been in court before. I'd be a little scared . . ."

"Oh, don't you worry," Covington said quickly, trying to endear herself. "I'll help you get ready, so it won't seem as scary. All you'll have to do is talk about seeing the woman, giving the police the description, and then recognizing her on TV. But it's very easy, because I ask you questions, and then you answer them. So there's nothing to memorize, it's just like we're having a conversation. But you don't have to think about that now, we'll have plenty of time to talk about it before you testify."

"Well, I suppose I should do whatever I can to help. But she seems like such a nice lady."

"Looks can be deceiving, Mrs. Walker. Very deceiving," Covington said, hoping she could convince Mrs. Walker—knowing this was the very problem she faced with the jury.

"What a shame. The poor girl must have been off her trolley."

"Well, that's certainly one way to describe her." Covington could barely contain her delight. "Anyway, you'll be contacted shortly by an investigator from my office. As we get closer to trial, I'll call you. But if you have any questions before then, please feel free to call me. Oh, and by the way, if Ms. Fielding's attorney calls you, be sure to tell him what you saw, just like you told me." As she replaced the receiver, Covington shook a clenched fist with an exuberant "Yes!" Gotcha.

Rebecca had just stepped out of the shower, a half hour of peaceful surrender to the warmth and comfort of the steamy water. One benefit of living in a condo was unlimited hot water. Jack had left for work hours ago and Tom was spending his afternoon scrounging for an office, so the pounding on her door could only mean trouble. Rebecca quickly threw on her robe and went to see who was there.

"Ms. Fielding?" boomed a familiar voice.

"Yes."

"Detective Henderson."

"Uh-huh," Rebecca said slowly. Yesterday he had sat across a table from her as she tried to explain what happened. But she felt that he was scoffing at her claims of innocence, implicitly accusing her of lying and worse. Tom said she was reading too much into Henderson's reaction. After all, if he didn't believe her, why would he allow her to be released?

"I'm here to execute a search warrant."

"For what?" Rebecca demanded before realizing he didn't have to satisfy her curiosity. "Look, I just stepped out of the shower. Could I have a moment to dress?"

Henderson doubted she could rappel down the side of the building, so he permitted this small accommodation. When she returned to open the door he handed her the warrant, then stepped in accompanied by three uniformed officers. The scope of the warrant took her by surprise. It authorized the seizure of items that constituted evidence concerning the killings of Eric Penhall, William Matheson, Bradley Knight, Steven Jaffe, Harold Riddell, and James Hempstead. Rebecca knew what that meant.

"You bastard! You were just snowing us, weren't you? You weren't interested at all in what I had to say about Hempstead. You already made up your mind. Well, I'm not letting you search until my attorney gets here," Rebecca spat out, her panic growing.

Henderson pointed to the search warrant, wondering why he had to explain the procedure to—of all people—a member of the D.A.'s office. "That's not what this little piece of paper says, Counselor," he said, his voice dripping with contempt. It made the frozen smile all the more unnerving.

Henderson directed the search, sending the officers to different rooms to seize the sought-after evidence. Rebecca frantically called each of Tom's numbers, finally reaching him on his car phone. Although he was halfway across town, it seemed he would have an easier time keeping his promise to be there before she knew it than he'd had keeping his earlier promise—that this would all blow over in no time.

When he arrived, Tom bolted into Rebecca's condo, demanding to know what was going on. One of the officers unceremoniously pointed him in the direction of a towering figure in a dark, double-breasted suit and colorful African-print tie. The face, in permanent scowl, must intimidate many hardened gangbangers, Tom thought, but he was too angry to be scared.

"What the fuck is this?" he yelled as he pointed to the searching officers.

"Now, is that any way to start a conversation?" Henderson asked with a smile.

"Listen, asshole, if you want to keep that badge, you'll tell me right now what the hell is going on here! My client has just been through a nightmare—kidnapped and assaulted, then arrested. We get everything cleared up and then I find you here trashing her place?"

Henderson moved closer until he was looming over Tom. "First of all, I don't know who told you that things were 'cleared up.' They're not. Second of all, I'm executing a search warrant, what does it look like? And third, don't ever think of calling me asshole again."

Tom ignored the clear physical disparity and refused to back up. "You heard her statement. She killed Hempstead in self-defense."

"Yes, it was a very moving statement. So harrowing. And just imagine how lucky she was to have that gun with her. That unregistered, illegal gun, with those nasty illegal hollow-nosed bullets. Now if you'll excuse me, I've got work to do." Henderson turned his back on Tom without giving him the chance to think of anything to say on Rebecca's behalf.

Tom watched one detective after another cart off what they considered to be incriminating evidence— a navy blue jacket, two books on serial killers, a half-empty box of bullets, a knife, and newspaper clippings of the murders. It was bad enough that they had convinced some judge to give them a warrant, Tom thought, but now they seemed to be finding what they were looking for. That realization troubled him, and his mind struggled to lock on a reasonable explanation.

The officers left without a word, which was fine with Tom, since he was too unsettled by what was going on to have anything meaningful to say. He remained in the living room feeling staggered and confused, like he'd just gone a few rounds with Mike Tyson. It took him a few minutes to regain his focus and realize that he had completely forgotten about Rebecca. When he found her, she was sitting quietly in her kitchen, as if she were oblivious to what was going on. She seemed so small, so fragile in an oversized white sweater and black leggings with tears staining her face.

"It's amazing what jerks cops can be when they're on the other side," Tom fumed as he leaned against the doorway.

"They're just doing their job," Rebecca offered, not really knowing what to say. She got up wearily and walked over to the sink and started loading up her dishwasher with everything the police had touched in the kitchen. She stood rinsing and stacking dishes mechanically, her mind trying to tune out everything else.

"Oh, great. Save me the Joan of Arc nobility. These people are trying to eat you alive. The least you can do is call them names." Tom started pacing as she tried to rid her kitchen of any trace of the police. He stopped and looked in Rebecca's direction.

"From now on, it's hardball all the way. We don't talk to anyone and we don't volunteer anything, and that includes Jack."

Rebecca lowered her head, Tom's words adding another layer to her loss. "Sure. The first man to believe in me, and now I have to stay away from him." She looked at Tom and saw that she had hurt him. "Sorry, I didn't mean it the way it came out. I don't know what I mean." Rebecca wiped away some tears with the sleeve of her sweater.

"No, it's all right," Tom said, walking over to pat her on the back. "Maybe you shouldn't listen to me when it comes to him. I wasn't that thrilled with you dating him in the first place. I guess I was jealous."

"Well, I suppose it doesn't matter now. Nothing does," she said with a heavy sigh. Tom saw her as too quick to give up, too easily falling into despair. She focused on the dishes, losing herself in the menial task.

Tom moved his arm around Rebecca's shoulder and gave her a gentle squeeze. "Please. Don't start talking like that. I can't have you falling apart right now."

She looked up at him, her face flushed with fear. "But, they think I did it. They think I killed all those guys, don't they?" She looked into his eyes, begging him for answers. "How did this happen? I thought everything was taken care of. I told them what happened. Why didn't they believe me?"

Tom looked away. "We don't know anything yet, so don't jump to conclusions."

"Please. Just be honest with me. This is serious. I'm in real trouble, aren't I?"

The phone saved him from having to admit that she was right. Rebecca grabbed the receiver with an irrational eagerness that had her hoping it was someone calling to apologize for the terrible mistake.

"Rebecca?" It was her secretary, Joan. She sounded flustered, her usual professional demeanor shaken. "There are all these policemen in your office. They showed me a warrant to search it. I wouldn't have let them in if they hadn't—you know that."

"Of course, Joan. It's all right. There's nothing we can do to stop them." Rebecca picked up a sponge and started to scrub the counter.

"But they're turning it upside down, they're going in all your files and drawers." Joan looked back at the officers, worried that they might think that she was aiding the enemy. She lowered her voice. "It just doesn't seem right. I wish there was something I could do to help you. And I don't believe what they're saying about you, I want you to know that. I'm sure this is all a huge mistake." Joan was someone forever locked in a time warp when loyalty and devotion were part of the job description.

"I'll be fine. Tom Baldwin's representing me." Did Rebecca imagine a gasp, or was Joan genuinely shocked? "I'll have him go down there to see what's left of my office. I'm just not in the mood to do that now."

"I understand." Joan's voice faded into sadness and then suddenly grew angry. "Listen—Ralph Simpson is strutting around the office like he owns the place, telling everyone how he knew it was you all along. I overheard him telling someone that he had been helping the police. I don't trust him."

"Don't worry about Ralph, he's an idiot. Anyone can see that." Rebecca hoped she was right. "Joan, you're a sweetheart. You have no idea how much your support means to me."

"I just pray everything will be all right."

"Me, too. I'll talk to you later." She hung up, dropped the sponge, and turned to Tom. "Well, they're not wasting any time. They're searching my office."

"There's nothing really there that can hurt you, right?" Tom asked, looking for reassurance.

"I don't think so. The only thing there besides my work files are the personal files I keep on the defendants. I suppose they might try to twist that into something sinister. I can't think of anything else."

"What kind of files are these?" Tom asked. He had a bad feeling that he was about to hear something that he really didn't want to hear.

Rebecca walked toward the living room to start straightening up the mess the police left there. Tom followed, waiting for her answer. "Just records on the defendants I've prosecuted," she said offhandedly. "You know, their court files and then my personal notes about them."

"Do these personal notes contain anything damaging? Anything we need to worry about?"

"Like, 'die, you shithead'?" Rebecca forced out a weak laugh. She knew she'd never make it through this if she forgot how to do that. "No, just my summary of their offenses, their trials, their probationary experiences, that sort of thing." She paused and looked a little uncomfortable. "And reports from some private eyes I hired to check into some of the guys." She saw the look of shock in Tom's eyes.

"You're kidding me. I've never known anybody to keep files like that. What were you doing?" And why didn't you tell me this before? Tom thought, furious. He was starting to lose his cool and he didn't mind if it showed. Lawyers hate surprises, especially coming from their client. Especially when their client is another lawyer who should know better.

Rebecca felt Tom's anger and raised her own voice defensively. "I felt more comfortable keeping records on my defendants. It kept me from having to just sit around and wonder what they were up to."

"Like a backup probation officer?" he asked, trying out this spin on it.

"Well, yes. But it was really more for my own comfort level. I just wanted to know what they were up to." Rebecca sat down on the couch she had just rearranged. She was tired and couldn't muster enough energy to defend herself. She did what she thought was right and never thought it could possibly be used against her.

Tom wasn't convinced yet that there were reasonable explanations for any of this, and he wasn't about to rest until he found some answers that satisfied him. "Look, will you be all right by yourself for a few hours? I need to find out what they seized out of your office. I want to know what's going on right now."

"Sure," Rebecca lied. She wasn't all right. She was scared, confused, and felt very alone. She didn't want him to leave. She was afraid to be by herself, but she didn't want to burden him right now. She needed him for the bigger battle to come. As he reached the door, she called after him, "Tom?" He stopped and turned, watching her as she seemed to go through an internal struggle about whether to say something or not. "Never mind," she said finally.

Tom walked out, afraid to find out what she wanted to say, still unprepared to deal with her truth.

27

Tom's new office was decorated like an executive suite compared to his old early-yard-sale digs at the D.A.'s office. The walls were dark wood paneling, the carpet a beige Berber, and all the chairs matched. He even had a nice view of palm trees out his eighth-floor window. He had the choice of working at his large, oak desk or at the small table in the corner and, if he scheduled the time in advance, could use the community conference room. But there were no waves or hellos as people passed by his office, and the only familiar faces were defense attorneys who just a week ago he'd considered the enemy. Yet Tom knew this was no time for recriminations—he'd made a choice, and he'd have to live with it.

He sat, trying to figure out what the police were up to and how he could counteract their attack, when his thoughts were interrupted by the shrill sound of the phone. He instinctively waited for his secretary to tell him who it was until he remembered that he was his secretary. "Tom Baldwin."

"Mr. Baldwin, this is Diane Covington. I'm returning your call about the Fielding matter."

"What the hell does your office think it's doing—"

"Whoa there, big boy. First of all, let's get something straight from the outset. You don't yell at me, and I won't yell at you. If you can't live by those rules, then we will only communicate in writing from here on out. Do you understand?"

So much for macho posturing. In less than thirty seconds, Covington had chewed him up and spit him out, and Tom knew it. He stifled a "fuck you" for Rebecca's sake, knowing that a few more of these calls and he'd be mainlining Maalox. "That's fine. But as you might imagine, neither my client nor I are in any mood for game playing."

"And what game am I playing?" Her voice—even and detached—further irked him.

Tom tried not to let Covington get to him, but his mounting frustration was easy to tweak. He didn't like his new role as a defense attorney and was already convinced he'd made the second biggest mistake in his life agreeing to take Rebecca's case. As a prosecutor he had called all the shots and was never caught off guard, but now it seemed that everything was happening beyond his control.

He doubted Covington would confuse his bluster for real power, but right now it was all he had, so he kept his voice loud and forceful. "You guys have served search warrants everywhere, and not just for the Hempstead murder. You've searched my client's house and her office for evidence concerning all of the child molester killings. What the hell is going on? She has absolutely nothing to do with those killings. She was arrested in a self-defense shooting of a man who happened to be a two eighty-eight felon and suddenly your office decides to come after her for all the child molester murders. Your office is invading my client's privacy and harassing her for no good purpose."

Covington grinned broadly. She lived for calls like this. "Please stop using the phrase 'your office.' It sounds so odd coming from you. Don't forget, until a couple of days ago, you were one of us."

Tom thought Covington's reputation as the mega-bitch from hell was both well deserved and a bit of an underestimation. "I was never one of you. I would never have put an innocent woman through this kind of harassment."

"Mr. Baldwin, I'm much too busy for this." Covington used the imperious voice she saved for ranting defense attorneys. Tweaking them was part of the fun of her job. It made up for the low pay and long hours. "Did you call for a reason?"

"I want access to the murder book."

"As soon as it's completed, you'll get it. We are still compiling and cataloging the evidence."

"When do you think that will be done?" Tom tried to keep his voice level. He stood up and started to pace his office and noticed his new office had a lot more space for nervous wandering.

"It's difficult to say, now that additional charges have been filed."

"What additional charges?"

Covington paused, savoring the moment. Too bad it wasn't a face-to-face, she thought. This would be worth watching. "We just filed murder-one charges against your client for the other five murders. We are seeking to consolidate these cases with the Hempstead case and intend to go forward with all six."

Tom stopped dead in his tracks. "Are you people out of your mind?" Tom's voice boomed. "Do you know what you are doing?"

Covington remained icily unaffected. "I think the

better question is what was your client doing? I'm
not sure you are going to like the answer."

Tom scoffed. "Right, like you have any evidence."

"Well, we'll make all that available to you at the
arraignment. Suffice to say that we have more than
enough to tie your client to each murder. As you
might imagine, Mr. Baldwin, this will change our
position on bail. I'm sorry."

Tom struggled to speak and leaned against the
windowsill. "I doubt you are," was all he could force
out of his tightened throat. His head was swimming.
He walked back to his desk and fumbled in his briefcase for an aspirin, knowing his problem was probably immune to medication. Why would the police
move this fast unless they had discovered something
big? He quickly realized that he was falling victim to
the where-there's-smoke-there's-fire mentality. And
he recognized that he was having trouble seeing
things like a defense attorney. For his and Rebecca's
sake, he knew he had better learn how to shift gears.
But then, after fifteen years as a prosecutor, it was
still hard for him to shake the belief that most defendants are guilty as sin.

Tom spoke firmly, keeping his doubts out of this
conversation. "Ms. Covington, I can't believe that
you're going to try to fabricate a connection between
the Hempstead case and the others. You know they
are totally unrelated. I'm sure you're under a lot of
pressure to get a conviction on those other cases, but
you're making a big mistake if you think you can get
beyond the prelim with this bullshit. My client is innocent and I can't believe that you're willing to sacrifice
her reputation because your office is in some great
rush to judgment. You can't possibly believe that she
committed those murders. I intend to hold you and
everyone else in the chain of command personally
responsible for this gross miscarriage of justice."

"Mr. Baldwin, please, save it for the jury. You do what you have to do and I'll do what I have to do. Now, if that's all, I have work to do." Covington hung up, getting in the final shot and irritating Tom further by depriving him of someone to vent his frustration on. He stood for a moment with the dead receiver in his hand before slowly sitting back down.

As soon as Tom hung up a copy of the new complaint was faxed to him. Even though it was expected, it nevertheless jolted him. What started out as a simple case of self-defense had become part of the most notorious serial killer case to hit Los Angeles in a long time—one already long a topic of the evening news, radio talk shows, and local tabloid TV, now likely to heat up even further with the addition of an attractive female suspect who some would say was simply doing God's work. Tom's goal in the case suddenly changed from keeping Rebecca out of jail to keeping her out of the gas chamber. He grabbed his jacket and slowly headed for the door to deliver the news in person.

The ride to Rebecca's was unfortunately too short for him to think of a gentle way to tell her about the additional charges. He was unprepared to see her, even more so to find her looking so eager and optimistic. He had seen this look before, when she was a brand-new attorney, brimming with excitement over what lay ahead. Her innocence and hope enchanted him back then. Today, it evoked only pity.

"Tom, I've been doing some thinking," Rebecca said as she let him in. "I'm not going to do myself or you any good if I just sit here feeling sorry for myself. If I'm going to get through this I just can't go to pieces every time something bad happens. I've got to stay strong. What did Yogi Berra say? It ain't over till it's over. It's going to be a long tough road, but everything's going to be okay. Right? I'm innocent, and that will ultimately come out."

Tom said nothing at first, knowing the damage his words would do. He walked slowly over to her kitchen table and motioned for her to join him. He took off his jacket and draped it over a chair, taking the opportunity to delay the inevitable. He was suddenly sorry he hadn't taken the coward's way out and told her about the additional charges by phone. It seemed as if he'd made a career out of hurting her, and out of always being there to see the hurt in those eyes. "Rebecca," he started softly. "They filed five additional charges against you. They're charging you with all of the child molester murders."

She silently absorbed his words, closing her eyes and taking deep breaths. She tried to remain placid, but Tom wasn't fooled. He knew what to look for. When she opened her eyes, he saw that they were now red-rimmed and brimming with tears. Exactly as they had when long ago he told her they were through. "This is all happening so fast," she said, her voice cracking.

"I know." He reached over and squeezed her hand.

"I must be the most naive, the dumbest . . ." She could barely get the words out between wrenching sobs. "I—I thought this would just . . . blow over, that if I told them the truth, they would believe me. I'm such an idiot!"

He walked over and put his arm around her, feeling her body shake. When her crying settled to a rhythmic murmur, he spoke. "We'll get through this. You've got to be strong."

Rebecca looked at him, confused. "Why me? Why is this happening? It's like a bad dream that just keeps getting worse and I can't seem to wake up. Why are they coming after me? What did I ever do?" Her words came out choked between sobs.

Tom didn't have any answers—at least none that

would help her. He sat back down across from Rebecca and took her hand. "I just wish I could understand why the D.A.'s office is pushing this so fast. Why are they so sure?" He dismissed the thought that it was a simple case of politics, though he knew too well that decisions were sometimes made with an eye toward votes and funding rather than justice. Yet he couldn't find an explanation for the D.A.'s office gunning for one of its own, except of course the obvious explanation.

Rebecca pulled her hand back and looked away. "I don't know," she said, disconcerted. She heard an accusation buried in his question but ignored it. She wasn't about to explain anything to him. She said she wasn't involved and that should be enough. It was his duty as her lawyer and her friend to believe her.

Tom sat for a minute mulling the recent events around in his head. "This may in an odd way work to our advantage," Tom said hesitantly. "You know, their proceeding on all six."

"Why? Because after they execute me for the first killing, you can brag that you kept them from executing me for the other five?" Rebecca snapped.

"I'll ignore that. I know that you're upset."

Rebecca's eyes narrowed as her fragile pain turned to anger. "Don't be so damned condescending. You have no idea how 'upset' I am." Tom steeled himself as she lashed out, her voice raised. "They're charging me with murder—six counts of murder. How can you just sit there like nothing's happening?"

"Do you want me to help you or not?" He didn't wait for a reply, fearing the answer. "We can work on your case or we can fight. I think our time would be better spent working. What do you think?"

Rebecca's face softened. The wall came halfway down. "You're right," she said gently.

Tom laid his hands out on the table. "Okay. Now, the reason I'm not troubled by the additional charges is simple. I think that by trying to prove too much, the D.A. runs the risk of cheapening the credibility of its entire case."

"How's that?" she asked, brushing away a tear.

"As I see it, with Hempstead, all they have to prove is that your explanation is bullshit. You admitted killing him. So the prosecution only has to impeach you on the self-defense claim. And since so far no one's come forward to say they saw him grab you, and since he had no weapon, the prosecution has a decent shot at a conviction on that case. But unless the prosecution can prove the other five, they weaken their Hempstead case. So we can get an acquittal on all the charges, rather than risk a conviction on just one."

Rebecca looked lost. She was in no position to argue the finer points of legal theory. "I just can't imagine how this can be good news. All the behind-the-back gossiping at the office, all the whispers about me—even Jack's partner suspected I was involved in the murders. And now, they've all been proven true. Everyone I know's going to go on TV to say how they suspected me all along. No matter what you say, this isn't good."

Tom sat back and loosened his tie and unbuttoned his collar. "I'm not so sure. If they had evidence against you for the other five, they would have had you arrested and your place searched before. You gave them the only evidence they have when you shot Hempstead. Aside from him, they have nothing on you except their suspicions, and that's not enough. I told the D.A. she's in another rush to judgment, but I don't think she appreciated my use of the phrase. But I think it sure fits."

"I hope you're right." Rebecca rubbed her hands

along both cheeks, wiping away the last tears. She felt drained and yet agitated at the same time and got up suddenly. She looked back down at Tom. "You want some coffee? I need to do something."

"Sure. Thanks."

Rebecca walked over to the kitchen and grabbed a bag of coffee out of the refrigerator. She headed for the coffeemaker, taking time with each step to focus on the mechanics—putting in the filter, scooping out the coffee, checking the water level—and keeping her thoughts away from the case. "Let's talk about something else for a minute, before I lose my mind."

"Like what?"

"I don't know, anything. I need to take a break from all this."

The shift seemed odd to Tom. "Okay." He watched Rebecca take the milk out and put it on the counter, next to the sugar bowl and two mugs and tried to come up with something to say, but he could think of nothing but the case and how he was going to handle it.

Rebecca leaned back on the counter. She'd thought of another topic. "So how did Claire handle the news of your first case as a defense attorney?"

Tom snorted. "Really well, for her. She left me a note at the apartment saying I have till the weekend to move out and that she wants a divorce." He reported the incident without expression, both his face and voice betraying no emotion. "If she really wanted me to suffer, she'd make me stay and listen to her bitch for the next twenty years about how I ruined her life. So, I guess I'm getting off easy. I knew she was looking for a way out. She just needed to find a way to put all the blame on me. I guess I was happy to oblige."

Rebecca's eyes filled with compassion and sadness. "I'm so sorry. I guess asking you to be my attorney was pretty selfish of me. I knew this was going to cause problems, but I couldn't see past the fact that I needed you. I couldn't imagine going through this with anyone else. But I didn't mean to screw up your life."

Tom stopped her. "Don't. It's okay." He stared at the stream slowly filling up the coffee pot. "At least I was lucky—we never had kids. Hell, we don't even have a set of matching bath towels. It'll be quick and simple, like pulling out a splinter. Really, it's the best thing that could have happened." Tom found the bag of Milano cookies Rebecca always kept tucked out of sight and brought it to the table. "You know, it's a little bit like the man who gets a congratulatory call from his attorney on his twenty-fifth wedding anniversary. He tells the attorney that he's the last person he wanted to hear from. When the attorney asks why, the man asks him if he remembers that on his fifth anniversary he called the attorney saying he wanted to kill his wife. 'You told me not to do it because I'd get twenty years in jail.' When the attorney says he remembers that call, the man screams at him, 'Well, I'd be getting out today.'"

Rebecca almost managed a laugh. "Well, I still feel bad."

"Don't. Right now, all I want to figure out is how to keep you out of jail. The arraignment is set for tomorrow at nine. We'll see what Covington's position will be on bail. I'll try to keep you out at least until after the prelim. But, be prepared for the worst."

"You know me . . . I always am."

A corner table in a dark restaurant. Cliché, but then so was their relationship, Valerie thought. "So what are we celebrating?" Valerie asked as she raised her glass to meet Hillerman's.

Hillerman took a small sip, followed immediately by a more serious emptying of his glass. "My dear, we are celebrating an absolutely glorious week. What else?" He poured himself another glass and watched the deep red wine swirl. "Ms. Fielding arrested on suspicion of murder. You know what that means? Our troubles are over. She's going down."

"What do you mean?" Valerie took a sip, then put her glass back down, wanting not to seem uncooperative, yet not feeling wholly comfortable with the celebration.

Hillerman picked his glass back up and held it in front of his face, as if studying its contents. "Oh, don't you see? Here she has been on this crusade against us, thinking she has all the answers and we don't have a clue. And now we'll be able to turn the tables. All those pencil-pushing bureaucrats who took her seriously are going to have to distance themselves from her so fast it'll make their pin-sized heads spin. It is going to be rather difficult now for them to criticize us. We should be getting more referrals than ever. We may even sail through accreditation now."

"What if they don't tie her to the other killings?"

He looked at Valerie through the glass. "Oh, they will, trust me. They will."

"How can you be so sure?"

Hillerman put his wine down and picked up the menu. "Years of experience, my dear, years of experience." He signaled the waiter, whose job that night was to be immediately available at all times. Hillerman quickly scanned the menu, ordered for them both, then thrust the menu at the waiter with a snap of his wrist and leaned forward, looking deep into Valerie's eyes. She expected a gentle whisper, but it turned out to be more of a hardened hiss. "All I want is a front row seat to her execution. How appropriate—

the executioner gets executed." Hillerman amused even himself. "Do you think there will be popcorn?"

Valerie cleared her throat. "That's a little harsh, don't you think?"

Hillerman stared at Valerie as he took another gulp of wine. He kept his tone light. "It's not like I'm suggesting that we bring Raisinets or anything like that. Besides, they would melt when they throw the switch. Better make it M&M's." He threw his head back as he laughed, spilling a little red wine on the tablecloth.

"I don't think that's very funny," Valerie said as she reached across to blot the small stain.

"Oh, please. For the last six months I've been jumping through hoops because of that woman's campaign to put me out of business. She deserves everything she's getting. I'm trying to run an honest business, provide a valuable service to the community, and all I get from her is a nonstop effort to malign both me and the work we do here. Now, you can understand why I've grown a little weary of the battle, can't you? So now it's time to enjoy the fruits. You can't blame me for that." He lowered his head slightly, looking innocent and helpless.

Valerie fiddled with her still-full glass. "No, it's just I feel a little sorry for her. That's all."

Hillerman looked past Valerie as he spoke, his eyes scanning the room, taking in at a quick glance the other women in the restaurant. "You know, it's one thing to feel empathy for your patients. You're paid to do that. But leave it at the office, sweetheart." He turned his gaze back to Valerie and smiled, his eyes gleaming in the light. He leaned over and patted her hand, looking at her as if she were the only woman in the room. "Let's not ruin the night. The way I see it, her arrest is actually going to save us quite a bit of money. I won't have to give Stan every penny I have to fight her anymore. That's why I can afford to take you out to a nice restaurant. So, see, it does no good feeling sorry for her. What goes around comes around, as they say."

Valerie looked away, a little uncomfortably. "I suppose," she said.

Hillerman picked up the bottle. "C'mon, drink up. There's no shortage of wine tonight." He topped off her glass.

Valerie sipped gingerly. She had learned not to try to pace him. His thirst for alcohol seemed interminable. "There never is."

He frowned. "Now, that was uncalled for. Good thing I'm too happy to be upset." He stopped to ponder for a moment. "You know, I've dreamed of shutting her up, but I never imagined it would work out so well."

28

As the news media's pool camera whirred into action, Judge Jaramillo looked up with a touch of sadness after his clerk read the next matter on this morning's arraignment calendar. Before his recent transfer downtown, he'd been on the bench in Van Nuys Superior Court and had the opportunity to preside over quite a few matters prosecuted by Rebecca Fielding. He fondly recalled having Rebecca in his court, an able, dedicated, and impassioned representative of the People. He remembered her intense commitment to the law and to the victims she represented. How distressing to have her standing on that side of the table.

Jaramillo spoke with just a trace of his East Los Angeles roots in his melodious voice. "Rebecca Ann Fielding, you have been accused of the crime of murder. It is my duty to advise you as to certain of your constitutional rights." He continued for one minute, ten seconds, by Rebecca's count of the clicks on the court's clock. ". . . Do you understand your rights as I have outlined them for you?"

"Yes," she answered, her voice deceptively strong.

"Are you represented by counsel?"

Tom spoke. "Ms. Fielding is represented by Thomas Xavier Baldwin, your honor."

Judge Jaramillo raised an eyebrow. Things were indeed upside down today. "Very well. You may arraign the defendant," he said as he nodded his head toward Covington.

Covington reached down and grabbed a stapled document and leaned across the counsel table to hand it to Tom. Then she asked, "Rebecca Ann Fielding, is that your true name?"

"Yes," Rebecca replied.

Covington continued. "Ms. Fielding, I have handed your attorney a copy of the complaint filed against you, case no. W573224. You are charged in this complaint with six counts of murder, to wit . . ." Rebecca stood dazed, the words from Covington too painful to hear. She concentrated on keeping her knees locked and her body steady, hoping when it was her turn to speak her voice wouldn't fail her. "Ms. Fielding, do you understand the charges as I have read them to you?"

"Yes," Rebecca answered solemnly. She felt herself weakening and gripped the counsel table for support.

"And have you discussed those charges with your lawyer?"

"Yes."

"At this time do you wish to enter a plea of guilty or not guilty?"

"Not guilty." Rebecca would not let her voice waver, speaking clearly and forcefully as she always did in court—knowing her plea would be the sound bite for the evening news.

The routine completed, Judge Jaramillo resumed. "Let's set a date for the pretrial conference and for the trial." He gave the attorneys dates that seemed amazingly soon to Tom, but a lifetime away for Rebecca. She wanted this nightmare over now. Setting the dates only reinforced how this wasn't going away.

After reviewing their calendars, both attorneys signaled that the dates were acceptable.

"Very well. And what about bail?" Judge Jaramillo asked. He took off his reading glasses and looked out at the counsel table. "With six murder charges pending, would I be correct in assuming that bail is not an option?"

"Yes, most definitely, Your Honor," Covington stated, eager to see Rebecca squirm.

Tom knew it was coming but was still stung by the lack of hesitation shown by Covington. He rose, knowing that he had an enormously difficult task—convincing the judge to ignore the law. "Your Honor, this is absurd." He paused for effect. "If Ms. Fielding were going to flee, she would already have done so—after we were notified that the additional charges were going to be filed. In no way does she pose a flight risk. There is simply no reason to believe that Ms. Fielding, who has served the People of the State of California so honorably for so many years, will not be here for every aspect of this case. Her whole life has been about participating in the criminal justice system. It is a system for which she has great respect and trust. She will be here because she believes she will be exonerated."

Covington's turn at bat. One fat one, right across the plate. Nothing to sweat. "Your Honor, Mr. Baldwin's argument ignores one crucial, dispositive point. Ms. Fielding has been charged with six capital crimes. Under the law, she is not entitled to bail regardless of her flight risk. Her so-called stellar career as a D.A. is simply of no consequence. However, even if it were, we must remember that the defendant knows the judicial system inside and out. Who better to exploit its weaknesses, and who better to know when and how to run? Furthermore, the defendant has no family in Los Angeles, no personal ties whatsoever. This simply is not a case suitable for bail."

Tom knew that Covington was right, but that was not going to stop him from making a record for the press, who were taking down every word being said. "I daresay there's never been a case like this one, where the district attorney's office decided to offer up one of its own as a sacrificial lamb on the altar of public opinion. I know of no precedent for a case where a top district attorney is being charged with multiple murders on the flimsiest of purported evidence. The public clamor for more convictions must not drown out our obligation to protect the rights of the accused and to proceed in a rational and fair manner. The law does not require idle acts. And absent a flight risk, denial of bail in this case would be an idle act. This is grossly unfair."

A voice came from the back of the courtroom. "Your Honor, may I speak?"

Judge Jaramillo looked up, surprised. "And who are you?"

"Detective Jack Larson." Jack approached the front of the court, stopping just short of the podium. "Up until yesterday, I was in charge of the investigation into the child molester murders." Covington glared back at him, her arms crossed defiantly in front of her. "Can I say something, Your Honor?" he asked.

"Well, now, Detective Larson, the People are capably represented by Ms. Covington. What possibly could you add?"

"I wanted to speak out on behalf of the defendant, Your Honor." A hush penetrated the courtroom like a layer of fog. "I will personally guarantee the defendant's appearance at any further proceedings." Jack looked at Rebecca. "She is not a flight risk. She is an honorable person, wrongly accused of a terrible crime. But she will stand to fight the charges and clear her name." He then turned toward Covington, meeting her gaze and absorbing the daggers she sent his way. "The People have nothing to worry about, except the embarrassment of proceeding against an innocent woman."

"Well, Detective, I must say that in all my years on the bench, this is certainly the first time this has ever happened. I appreciate your comments and your sincerity. However"—Judge Jaramillo paused to choose his words carefully—"while the defendant is well known to this court and has had a long employment relationship with the district attorney's office, I nevertheless have to say that I agree with the prosecution. This simply is not a bailable offense, Detective, regardless of how well known the defendant is or how long her record of service with the county. In my court, justice is blind and all defendants are treated the same. Therefore, as the statute mandates, the defendant will be denied bail and remanded to custody. I think that is all for now. Anything else, Counsel?"

The only thing the attorneys could agree on was that they had nothing more for the judge. In unison they said, "No, Your Honor," and were sent on their way.

Tom turned to say something comforting to Rebecca, but knew his words seldom worked that way. "I'm sorry. I'll come see you after Covington shows me what she's got."

Jack approached Rebecca and mumbled, "I tried," from the railing behind the counsel table. Rebecca mouthed, "I know." Jack heard the sound of the handcuffs snapping into place and saw Rebecca shiver slightly from the cold steel. He stood immobile as she was taken away, a panicked look crossing her face. He absorbed her terror like a blow to the heart. Rebecca felt herself being pulled out of the real world, to be taken to the very place she had championed for others. She tried to speak but her voice wouldn't oblige. Her eyes conveyed what she couldn't say. Tom could do nothing but watch as she was led away.

As Jack stood reeling, Covington came over. "Nice speech, Detective. But then, you've always been a sweet talker, haven't you? Or don't you remember me?"

Jack had been stunned when he first learned who the prosecutor would be but had kept it to himself. Now he feared that his own indiscretion was giving Covington an extra motivation for going after Rebecca. "No, I remember you. But this isn't about you or me. If you have some gripe with me, don't take it out on Rebecca."

"Oh, please, don't flatter yourself," Covington said. "I'm not taking anything out on Ms. Fielding. I'm just trying to seek justice. You remember that, don't you, Detective? That's when people get what's coming to them. And it's my job to make sure that happens here. Now, if you'll be so kind." She hurried past him for her statement to the press. Even watching him twisting uncomfortably wasn't worth missing a photo opportunity.

The leather clothing shops, body piercing boutiques, and men walking hand in hand were something out of the ordinary for Larson, but then West Hollywood is no ordinary town—it's the self-proclaimed homosexual capital of the world. Had Larson been in a better mood, he might have found the scenery amusing. But he had a job to do, and Frank was as good a starting point as any. Larson scanned the mailboxes, half-expecting to see the residents listed as Mr. & Mr., until he found Frank's name. Larson went upstairs, located 204, and knocked on the door, the cheap, weathered plywood giving with each rap.

"Who do you think that could be, Cleo?" Frank whispered as he opened the door just wide enough to pull the chain taut. He peered through the crack. "Well, I'll be dipped in shit. Detective Larson, what a surprise. Oh, calm down, Cleo, it's okay, it's a friend of ours. Hang on." Frank picked up the nervously purring calico mix and swung open the door. "I hope you don't mind. I was just getting dressed and I haven't put on my face yet."

"That's quite all right." Even a hardened cop like Larson was still startled to find Frank in a too short pair of cutoffs and a halter top.

"C'mon in. I won't bite, unless you're lucky," Frank teased as he led Larson in. "Here, come, come sit on the couch. Would you like something to drink, maybe some iced tea? It's homemade and fab-u-lous." He flashed his best smile.

"Sure, thanks, Frank—it's okay if I call you that?" Larson looked around the small apartment, expecting feathered boas and red velvet curtains. Instead, he was surprised by the tastefully furnished living room with a blue damask sofa behind an oblong metal-framed glass coffee table, on top of a handsome Oriental rug. He sat on the couch and adopted as relaxed a pose as he could muster under the circumstances.

Frank stood pouting for a moment, before mumbling a hurt "I suppose" as he made his way into the kitchen. He returned with a tray of tea and cookies, almost as if he and the girls were about to set off on an afternoon of gossiping. "I guess I was wrong about Hillerman. Oh, well. You can't be right all the time, I suppose." Frank sat down with some effort, pulling on his shorts and adjusting his top. "So why are you here if you arrested the killer?" Frank leaned forward and grabbed a cookie.

"Because I don't think the killer has been arrested." Larson watched Frank for a reaction. "Yet," he added.

Frank stopped in midbite and dropped his cookie. "I—uh—I don't get it," he finally managed to say. "I thought you were the lead detective."

"I am."

"Oh," Frank said, looking down at the cookie in his lap. He picked it up and brushed away the crumbs. "Look at the mess I made."

Frank leaned forward, filled his glass almost full of iced tea, and took a leisurely sip. Larson didn't know what to make of Frank's demeanor. Since the microscopic testing on the blonde wig had been inconclusive, he still didn't know if Frank was a suspect, a font of useful information, or just a lonely guy who wanted to stir up trouble. Yet he had nowhere else to turn. "So why don't you tell me your theory about Hillerman again. It just doesn't seem to fit."

Frank let out a sigh. "Honey, believe me, it fits," he protested.

Larson wasn't used to being called "Honey" by a man, but if it would help free Rebecca, he'd let Frank kiss him. "Why would he kill his patients? I don't get it."

"It's so obvious." Frank crossed his legs, bouncing his pink pumps under Larson's nose. He noticed that Larson was staring at them. "You like?"

"What's not to like? They're perfect on you," he said, a little too sarcastically.

"Ouch. Meow to you, too."

Larson let it pass, since he wasn't entirely sure what it meant. "So, tell me again why you think Hillerman's so obviously the one."

"Because look who's been killed so far. Looooosers," Frank sang.

"Yeah, so?"

"What can't Hillerman afford to turn out on a regular basis?" Frank waited like a game show host for the contestant's answer. When Larson didn't play

along, Frank answered his own question. "Losers."
He beamed, pleased with his insight, then turned
serious. "Why the glazed eyes? Where'd I lose you?"

"You told me that before. I still don't see it. Why
would that mean shit to Hillerman?" Or to you, for
that matter, thought Larson.

"Because," Frank sighed, exasperated. He shook his
head, then blew a few random strands of hair off his
face. "You don't get it. I'll spell it out for you. Twenty
years ago the libs said treat, don't punish, bless their
bleeding hearts. But now the pendulum has swung
back. Now they want proof this stuff works, or all of us
are headed for the steel resort. So they look at Oakwood
and they say, fine, you're the biggest, you want to stay in
business, then you're going to have to prove how successful you are. If you do, you get a big ol' stamp of
approval, and the money'll keep flowing in. But, if you
don't, you're out of business. Well, Hillerman just
about had an aneurysm when he was denied accreditation last year. It could mean the end of Oakwood."

"What are you talking about?" This was news to
Larson, who had heard rumors of Oakwood's problems but never anything so specific before.

"I'm not supposed to know about this, but since
you were too lazy to do your homework . . ." Frank
leaned forward and lowered his voice. "All right,
there was this big to-do, all these white shirts coming
by to check things out. Hillerman was a gas, strutting
around there like a peacock in heat. Then, instead of
accreditation, he gets slapped with probation. How's
that for a kick in the ass? I got a copy of the letter.
Don't ask me how, but I did. He had one year to get
his act together or adios."

Larson thought for a moment about what Frank
was saying. "So he kills the losers, and all that
remains is the winners. Hillerman gets his accreditation, and everyone else lives happily ever after."

"Right. Now you've got it." Frank raised his glass in a toast and Larson smiled awkwardly in response.

"Do you still have this letter?" Larson asked.

"What would you give me for it?" Frank smiled.

"Frank," Larson began, exasperated, "I don't buy evidence. We're talking about murder here and about an innocent woman behind bars while the real killer goes free. If you have something on Hillerman, it's your civic duty to give it to me."

"Here, here," Frank said as he clapped his hands. "What a noble speech."

"I guess I could also beat the crap out of you," Larson said, only half-jokingly.

"Oh, don't have a cow, big boy. Sit here, I'll be right back."

Larson sat uncomfortably, not quite sure what Frank had in mind.

Frank returned with a piece of paper in his hands. "It's lucky for you I like you. Here"—Frank dramatically flung it at Larson—"this is for you. But, please, you must keep my name out of this. I still have to go back to Oakwood and I don't want Hillerman on my butt. You and I know what it could mean if Hillerman doesn't like you." Frank dragged his index finger across his neck.

Larson read the letter, fairly damning in its curt rebuke of Oakwood. "This is pretty hot. Hillerman sure doesn't act like someone with his feet to the fire."

"Don't let him fool you. Hillerman hides many things."

"Like what?"

"Like the fact that he's porking Valerie."

Larson recoiled slightly, the picture in his mind too nauseating. "You're kidding. He's old enough to be her father."

Frank winked. "You know how those father-daughter relationships can be."

29

With the preliminary hearing less than two weeks away, Tom was getting his first look at the evidence the prosecution intended to present to convince the judge to hold Rebecca over for trial. Covington strode into the conference room, oozing an arrogance typically reserved for the victory party. She theatrically dropped a box containing file folders on the conference table, and stood back, arms crossed, looking decidedly imperious.

Tom looked up, unimpressed. "And just what do you want me to do with that?" he asked belligerently. He resented the show.

"You can do whatever you want, but I'd suggest that you read them. I think you'll find them very interesting," said Covington, a smug look on her face. It irritated Tom how certain Covington seemed about her case, and it worried him that perhaps her confidence was justified.

"Let's, as they say, cut to the chase. Leaving aside Hempstead, how are you intending to tie Rebecca to the other murders?" he asked.

"All right, Mr. Baldwin, let me lay it out for you." Covington sat down, leaning forward, arms on the table, only too happy to oblige. Tom took a seat across the table from her, and reclined in his chair.

Covington smiled confidently and began. "Motive, of course, is the easiest. Each of the deceased represented a major loss for your client, one that affected her personally and professionally. Her obsessive hatred was obvious from the detailed files she maintained. As you will see, your client kept better records on these men than the IRS does on tax shelters." She paused, wanting each bit of evidence to sink in. "Her records include their home addresses and phone numbers, their work numbers, notes from conversations with their probation officers and therapists, the names, addresses and phone numbers of the women they dated, requests to the DMV for information on them, calls to local police departments to confirm they registered, much more data than I or any other D.A. I know ever keeps on a defendant." Tom's reaction showed he could be included in that list, she noted with pleasure. She continued, speaking slowly, for maximum impact. "And this goes for each of the deceased, with information on them updated virtually to the day of their deaths."

Covington leveled her gaze and was pleased to note the slight furrowing of Tom's brow. "Just to show you I'm not tap-dancing here, your client has an entry in her calendar that shows Eric Penhall's change of residence, two weeks before he was killed. Why, over four years after he was prosecuted, would your client need to know that he'd moved?" It was obvious from her self-satisfied expression that she thought she knew the answer. "We have notes of her phone calls with Matheson's therapist about his poor progress in therapy, including her final note to herself:

'How can they let this guy off probation?' I guess she found a way around that," Covington said disdainfully.

Tom rocked slightly in his chair, trying to maintain an air of disinterest. "This is all fascinating. You've established that my client is passionate about her work. What a news flash. Where's your evidence, Counselor? Where's your case?"

"You want the details? Fine." Covington was not impressed by Tom's swagger and was ready to begin her onslaught. "We have a match on the fibers of her blue suit jackets and fibers found on the front door to Matheson's apartment, fibers apparently left there by your client as she pushed open the door to the apartment. We also have long, blonde hairs that were found at Matheson's that are similar to your client's. And, finally," she added, leaning forward for added effect, "two pieces of the puzzle that together will nail your client. We have a partial palm print found on the door jamb to Matheson's apartment that they previously had been unable to identify. It was left there by Ms. Fielding. And we have Mr. Riddell's neighbor, Mrs. Walker, who positively identified your client as being seen just outside of his apartment the night he was killed." She sat back and looked for a reaction and thought she saw a chink in Tom's armor. She bore in.

"You want more?" she continued. "You know we don't need any more than that, but I have plenty more." As she spoke she ticked off each item on her fingers. "In the case of Knight, we have more hair, which has already been established as matching the hairs found at Matheson's. And we have in her date book a notation of Mr. Knight's standing appointment at the acupuncturist. You have to ask yourself, why did she have that?" Her voice filled with condemnation. "Steve Jaffe lived in such a remote area even his probation officer was unable to locate him, and yet your client had not just his address but the directions to his house in her files." Covington's self-satisfied smile spoke volumes, and none of them good for Rebecca.

Tom called on his years of playing hold-'em and tried to maintain a fairly nonchalant expression. When she had finished, he looked down at the files, then back up at her, his face brimming with incredulity. "That's it?" he asked in feigned amazement as he started laughing. "You've got to be kidding! What you've told me shouldn't have been enough to get a search warrant, let alone a criminal complaint. I'm stunned some judge signed off on this. What you're telling me is the killer has blonde hair and may look something like my client, and may have similar common clothing items in her wardrobe. That's your case?" He looked disgusted. "You have no case. This is all bullshit. My client is being rail-roaded so that the police department and D.A.'s office can deflect criticism that they haven't taken these cases seriously. And when she is exonerated later, you can chalk that up to our flawed criminal justice system. You'll blame the jury for being too stupid to understand the evidence. She'll be ruined to save the reputation of the department." Tom stared at Covington, who refused to flinch. "Can you live with that?"

Covington spoke softly. "Mr. Baldwin, you are going to have to live with the fact that your client is a murderer. I believe you will have the tougher time of the two of us." She leaned forward again, her voice becoming harder. "Your client has some serious problems. She has disgraced this office and you should be as disgusted as I am."

It was obvious the conversation was over, although the fight had just begun. Despite his bluster,

Tom left the meeting shaken—by what he'd heard and by what he'd seen. He hoped it hadn't shown, but he left with more questions—and doubts—than answers. What were Rebecca's prints doing at Matheson's? Everything else could be explained away. Eyewitnesses don't have perfect recollection. Fibers are no guarantee; they are often common enough to point to a number of people. Many people share the same hair type. But why had Rebecca been at Matheson's apartment? And why hadn't she mentioned it to him?

As he rounded the last corner and reached the top of the hill, Tom was stunned by the grotesque nature of the situation. He was visiting Rebecca in jail. A stranger scenario was difficult to imagine. Or was it? He ushered the doubting thoughts out of his mind with a quick shake of the head—they would serve no useful purpose here. His substitute thoughts, however, were no more comforting. A sick feeling came over him at the thought of Rebecca living in such a shatteringly cold and lonely place. But Tom didn't fully appreciate how harrowing the desolation of jail was for someone like Rebecca for whom solitude brought no peace, only the intrusion of brutal memories.

He walked to the guard's station, his eyes straining up to the gray sky, hoping that inspiration was buried somewhere within the clouds. The women's jail was deceptively pleasant-looking from the outside, a small grassy area off to the right and freshly painted exterior giving the impression more of a community college. But the thin barbed wire curling around the tops of the fences and buildings brought reality back into focus. He wondered whether he'd ever be able to escort Rebecca through the gate to freedom, or whether this would become her permanent reality.

Once beyond the perimeter gate, he was led into the attorney conference room, where he stood waiting for Rebecca, still hoping for the inspiration that would help him find a way to tell her of his meeting with Covington while at the same time not unduly alarming her. A fine line indeed. Unfortunately, Rebecca arrived long before the inspiration. The sight of her in prison garb was a jolt. He closed his eyes for just a second, but long enough for her to sense his shock. She saw herself reflected in Tom's momentary revulsion, and it scared her.

He sat down, slowly laid his briefcase on the desk in front of him, and looked over at Rebecca, not sure what to do. As a D.A. he'd had few opportunities to come to jail as a visitor and the protocol seemed to elude him. After an uncomfortable pause, he picked up the telephone, and when Rebecca put her phone to her ear, he began. "I'm sorry it took so long. Are you okay?" he asked, knowing it was a stupid question as it left his lips.

"Tom, you've got to talk to the judge again." Rebecca's voice was crackling and brittle. "There has to be a way," she pleaded.

He was angry with her for asking him to do the one thing he had no power to do. Something she knew he couldn't control. "I'll try, but I don't think I'll have any luck. You know the judge's hands are tied. But we can keep pushing the case along—no delays, no continuances. The sooner this is all over the better, right?"

She looked down sadly. "Unless we lose, in which case, it doesn't really matter when things happen."

He tried to meet her gaze, to connect with her—to force her not to let doubt and fear take over. "No, you can't think that way. I've got some time to poke plenty of holes in what she's got. We're not going to lose," he insisted, belying his doubts.

"I want to trust you, but they've already been able to convince the judge they had enough to hold me over. The district attorney thinks I'm guilty, the public thinks I'm guilty—how're we going to turn that around? No one wants to listen to me. I've told the truth and no one hears me." Rebecca looked up into the bright, fluorescent lights and shook her head, dejected.

Tom worried that she was slipping away, falling into an abyss of despair. He needed her to stay strong; this was not a battle he could win alone. "I hear you, and what we need to do now is make twelve other people hear you. In the meantime, what can I do to make this easier for you? Is your cell okay? Do you want to move? What do you need?"

"I need to go home." The words came rushing out in a torrent of tears that took Tom by surprise. Rebecca dropped the phone and sat sobbing, her head resting on her arms. Tom watched the movement of her trembling shoulders, first rapid as her crying began then slowing down as her tears subsided. When she was ready, she picked the phone back up. "I'm sorry," she whispered.

"No, I'm sorry, Rebecca. I wish I could do more. I'm doing the best I can."

"I know." Rebecca wiped away the tears on her reddened face. "So did you meet with Covington?"

"Yeah, earlier today. What a bitch."

Rebecca bit her lower lip nervously. "What does she have?"

Tom thought it best to soft-pedal the evidence to Rebecca. "Not too much. Mostly it's circumstantial evidence."

Rebecca managed a weak smile. "Tom, look who you're talking to. Most evidence is circumstantial."

"I know, I know." He paused, trying to find something to say that would comfort her. "Well, I've been watching the news and I'll tell you, you've got a lot of popular support. Most people didn't even want the police to catch the killer and now they want the D.A. to set you free. You'd be amazed how much backing you have from a lot of different groups. It's got to be driving the D.A.'s office crazy. First they're criticized for not successfully prosecuting murder cases, now they have their next big high-profile case and they're being criticized for prosecuting it at all. The public thinks the child molesters got what they deserved and you're their hero."

Rebecca's face turned hard. "Don't you understand? They support me because they think I did it. All this public support you're talking about is for the killer, not for me." She looked at Tom curiously. "I'm not their hero, their hero is the real killer. I'm not Ellie Nessler, I'm no hero. She shot the man who molested her son—I didn't shoot those men. Why would I be comforted knowing everyone thinks I'm guilty before the trial, even before the prelim? What chance do I have to prove my innocence if the deck is stacked against me from the start?"

Tom looked flustered. "I—I didn't mean it that way. I just thought . . . well, it's better to be popular than not. It's better than if the public was against you. Don't you think?"

"No, I don't. It's better if everyone believes that I didn't do it. It's better if the D.A.'s case is weak. It's better if the police catch the real killer. That's what'll help. Not for me to be the poster woman for punishing child molesters." Rebecca recognized Tom's reluctance to discuss her case directly and took it as a sign things were not good. Yet she wanted to hear it from him. "So tell me what evidence they have, 'cause that's the only thing that really counts."

Tom took a deep breath. "Okay. Here's what we're facing for the prelim. We gave them Hempstead and they're building their whole case about the similarities between him and the other victims. There are a few pieces of evidence that they're using to tie you to the other killings—primarily the fact that you and the killer apparently look pretty similar. They recovered some long blonde hairs at the scene of both Matheson's and Knight's murders, which they claim match yours, and they have an eyewitness who saw someone who looks like you at the scene of the Riddell murder. And then they have your personal files on these guys, which aren't terribly helpful to our cause."

"And, of course, they will have no trouble establishing motive," Rebecca offered.

"And boy, don't they know it. But motive isn't enough. A lot of people had a reason to kill these guys. Frankly, I can't see a jury believing that simply because someone prosecutes child molesters for a living they would turn around and kill them. They're going to have to show more. But I have to tell you, motive wouldn't be such a problem if you hadn't been so public about hating these guys."

"So I should have organized a 'take a pedophile to lunch' program, then I wouldn't be in trouble now? I see, so it's all my fault," Rebecca said, her voice raised to the point that the guards took notice and the talking couple in the next cubicle shushed her. "I wish we could have some privacy."

"I know." Tom looked over to see if the guard wrote down anything or called a supervisor. It didn't appear so. "Now, listen, I'm not going to let you twist my words around just so you can get mad at me. All I said was that you practically handed them motive on a silver platter. I'm sorry if that upsets you, but it's something we're going to have to deal with."

"Well, what was I supposed to do, lie and pretend I wasn't angry these animals walked?" she asked in a raspy stage whisper. "Just throw up my hands and say, 'Oh well, that's how the system works'? How can anyone with a conscience ever get used to such injustice? Children's lives are destroyed and the best the justice system can do is tell the offender 'Don't do it again or next time we'll punish you'? Of course it upset me and I tried to change things. But, that doesn't make me a killer."

"No," Tom conceded, "but when your job is to prosecute these men, I guess the feeling is that you should get used to the way things are. It's not healthy to get angry when the system doesn't operate the way you want it to. If I had gotten upset every time a jury handed down an irrational verdict or every time a judge gave a sentence that seemed too light, I'd have an ulcer the size of Montana. Most of us learn to roll with the punches and not to take it so personally."

Rebecca clenched the receiver tightly. "Well, I guess I was a failure then at that as well, because I never learned how to just shrug it off and accept that sometimes the system really stinks."

"We can all agree that things should be different. But what I'm faced with now is making sure the jury doesn't think that you decided to change things at the end of a gun. And it forces us to explain why you kept such detailed files on the men you prosecuted, especially those who turned up dead." He paused, measuring his words. Yet he couldn't hold back what he was thinking. "Rebecca, even I was amazed when I read those files. I've never known anyone else in the office who kept tabs on their defendants after the case was over. What were you thinking?"

How could Rebecca possibly explain herself? She did what she did because she thought it was the right thing to do at the time and gave no thought to how it might look. Only now that she was an accused killer did her acts of diligence take on a sinister appearance.

"Tom, I don't need you getting mad at me now. You're supposed to be on my side." Her voice cracked and she closed her eyes.

Tom held the phone firm in his hand. "I am on your side, and don't ever worry about that."

She nodded a tenuous acceptance. "I'm sorry."

"Don't apologize. Just remember, I'm more than your lawyer. I'm your friend. I may question some things that you have done, but you are going to get the best defense anyone can give you."

"Thanks. I think that's good. Unless you mean that no one can win this case," Rebecca said with a weak smile.

"Well, at least you haven't lost your sense of humor. You'll need it. We have a lot more bad evidence to deal with."

"Like what?"

Tom leaned forward to whisper—a meaningless gesture he realized when he looked over at the phone in his hand. "Like your prints at Matheson's apartment. How did they get there?" His voice betrayed his frustration.

Rebecca paused, taken aback by Tom's accusatory posture. "I just went there to check up on him."

"So you really went there?" He tried to hide his shock, but his eyes brimmed with disbelief.

"Yes."

"When?"

"A little while before he was killed."

Tom slammed his hand on the desk and the guard practically jumped out of his seat. Tom waved him off with a weak "sorry." "This is the craziest thing I ever heard, a prosecutor out visiting a former defendant," he snapped.

"I don't think so," Rebecca said defensively. "I wasn't visiting him, I was just following up on some things I'd heard, checking to see if he was violating probation. I don't see what's so sinister about that."

Tom reluctantly let the matter drop. It was too late for debates, he'd just have to deal with the evidence as it stacked up. He tapped his pen nervously as he prepared to broach a new topic. He figured the conversation couldn't get much worse at this point. He fumbled for his words. "Rebecca, I—uh—was wondering something. What do you think about getting an evaluation before trial? You know, a psychological evaluation." He looked hesitantly at Rebecca, nervous about what he suggested, nervous about her response.

She returned the glance, hurt by the insinuation. "What am I supposed to say now? 'Sure, let some shrink psychoanalyze me, let's just open up my entire life for everyone to trample through. I want my innermost thoughts to be headline news'? No, I'm not going to agree to that. I am perfectly sane."

"Even if it means the difference between life and death?"

"That's right!" She looked at him, unyielding in her convictions.

"But, with your history . . ." Tom groped for the right way to say this. "It would not be inconceivable for your work to have gotten to you. It might be something you're not even fully aware of. Maybe we should have you see someone, just to explore this."

Rebecca dropped the phone and got up suddenly, forgetting she had nowhere to go. She sat back down slowly and picked up the phone. "No. No examination. I'm perfectly aware of my 'history' and it's not a problem. I'm not going to fabricate some defense just to make it easier on you."

"I'm not suggesting that." He was feeling the heat.

"That's not why I brought it up. I'm just doing my job. You know, representing you to the best of my ability. Any attorney you hired would have said the same thing to you. If you killed the others, we can use your . . ." He struggled for the words. Rebecca's eyes narrowed in pique and he wanted to avoid her ire. ". . . what happened with you and your father, you know, to plead temporary insanity. I don't want you jumping down my throat, I just want you to hear what I have to say," he pleaded. "It's my job to give you the best defense I can. I want to make sure I'm doing just that."

"Tom," she started, fighting to keep her voice level. "I am not going to claim to have done something just because it opens up a good defense. I didn't kill the others. And I'm not going to bring up the past to make myself a sympathetic accused. I've seen that game played before and I'm not going to be part of it. I don't want sympathy and I don't want the support of millions. I've told you what I know and you're just going to have to work with that. But if you try to play games with me, you'll regret it. Do not put me on the stand and then ask me about my 'history.' It's not relevant and I'm not going to discuss it."

"You may not, but if the D.A. gets ahold of it, she's damn well going to raise it, and not sympathetically—I can promise you that. But you're the client. You call the shots." His irritation with her was plain to see. "All right, let's drop it."

"No, I'm not going to drop it. My 'history,' as you call it, is no one's damned business. I never wanted anyone to think that I had any psychological axe to grind, because I didn't."

Tom leaned forward, the phone clutched so tightly his knuckles went white. He needed to ask the question that hung unasked in their discussions. "Then why did you choose to prosecute them? Why did you choose to practice in that arena, having to be exposed to that every day? Wasn't it hard for you?"

"No . . . At least not when I won. In those cases, I felt powerful, like . . . superwoman. I was able to make those creeps pay for what they did. I gave the children the rest of their lives. I helped bring about justice." She knew she couldn't make Tom understand—he'd never looked into the face of what scared him the most. But she had. And that's what had kept her going. "It's a pretty heady feeling." Rebecca sat for a moment, turning somber as she reflected on the other feelings—when you stared into evil, and evil won. She knew it was Tom's unenviable job to convince a jury that those feelings didn't turn her into a killer.

"But what about when the creeps didn't pay. What then?"

She chose not to take the question head on. "I'm not this poor loser that they're painting me to be who turns into a homicidal maniac just 'cause a couple cases don't go her way. Even when I lost a case, I knew that I had still done some good. I was able to be there for the victim, to let them know that I believed in them and that I knew it wasn't their fault. I know that for me it would have helped knowing someone, especially some grown-up, was out there who cared about me, who believed me, who wanted to help me. The feeling of isolation, that it would never end, that no one cared, was almost worse than the abuse itself."

Tom sat there looking helplessly at Rebecca. "I never know what to say at times like this."

Rebecca was touched by Tom's willingness to even talk about the subject with her and the genuine look of sadness in his eyes. "You don't have to say anything. What you'll never know is that what I need most is just to be heard. That's what hurts as much as the abuse, not being able to tell anyone. Or finding the courage to tell and having no one believe you. That's why I don't want to make up a defense. It's important for me to tell the truth and be believed. Almost more important than getting out of here."

Larson had just made it inside the doors of the Oakwood when the gray skies finally sent the promised rain. He was glad the weather was finally starting to change for the worse. The bright sun had seemed like a cruel joke. Finally he had a day that fit his mood, one not likely to improve after his meeting with Hillerman.

Hillerman was more jovial and welcoming than in the past, actually greeting him with a hearty handshake. "Well, well, Detective Larson, I'm certainly surprised to see you here. I thought the case was closed. Isn't the vigilante D.A. safely behind bars? You haven't let her escape, have you?" Hillerman ran straight through the stop sign painted on Larson's face. "My clients were just starting to sleep well at night again."

"I find it hard to believe after what they did to get sent here, your clients ever get a good night's sleep. I would have assumed they'd be haunted day and night with the knowledge of what slime they are." Hillerman's face sagged, Larson's bluntness reviving their conflict. "But that's not what I'm here to talk about, Dr. Hillerman."

"Oh? Well do enlighten me, Detective," Hillerman said insolently. "To what may I attribute this return engagement? And where is your spunky little sidekick?"

Larson deflected mention of Randazzo, taking his seat without looking over at what would have been her chair. The loss of his partner was still too difficult to consider. "My investigation continues until there is a verdict. Now, there is still some information that you owe us, and your attorneys have been fighting us tooth and nail. That makes me wonder, you know what I'm saying?"

Hillerman had expected this would be a pleasant meeting, now that the police considered the killer caught, but he was quickly realizing he was wrong. "Detective, you obviously do not understand the position I am in. It's not that I don't want to give you the information. I simply have to protect the privacy of my staff and that of the patients. Perhaps you should be talking with my attorney."

Larson's eyes narrowed and he sat forward, a sudden move that caused Hillerman to recoil. "And perhaps you should tell me just what you're hiding, Hillerman. I'm sick and tired of being jerked around by you. I want to know where your therapists come from, their references, what you know about them. I want their work schedules, their vacations, their daily logs. I want not just the sanitized reports about your patients, but all your notes. Especially about Frank LaPaca. I asked you for his file weeks ago and what have I received? Nothing. Why is that?"

Hillerman's pasted-on smile dropped and he reverted to his insufferable posturing. "I don't know what you are implying, Detective, but I do not like the tone of your voice or the nature of the accusations."

"Oh, I'm so sorry if I am offending you in any way," he responded sarcastically. "Why don't I tell you what I've been able to find out without your help? Maybe we should first discuss why you've hired a convicted sex offender to be a therapist here. Or, I'd be happy to discuss the circumstances of Dr. Rubin's leaving. Or perhaps you'd prefer to discuss why you're listed in Ms. O'Toole's school application as her treating physician? And I hear that you and Ms. Kingsley are an item. That's some relationship you have with your staff. So, where do you think we should start? Of course, if you're tired of speaking with me, I'm sure the psychological licensing board will be happy to discuss this with me."

The wind shifted outside, blowing the downpour against Hillerman's window. The noise of the onslaught echoed inside the room and sent a chill through Hillerman. "Detective, you are treading in a very delicate area you simply do not have the background to understand. First of all, my relationships with my employees are none of your business. Both Anita and Valerie are valued members of the Oakwood team and contribute handily to our work here."

"That's fine and dandy, but what does that have to do with acting as Anita's doctor?" Or Valerie's lover, for that matter, he thought.

Hillerman was determined not to say anything he might regret, but the strain of controlling his impulses was starting to show. "I think you are mistaken. I am not a medical doctor, I am a psychologist, and I am not about to discuss my professional relationships or my professional decisions with you."

"Do you know that Ms. O'Toole is on medical leave from school for depression and that she describes herself as under your care for—what did they call it—oh, yeah, mood disorder? Do you have a habit of employing mentally ill people as therapists?"

Hillerman's laugh echoed against the rattling window. "You should not be so eager to display your lack of knowledge, Detective. Ms. O'Toole does not suffer from any mental illness. A person can be fully functioning in one area of their life and still have other areas they would care to work on. Ms. O'Toole realized that school was becoming too demanding and we both thought it best if she concentrate on her internship right now and finish up with her formal education when she's ready."

"So you think she is fully capable of treating others while she's too unstable to continue with school?" Larson demanded.

Hillerman bristled, feeling misconstrued and under attack. "I said nothing about her being mentally unstable. I can assure you that it poses no concern to me whatsoever. She is an excellent therapist and is doing fine work with her groups. I wish all our therapists could do as well."

"And what about Mr. Green's police record? Don't you screen people before you hire them? I mean, it's got to look bad—a convicted sex offender treating sex offenders. Kinda like the slime leading the slime."

Hillerman's entire body clenched with the effort not to throw something at Larson. "Detective, as even you must be aware, people who have overcome problems in their own life can make a wonderful contribution to helping others make similar changes. That is the whole precept upon which AA is based, that only those who have been there can help others. Mr. Green's problems were in the past, youthful indiscretions gone awry. Now he is a valuable aid to help others overcome their antisocial sexual predilections."

"Yeah, I'm sure." Jack looked out the window. The water was coming straight down now, visible as discrete drops, the heavy downpour going as quickly as it came. "Tell me about LaPaca. Why haven't you sent us the computer run to show his group participation? We asked weeks ago whether Frank was ever in the groups of the other murder victims. Where are the records? Why the delay?"

"Oh, I'm so sorry. That request never made my desk. I can get that for you. See? We have nothing to hide." He forced a smile.

"When will I get it?"

"I'm sure I can get it to you within the week," Hillerman promised.

"And the other information?"

"Soon."

"Look, Hillerman, I'm not playing games. Have that information on my desk or I'll be back." Larson stood up. "Don't get up, I'll let myself out." He walked through the door into the hall and was gone.

Within seconds, Hillerman was on the phone with Stan. "I don't want to have to put up with this idiot cop. It was a shakedown. I want you to do something to keep him out of here."

"Why do you think he was there?"

"I don't know. There's already been an arrest, for Christ's sake. But I didn't like it. He knew more than he should."

"Like what?"

Hillerman did not want to share his personal business with his attorney—he certainly didn't want to be lectured about the legal pitfalls of sleeping with his employees. "That's not important. Just keep him away from here."

30

Jack placed his hand on the glass partition and Rebecca put hers up to match his, both a little embarrassed by the futile gesture yet not knowing what else to do to try and connect. As Rebecca tried to imagine Jack's touch, the barrier between them became too much. She quickly brought her hand down and picked up the phone, hoping the sound of his voice would bridge the gap.

Jack spoke first. "Hey, cutie." The familiar greeting belied the grim setting.

"It's good to see you. It's really good." She looked into his eyes, the same eyes she started falling in love with a million years ago before this all happened. She noted no distance, no distrust, and gained strength from the sight.

"I've missed you." Jack felt as if he were shrouded in a fog, but he struggled to at least appear strong for Rebecca.

"Me too."

Jack had tried to prepare himself for the visit, yet he wasn't ready for the feelings that enveloped him as he looked at Rebecca. "I don't even know what to say. I can't believe I'm sitting here across from you like this. This is such a nightmare. I just want to burst through this glass and grab you and take you out of here."

Rebecca smiled sadly. "I wish you could. I just wish you could hold me, if only for a minute. But just having you here, knowing you're still here—I can't tell you how much that means to me."

Rebecca's first smile felt like a warm embrace to Jack. "I'll always be here. Nobody can keep me away. And somehow, we're gonna get through this. I need you to be strong and to believe that we will make it. You've got to trust me on that. I'm not going to let you down. The rest of the LAPD can kiss my ass, but I'm not about to stand by and watch them try to build a case against you. They are dead wrong, and I know it, and I'm gonna prove it."

Rebecca looked doubtful. "But, how? What can you do?"

"Hey, I'm the lead detective on this case, remember?" Jack said with a melancholy smile. "Or at least I used to be. That can't stop me from continuing with my own investigation. I've got some good leads." He hoped he sounded convincing.

"Like what?"

"Like—listen to this. Do you remember a guy by the name of Frank LaPaca?"

"The transvestite?"

"Yeah, that's him. Or her. Anyhow, he came by the station awhile ago to tell me that he knows who the killer is."

"And who did he tell you it was?"

"Hillerman."

"Hillerman? As in Hillerman from the Oakwood?" Rebecca looked surprised.

"Yeah."

"That's ridiculous," she said. "You know why he told you that, don't you?"

He felt a wave of disappointment coming over him. "No, why?"

"Because about six months ago, maybe a little more, Hillerman recommended that Frank's probation be revoked. The case is winding its way through the courts. But once it gets before a judge, it's pretty clear that Frank is going back to jail, and for some time."

"So what you're telling me is that he has a reason to hate Hillerman." And try to set him up, Jack thought.

"With a passion. In fact, twice he's reported Hillerman to the State Psychological Association."

"For what?"

"I'm not really sure." Rebecca looked off to the side, as if mentally flipping the pages of a notebook to find the right entry. "I think one time he claimed that Hillerman was harassing him and the second time he claimed that Hillerman had disclosed patient secrets."

"What did the board do?"

"Both times they ultimately dismissed the charges. But from what I heard, they really put Hillerman through the wringer. Anyway, after the second time, coincidentally, Hillerman writes a real unfavorable report about Frank." Rebecca sounded stronger as she talked about the case, and for a moment both of them forgot where they were.

"And did he say in that report that Frank's probation should be revoked?"

"You got it."

"Sounds like the two of them are in quite a pissing contest."

"It sure looks that way. But I don't see how that's going to do me any good." A somber look came over

Rebecca. "Jack, I know you're trying real hard to get me out of here and I want you to know that I really appreciate it. . . ." Rebecca struggled to finish the sentence.

"No," he said sharply. "I know it sounds like a whole lot of nothing, but there's got to be something there. Too many things point in that direction. Now, I haven't yet figured out who's setting up who, but I know I'm getting closer. You just have to believe me. I'm gonna get you out of here."

She wanted to believe that he could deliver on his promise, but everything she knew and everything she felt told her it was impossible.

Tom had finished preparing for tomorrow's preliminary hearing and was getting ready to leave the office and head over to see Rebecca. He felt somewhat uncomfortable with what he had accomplished in the last two weeks, although he kept reminding himself that preparing for a preliminary hearing was markedly different now that he was a card-carrying member of the defense bar. While prosecutors have to make an affirmative showing of probable cause at the prelim, smart defense attorneys merely sit there and poke holes in the evidence. Since there was no way that a judge would dismiss Rebecca's case at the prelim stage, Tom's goal was merely to find out everything the prosecution knew and maybe a few things that they didn't.

As he headed out the door, Tom grabbed a few dozen letters of support that he thought would cheer up Rebecca. The letters—which were now starting to number in the hundreds—came from across the country, mostly from women, applauding her courage and dedication. Unfortunately, Tom knew that none of these fans would ever make it on the jury, but he hoped Rebecca would be comforted nonetheless. Some of the letter writers, like Laurie Jenkins, Matheson's victim, came out and actually thanked Rebecca for what they thought she had done. Tom decided to leave those at home, knowing they wouldn't provide much solace, since they presupposed Rebecca's guilt.

But as soon as Tom reached the door, the phone rang. Since he had only one case, and he'd already spoken with Rebecca today, Tom figured it had to be Covington. He grabbed the phone reluctantly, doubting Covington was calling to see how he was doing.

"Well, Counselor," she began, her voice artificially bright, "did I catch you at a bad time?"

"Nope," Tom lied, not wanting to give her any satisfaction. He took the offensive. "Just sitting here wondering how you're going to get by the prelim without any evidence."

"Don't need any."

"Oh, have the rules of evidence changed in the last day or so?" Tom was proud of his snappy retort.

"Nope, just the rules of the game." Covington was even prouder of hers.

Tom sensed he was going to lose this one. "Listen, I'm too tired for one of your games." *Especially since I never seem to win one,* Tom thought to himself. "What are you talking about?"

Covington could barely contain herself. "I just called to inform you that you won't have to appear tomorrow at the preliminary hearing. It's been canceled."

"And why is that?" he asked, more than reluctant to hear the answer.

"Because the grand jury just handed down six indictments against your client for first-degree murder." Covington found the dead silence on the other end completely satisfying.

"What the hell are you talking about?" Tom finally stormed when he regained the ability to speak. "I've never been told anything about a grand jury investigation." Tom quickly moved from irritation to full-blown anger, his voice blasting across the phone lines. "How dare you convene a grand jury and not tell me? Just who the fuck do you think you are?"

Covington was mildly amused by the macho bluster. But not as happy as she was going to be when she stuffed him at trial. "Mr. Baldwin, I am just using all the procedures that the law provides. Would you expect me to do any less? I just thought you might find it interesting that the panel had no trouble reaching its decision. It moved very quickly."

Tom fumed. "Ms. Covington, I'm sitting here with a thousand letters from people who do not even know Rebecca and yet they support her one hundred percent."

"Is that going to be your defense?" She let out an ugly little laugh. "When I'm done with Rebecca, everyone will realize she is far closer to Son of Sam than she is to Joan of Arc."

At this point Tom didn't know what was true. His gut told him no jury would convict anyone of killing child molesters, and yet his head told him never to try to guess what a jury would do. But he wouldn't let Covington sense his doubt. "Good luck finding a jury who'll convict Rebecca. You'll never find twelve people who don't think your so-called victims got just what they deserved."

"Do you honestly believe that the judge will ever let any vigilante mongers on the jury? No way. Just good folk who believe murder is murder, regardless of who the victim was. Your client's going down in a big way. Get used to it." Covington paused before delivering the coup de grace. "One other thing. The death penalty review panel here has recommended that we seek the death penalty." She wished she could see his face, but for now it was enough hearing his silence.

Tom sat motionless at his desk, paralyzed by the sting of Covington's words. He finally propelled himself into action, motivated by the fact that he had better tell Rebecca the news before she learned of it through the jail's intricate rumor mill. He gathered his things and headed off to jail. Slowly winding his way east on the 10, in its usual bumper-to-bumper crawl, he drove automatically, his mind focused not on traffic but on how Rebecca would take the news. While the indictments only established the inevitable a little sooner, it was still a psychological blow to realize that at least fourteen strangers thought Rebecca was capable of first-degree murder.

As Tom walked into the small cubicle where she sat waiting, his eyes belied the message his smile tried to convey. "What's wrong?" she asked apprehensively.

He deflected the question. "I brought you some of your mail. There are an awful lot of people out there who support you. And not because they think you're guilty," he stressed.

"Sure." Rebecca wasn't buying it.

"No, it's true," Tom hedged. "People appreciate all the work you've tried to do for molested children. You'll see when you read the letters. Some of the kids you've worked with in the past wrote to you. Some of the families as well. And a lot of other people who don't even know you wanted you to know they support you. You've got a lot of friends out there."

Rebecca inclined her head slightly, accepting some of the support. It was better than being hated, after all. "Thanks. I'll read them later." As Rebecca looked at Tom, she sensed some apprehension on his part. "It looks to me like there's more on your mind than favorable letters. What's wrong? Worried about the prelim?"

Tom put his head down, shaking it slightly, while praying for strength. Why was he anointed as the conveyor of all bad news? "Rebecca, there's not going to be a prelim." A pause, let it sink in. Another deep breath. "There was a grand jury investigation going on all this time. You were indicted this afternoon."

Rebecca looked lost. "How did we not know? Who'd they call?" she asked, her voice pleading.

"I don't have any of the details yet. I just found out as I was walking out the door. But, there's more." Tom let out a heavy sigh, telegraphing his distress to prepare her for the worst. "Covington told me they've decided to seek the death penalty. There's no way they'd get it. We're gonna win, but even if we don't, no one's going to sentence you to death. I don't want you to worry. It's just all bluster, just bullshit posturing." His words came out in a rush, as if he could talk Rebecca out of her feelings.

"Oh my God, Tom." She gasped. "I never really thought . . . Are you sure?" Her voice trembled, her eyes entreating Tom to say something soothing. She felt as if she'd been punched in the stomach, a deep aching consumed her from within. There had to be a mistake, a horrible mistake.

Tom shrugged helplessly as he watched Rebecca go through her own personal agony, a few feet away, and yet miles apart. The surroundings demanded he merely sit there and watch. It was like watching a person die from a snake bite—slow, inevitable, painful. So he did what little he could, trying to offer words of support that he feared weren't true, hoping she wouldn't see through them. "Rebecca, you know that it's just what they have to do for their own PR. We can't focus on it. We have to focus our attention just on the trial. We have a lot to do and not a lot of time to do it. I need you to stay strong. I told you what I had to, but you can't let it get you down. We can push on, we can beat them if you're willing to fight. Can you concentrate? Can you just put what I've told you out of your mind?"

"Sure. Just put it out of my mind. How do I do that, Tom?" she asked, her desperation weighing heavy in the air.

"I don't know. But I know you'll be no use to me if you don't. Don't give them that advantage." He thought it best to quickly move on. "Now, I've been working on the pretrial motions. I want to file a series of suppression motions. I'm challenging both search warrants, I don't see how they had probable cause to search your office or to search for evidence of the other killings. Are you with me?"

"Yes, okay," she said, sniffling back the next onslaught of tears, brushing the residue away as she pretended to have it all together.

"Thatta girl. Okay. Look, we need to work on your alibis." He flipped open his file, shaking his head. "It amazes me that so far we haven't been able to place you anywhere where someone might have seen you or talked to you. Nothing, except for maybe Jaffe. If the coroner could fix his time of death to that weekend at your sister's, that would be big."

"Don't work too hard on that one, Tom." He looked at her strangely. "I came back early." She said it so quickly, Tom wasn't sure he'd heard her right.

"What do you mean?"

Rebecca spoke reluctantly, her eyes downcast. She could see in his face what this news meant. "I didn't stay the whole weekend. I came back on Saturday. In the morning."

Her words shook Tom. "Shit! I thought this might be our ace. When were you thinking of mentioning that to me?" He couldn't stop his mind from jumping to very damning conclusions.

Rebecca looked at Tom and saw the doubt had returned and she struggled to regain his belief. "I didn't know it was important. Since they can't tell us when he died, I didn't know what good it would do. It doesn't cut either way for us."

"You know, I think you oughta let me decide that." Tom sat there mumbling under his breath. "Fine, so we won't have an alibi." He took a deep breath and felt his chest pounding. "Let's go back to how we can win this."

Rebecca nodded.

"Okay, I want to get our own scientists looking at the blood and hair. This raises an uncomfortable question. . . ."

"I know. You need more money. Well, I have no one to leave my money to, Elizabeth doesn't need it. So you can have whatever you need."

Tom didn't like the way she said that, as if she were someone who didn't see a future for herself. "Listen to me. We're going to win, so I don't want you to go broke. And, anyway, you probably don't have enough money—those forensic guys don't come cheap. And we're going to have to challenge the scientific evidence. If we don't, we're just handing the case to them. We need a fund-raiser. With all the support you're getting, I'm sure we can raise some money for your defense."

The thought made Rebecca uncomfortable; she didn't want to be anyone's poster girl. She shook her head. "Elizabeth offered her help. Just let me know how much you need and I'll ask her."

"You know, I could help you out somewhat, but I hate suggesting what I'm about to."

"What?"

Tom looked around uncomfortably. "If I could move out of the Motel Six, I could get along on less money. I was about to go find myself an apartment, but I thought that maybe, to conserve some money, maybe I could move into your condo for the time being. It'll save me the expense. I'll only need enough to feed me, and these days my appetite's pretty low. We can use the extra money for trial prep instead, getting the displays, blowups, experts, trial consultants, that kind of stuff."

Rebecca nodded slowly. "Sure. It makes sense."

"Thanks. I was afraid I was going to upset you."

"No, it's okay. I think I'm numb right now. It was probably a good time to ask. Just do me a favor. Don't have any fun there, okay?"

Finally, a promise he knew he could keep. "I'm not going to have any fun till you're out of here."

Randazzo came in late, knowing today would be difficult. She had brought a peace offering—a raspberry-filled donut—even though she knew that the rift between her and Jack might be beyond repair. As Randazzo settled down at her desk, she could feel the heat coming from Larson. She tried to ignore him, going through her message slips and getting up to fill her coffee cup. But when she sat back down, he was still staring at her. "What is it? You're gonna burn a hole right through my clothes. Just stop it. Turn those things off."

"What are you bitching about now?"

She pointed at him. "Those radar eyes of yours. What are you all pissed off about?" A stupid question. She knew, but she didn't want to hear it.

"What am I pissed off about?" He sat back and assumed his most hostile posture. "How was it that I never heard about the grand jury investigation? How was it my partner apparently goes down for a command performance and just forgets to tell me?"

Randazzo rolled her chair over to his desk. "Jack, maybe you never paid any attention to the warning they give you before you testify, but the grand jury is supposed to be a secret. It meets in private. You're not allowed to discuss your testimony with anyone."

Larson put his hand on his chest. "I'm not anyone, I'm your partner," he said, more hurt than angry.

"You know me, if someone swears me to secrecy, that's it. I'm not gonna go to hell just because we're partners and you don't want me keeping things from you. I swore on God, and that means something to me." Jack flicked his hand at her, dismissing her excuse. This wasn't the way it was supposed to be. They were supposed to be a team, working together, sharing everything. But no more, Randazzo thought. Now they were like strangers. "Don't think I didn't feel bad. I hated not being able to tell you. I kept hoping you'd be called, so we could talk about it."

Jack threw his hands up in the air. "No, I just find out like everyone else, turning on the tube. God, they're full of themselves. Their big announcement. They should have provided background music, maybe 'I've Been Working on the Railroad,' 'cause that's what's happening to Rebecca—she's being railroaded." He wagged his finger at Randazzo. "I'll tell you someone has it in for her. It's a fucking farce." She couldn't remember ever seeing Larson this mad. He was sitting at his desk and yet he seemed to be in constant motion, unable to find comfort in his own skin.

"No, it's the fucking justice system. It just never bothered you before. Remember back when you thought all defendants were guilty?" Randazzo said gently.

"Well, it's a crock. I can't believe they're going to

trial against Rebecca. It's ludicrous. And seeking the death penalty. Are they crazy? This is Rebecca we're talking about. I don't understand what's going on." His hands flew up again.

Randazzo didn't know what to do, so she went back to her desk, grabbed the bag, and offered it to Larson. "Here, I bought you one. That should help a little."

He shook his head. "No. This is something even a donut can't solve."

Randazzo tossed the bag back on her desk and sat quietly for a moment. "So, have you come up with any alternate theories?" she asked finally.

"Yeah, as a matter of fact, I have." Larson said it with confidence, yet just as quickly seemed to lose his resolve. He shrugged. "I just don't know where to go with them."

"Well, keep on plugging, maybe something'll turn up. If I can help in any way—"

Larson broke into a broad smile. "I thought you were lined up with the prosecution?"

Randazzo looked surprised—and a little hurt—by his statement. "You seem to forget that first and foremost I'm a cop. All I wanted from this case was to solve it and find the killer. If Rebecca isn't the killer, then we should keep looking. If she is, well . . . we'll deal with it. Right now the evidence against her looks pretty convincing to me. But if you come up with something else, great. I'll tell you one thing." Randazzo looked back to the chart on the blackboard, the one with Rebecca's name at the top, then turned back to Larson and shook her head. "This didn't go down the way I expected."

Larson was caught off guard by her simple statement and realized tears were welling in his eyes. He felt exposed and vulnerable—embarrassed by the raw emotion. He turned his head away suddenly, shielding Randazzo from his hurt. "Me neither," he muttered.

31

After a while, Rebecca had little trouble falling into the prison routine. Regimented, repetitive, inflexible, somewhat like law school only without the nachos and beer, she joked to Elizabeth. She had no choice but to make light of her situation. It was either that or go mad. As a high-priority inmate, signified by her ominously dark red smock, she was somewhat isolated from the other inmates. She occupied an entire corridor in the high-power section—six cells, twelve cots, one occupant. Meals were served in her cell. One exception to the isolation was negotiated by Tom, who made sure she could spend unlimited time in the library, allowing her to help with her defense. It helped keep her mind busy, so she wouldn't have time to think that soon she would have what would be quite literally the trial of her life.

It was only at nighttime, when she was alone but unable to embrace the comfort of sleep, that the terror began. The persistent thoughts boring into her head—the fear that she'd never be able to convince the jury of her innocence, the fear that at best she was preparing for a life without freedom, and at worst a life cut short by this surreal plunge into the justice system. The fear that her fate was no longer in her own hands. A new perspective on an all-too-familiar system, she thought.

As Christmas Day dawned, Rebecca found herself oddly relieved. Certainly no one expected her to be festive. Rebecca used to hate all that holiday cheer and others' insistence that she share in their mirth. This year, there was none of that. As bleak as it seemed to some, she knew that it wasn't her worst Christmas, by far. That distinction went to her tenth Christmas. Since her father was busy with his fifth eggnog and a too loud sing-along with Bing Crosby's "White Christmas," Rebecca's mother had gone ahead and tucked her into bed for a change. That was traditionally her father's job. In a burst of courage, hoping that the goodness of the season might provide some protection, Rebecca told her mother that her father had been molesting her for years. When her mother looked at her, disbelieving, Rebecca gave her some details, hoping that would help her to understand. Instead, her mother slapped her and then berated her for trying to ruin the holidays. She stormed out of Rebecca's room and threw out her presents. Rebecca could see the dented packages on the front lawn from her bedroom window. She heard the laughter and singing downstairs and waited for her father's visit. When he finally came upstairs, drunk and angry, he ripped off her nightgown and sodomized her. "Bad little girls get it in the ass," he told her through clenched teeth. He pulled hard on her hair till she cried and then hit her for crying. "You keep your fucking mouth shut or I'll really give you something to cry about," he snarled.

The next morning, Rebecca heard the presents being opened and Elizabeth's laughter, forced and artificial. She smelled the turkey cooking in the oven, and she could hear the Christmas specials on TV. Rebecca had wanted to stay up in her room all day, but her father came in, smiling. "Don't be a little Grinch. Come on, and let's have fun." He brought one of her retrieved presents, still wet from sitting on the lawn all night, and, after forcing her to give him a "special" Christmas blow job, he let her open her present. She had earned it, he told her. No, this wasn't her worst Christmas.

Jack was first in line for visiting hour. He sat down, and laid an envelope on the desk in front of him. "Hey, gorgeous. Merry Christmas." His voice sparkled across the phone.

"Hey, handsome. Merry Christmas to you, too."

As he looked at her, so beautiful, so fragile, and yet so strong, Jack's heart began to ache, what was left of it anyhow. "Rebecca, I've been doing a lot of thinking, about you and me, and it occurred to me that I may never have told you something very important. Something that I feel every minute of the day." The words came out quickly.

"What are you talking about?"

"I almost don't want to say it. I don't want this to be the first place you hear it." Jack paused, gaining strength from her. "Rebecca, I love you. I've loved you from the moment I saw this hard-nosed D.A. blush when I mentioned a second date. You think you're so tough, such a hard ass, and yet I could see right through you to the caring, gentle woman inside, the one who's funny and sweet and just wants to be happy. I love you, Rebecca. And I don't want to lose you."

Rebecca lost herself in his warm eyes and started to cry. "Well, I'm not going anywhere." She said it automatically, and it took a beat for both of them to notice the humor in it. "And I love you too, Jack. Just my luck the first time I get up the nerve to say it, I'm separated by four inches of Plexiglas."

"Nothing can separate us."

Rebecca felt her face flush, as Jack's words dissolved the barrier between them. "I'll keep telling myself that."

"Well, I want you to believe me. So, I got these." Jack opened the envelope and put a piece of paper up to the glass. Rebecca leaned in to read what turned out to be an airline reservation, date unspecified, for two traveling from LAX to Kauai. "When I get you out of here, I'm taking you to Hawaii. It can be our honeymoon."

Rebecca was caught off guard. She looked up at Jack and felt her heart quicken. "Did you just propose to me?"

"I think so."

Rebecca sat still for a moment, her eyes downcast—afraid to meet his gaze. She wanted so much to pretend, to believe that a simple yes could make everything better, but she knew it wasn't that easy. Yet to say no would deny all her feelings for Jack. "I don't know what to say."

"How about 'yes'?"

She looked at Jack, wanting nothing but to hold him, and shook her head slowly. "Jack, this is sweet and all, but I don't want to be unfair to you. If I don't get out of here, you have to live your life. I don't want you to feel obligated to stand by me, in case things don't work out. I can't make you put your life on hold for me."

"Without you, what kind of a life would I have?" It was a simple statement of fact.

"Don't say that."

Jack wasn't going to accept anything short of a yes, convinced that if she agreed to it, it could come true. "Well, you can't refuse my present. It's impolite. Now,

promise me you'll go. I want to have something wonderful to shoot for. Dreaming about running on the
beach with you will help me get through this. It
might help you, too."

"I want to say yes, but I don't want to make a
promise I might not be able to keep." She wiped the
tears out of her eyes. "At this point, it's pretty much
out of my hands."

Tom arrived in the afternoon, mad at himself for
forgetting to bring her a present, yet aware that the
one thing Rebecca really needed from him was her
freedom. He rushed into the conference room, his
hair badly in need of a cut, his face gaunt and
unshaven, dark circles surrounding his bloodshot
eyes. He obviously wasn't getting enough sleep,
and Rebecca doubted he was eating regularly, yet
somehow he seemed more alive than she had seen
him in years.

She picked up the phone. "You've got to take better care of yourself, Tom. How are you going to win
my case looking like that? You look more like a
defendant than an attorney."

"Don't worry about me. I'll get a beauty makeover
before the trial. Anyhow, without a continuance, I
have a shitload of work to do and we're coming
down to the wire. So personal care just has to wait."

"How are things going?" she asked tentatively.

"Swimmingly," Tom said somewhat sarcastically.
"Since your defense is based on misidentification,
I'm kinda hamstrung in what I can argue. I'm stuck
with, 'It wasn't me, I wasn't there' five of the six
times. But without a solid alibi, I've got my work cut
out for me. It's been impossible to try and figure out
where you were and what you were doing when each
of these guys were killed. Now if you were going to

plead self-defense or diminished capacity, I'd have something to work with."

Rebecca's eyes narrowed. "We've been over this. I didn't kill the other five and I can't claim that I did to give you something to argue."

"I know, I know." Tom sighed. He wished that for just a minute they could switch places so that she could see the case like a lawyer and not like the accused. "It just amazes me how many people think you're guilty and yet think you should get off."

"Are you one of them?" she asked, trying in vain to meet his averted eyes.

"No, of course not. I mean, I wouldn't blame you if you had. I certainly could understand if you lost it. And from a defense standpoint, it would be a whole lot easier on me if I could get up there and say, 'Yeah, she did it, but so what?' I think that's how most people see it."

"Well, I'm sorry I'm blowing your best defense, but I'm not going to say I did it and they deserved it. Because that would only be half right."

"Which half?" Tom closed his eyes, as if to shut off her response. "No, don't tell me. I don't want to know. Okay, look, I think it might be helpful if we could suggest another suspect. I don't think it's going to be enough for us to simply say you didn't do it. We need to point the finger in another direction. Let the jury believe that by convicting you they'd be letting the real killer go free."

"Jack's been working on something. He's convinced the killer's at Oakwood, but he can't sort out who it is yet. And no one is giving him any help. I don't know if he's really on to something or if he's so desperate to get me out of here he'd be suspicious of Mother Teresa."

Tom smiled. "Yeah, he's been keeping me filled in. He calls me from home or from pay phones so no one knows he's talking to me. You got a good one in him, you know."

Rebecca smiled and nodded. "I know. Unfortunately, everyone except you and Jack thinks I'm guilty as sin. As far as the rest of his department is concerned, they've solved the case, so he's pretty much on his own. I can't imagine it's a great career move for him to be working to clear me while his boss goes on TV saying I'm the killer."

Tom was saved from coming up with a comforting rejoinder by a rap on the door. "Mr. Baldwin," the guard announced, "there's an Elizabeth Fielding here to visit the prisoner. She's on the list. Do you want her to come in?"

Tom threw his head back and let out a groan. "Just what I needed." He exhaled loudly. "Sure, send her in." He stood up with great effort and tried to assume a pleasant pose.

Elizabeth walked past Tom and sat down. "Hi, Bec," she echoed through the phone. "How are you doing?" She cringed. "I'm sorry, that was dumb."

Rebecca was starting to feel like a hospitalized terminal patient whom everyone tiptoes around, never knowing what to say. "No, that's okay. I'm fine, really. Thanks to Tom, he's keeping my mind on the trial, so I don't have too much time to think about being here."

Elizabeth turned to Tom. "How's it coming?" she asked, more a demand than a true question. Civility toward him was always difficult for her to muster.

"We're working hard. I'm doing my best to get your sister out of here."

"Just don't blow it again. There's too much at stake. This is Rebecca's life we're talking about here," Elizabeth said harshly.

"I'm well aware of that, Elizabeth." This bickering was not doing Rebecca any good, Tom thought to himself. Better do something to head off the inevitable clash. "Elizabeth, I need to ask you something about the trial, outside. I might need you to testify." He turned to Rebecca, put on his warmest phony smile, and spoke into the phone. "We'll be right back."

Tom and Elizabeth walked out of the room together, and as soon as the door closed he leaned in on her, his voice filled with exasperation. "For God's sake, Elizabeth—no, make that for Rebecca's sake— will you just fucking mellow out on me? I know how you feel about me. The whole world knows. You took out an ad in the *New York Times* as I recall. But please, put it aside for Rebecca."

Elizabeth folded her arms. She considered keeping quiet for her sister's sake but convinced herself that she was doing this for Rebecca. "I just find it very difficult to see you in the position as her savior. What's to keep history from repeating itself?"

"Because it won't," Tom said sternly. "I may not be able to run my personal life, I may be a total failure as a lover and a husband. You won't get too much argument on that. But goddammit, I'm a good lawyer and I intend to win this case. But I can't do that if you upset Rebecca or get her to doubt me. She has to have faith in me and in my ability to get her off. Don't undermine that."

Elizabeth did not want to be told what to do by Tom of all people. She looked away, focusing on anything but Tom, yet having nowhere to stare in the barren hallway. She turned to him finally, scowling. "It just makes me sick to think of Rebecca putting her trust in you, of all people," she said, her disdain worn like a badge of honor, her face flushed with anger. "I just never understood how she stayed friends with you after what you did to her."

"Oh, put a cork in it," Tom chafed. "I don't know why you hate me so much. You act like I dumped you instead of your sister. It's been years. Get over it already."

"There's no time limit on breaking someone's heart. You should never be forgiven for hurting Rebecca. I don't care how many years pass. She trusted you. She gave you her heart and soul, and I never thought she'd be able to do that with anyone. I used to listen to her talk about you—she was so happy, so in love. And you just yanked it all out from under her." Elizabeth's eyes were hard, her lips pulled tight.

Tom wheeled on her, ready to pounce. He was done with being her whipping boy. "You know, you talk as if no one ever broke up with anyone else before. Not all relationships continue. Some break up. It's not this big trauma you're making it out to be. I'm getting blamed for a lot of shit I had nothing to do with. When is this dump-on-Tom crap going to stop? I'm sorry you grew up in that house, I'm sorry your father molested Rebecca, I'm sorry if you feel guilty about the fact that you were spared, but none of it is my fault, so stop dumping it on me."

Elizabeth started shaking, her voice tight and angry. "What did you say? Don't you ever talk to me about my family. You don't know anything—"

Tom was done playing the gentleman. "I know that you were so fucking grateful that Rebecca came along and took your father off your hands. I know that she was your salvation. I know that you just laid in bed night after night, hearing him going into her room next door, so thankful for the gift of a little sister, so grateful that he was leaving you alone—"

"You fucking bastard!" Elizabeth barely got the words out, her voice trembling with a rage deep within her soul.

Tom moved in, inches from her face. "No, Elizabeth.

I wasn't the one who sacrificed my sister, who played along pretending everything was all right when Rebecca was being torn apart. You're the bastard."

Elizabeth slapped Tom so hard in the face that the noise startled the guard stationed nearby. "What's going on here?" he demanded as he walked toward them. Elizabeth was breathing hard, still shaking with anger. Tom stood firm, glaring at Elizabeth while muttering a faint "Sorry, no problem here." The deputy looked at them both, offered a "Let's make sure of that," and returned to his post.

Tom continued, forcing his voice to stay low. "I know the truth is hard to take. But maybe it's time you faced it. You're not mad at me, you're mad at yourself. You're the one who let Rebecca down."

Elizabeth stood looking at Tom, wanting to strike him again, to keep hitting him until she could no longer hear his words. How dare he tell her what she should have done, what did he know about what choices she had? She wanted to scream at him, to tell him he was wrong, that he didn't understand. And yet she didn't want to face that he might be right about one thing—that he had been a safe repository of too much pent-up anguish, of feelings no child should have to live with of fear and shame and hopelessness. It was too much to consider, too much to admit, so she pushed his words aside. "Just look me in the eyes and tell me you'll get her out."

Tom was stunned by the change in Elizabeth as well as by the directness of the question. He hesitated to answer it, knowing a false promise wasn't what she wanted to hear. "Elizabeth, I swear to you that I will do everything in my power to get Rebecca acquitted. You forget, I gave up a lot to take this case. I gave up just about everything I had. I wouldn't do that if I didn't believe in her and her case."

She nodded her head slowly, accepting his words,

knowing it was all she could get as a promise. "Okay, fine."

He stood looking at her, baffled as usual by what to do next. He extended his hand, a feeble demonstration of reconciliation, but it was all he could think to do. "I'm sorry, it's the pressure, I didn't mean—" Tom scratched his head and felt pretty stupid.

"No, it's okay, really. We're both upset. We just decided to take it out on each other." Elizabeth looked down at the floor, then up at the ceiling, doing an excellent job of avoiding Tom. It felt odd to have a polite exchange with him, but she no longer had the choice to just resent him from afar. He had no right to say what he had said, but he had done it for Rebecca. His commitment to her was clear, and right now that was all that mattered.

"I'm sorry, too," Elizabeth said. "I guess this is what happens when you let feelings just fester over time, you say a lot of harsh things. It's not a pretty sight." She managed a smile, which Tom returned, as if greeting an old friend. "We've got to stick together if we're going to get through this. A lot's been said. Let's put it to rest, for Rebecca. And for us, too." Elizabeth suddenly reached out and embraced Tom, and the two of them held on to each other for strength, for comfort, for hope. A great burden had been lifted from their shoulders. The guilt that bound them was now out in the open. For the first time in a long time, Tom was free to deal with the future and Elizabeth was free to deal with the past.

They let go of each other. "Well, we should get back," Tom said. "We've been gone long enough, and she's probably wondering what's going on." Elizabeth straightened her back and lifted her head to compose herself, then nodded her readiness to him. He smiled warmly and took Elizabeth by the hand. "Let's get back in there and give her a good visit. She deserves it."

Elizabeth squeezed his hand and gave it a little shake. "You got it."

Walking back in together, smiling, hand in hand, they could instantly see the positive result their pact had on Rebecca. She beamed at the sight of the two of them together, friendly, on her side. Burying the hatchet, and not in each other's head. If their truce was possible, anything could happen. Including her freedom.

32

Jack dragged his feet for the long walk down the hall leading to Chief Bellamy's office. He wasn't up for the command performance, but he had little choice in the matter. For someone who'd steered clear of trouble his entire career, making fewer waves than a pebble dropped in the ocean, he was about to meet the chief in an unfamiliar role, as someone at odds with the department, a potential troublemaker at a time when the department had plenty of trouble already.

The door was open and the chief was alone inside, standing by his massive desk. Larson walked in a little hesitantly. "Chief, you wanted to see me?"

Bellamy walked up and greeted Larson with a hearty clasp on the back. "Yes, Jack. Please, come in, sit down." He sat reluctantly.

Bellamy grabbed a small humidor from the top of his desk, opened it, and extended it to Larson. "Cigar?"

Not a good sign. Bellamy usually preferred quick on-your-feet talks, not meetings long enough to smoke a cigar. "No, thanks." Larson felt uncomfortable, the setting bringing to mind his occasional youthful visits to the principal's office. "What can I do for you, Chief?" he asked.

"Now you know that the department thinks very highly of you . . ."

"But?" Larson was not in the mood for pleasantries. He knew this wasn't a social visit.

Bellamy leaned back on the front of his desk, towering over Larson. "But it has come to my attention that you've been still working on the child molester murders. And not as part of the prosecution team, I might add. Now, as you might imagine, that doesn't look too good for the department, one rogue cop continuing to investigate a case the rest of the entire department, along with the entire district attorney's office, believes has been solved. I understand you're unhappy with what has happened, but I think your relationship with Ms. Fielding is clouding your judgment."

Larson sat forward. "Chief, with all due respect, my relationships are none of your damn business," he snapped, noticeably irritated. Right now he didn't care that Bellamy was his boss or that he might lose his job and his pension. All he cared about was freeing Rebecca.

Bellamy restrained himself, yet was clearly not amused by Larson's impudence. "Jack, I think you should calm yourself down before you say anything that you might regret. In case you forgot, I run this department, and I will not tolerate anyone speaking like that to me. And I also will not tolerate dissension in the ranks." Bellamy stood up suddenly then walked around to sit behind his desk, resting his clasped hands in front of him. "We have our suspect, and if you want to keep working on the case, fine, you can help the prosecution during trial. You will not, however, continue your one-man crusade, harassing people because you don't like how this case has turned out." He jabbed a thick finger toward Larson.

"Chief, I'm sorry, but I don't know what you're talking about. Who am I harassing? All I'm doing is following up on a few leads," he protested.

"That's not how Dr. Hillerman and his attorney see it. They've complained that you're bothering Hillerman and his patients, continually questioning them even after there's been an arrest in the case. Visiting one of his patients at his home. Believe me, the last thing I want is to get any more calls telling me that you, me, and the department are going to be sued for harassment unless I pull you off this case. I don't know what you've got against Dr. Hillerman and, frankly, I don't really care, but you have no reason to be bothering him. He says you're asking too damn many questions that are none of your business." Bellamy's face hardened into a scowl—gone was the disarming smile the public was used to seeing. Larson knew that this face wasn't good news for whoever saw it. "Jesus Christ, Jack, you've been continuing the investigation as if we haven't made an arrest and aren't scheduled to go to trial on the case. How am I supposed to respond to that?"

"You could respond that I'm doing my job, and that my job is to investigate all leads whether or not it's convenient for Hillerman and his attorney. Sure seems to me they must have something to hide if they're so sensitive about a little questioning." Larson was beyond exasperated, feeling repelled in his efforts to save Rebecca. But he tried to maintain his composure, hoping somehow to reason with Bellamy and leave here with permission to conduct a discreet investigation. "What am I supposed to do, ignore the facts?" he asked calmly. "That patient I've been 'bothering,' Frank LaPaca, he came by the station before the arrest to tell me that he had evidence that Hillerman was the killer. Now was LaPaca telling me that because he was on to something, or was he there because he wants to cause trouble for Hillerman? Or is LaPaca the killer? I don't know, but I'll never know unless I continue to investigate."

Larson was making no headway—the chief seemed as unconvinced as when he started. Evidently, the only words he was prepared to accept were, "You're right, I'll stop." But Larson couldn't say those words. He knew the answer lay somewhere other than with Rebecca. "Look, the killings started just after Hillerman recommended that LaPaca's probation should be revoked. Revenge is a pretty strong motivator, don't you think? Speaking of revenge, how 'bout we look at the pissing contest Dr. Hillerman is engaged in with Dr. Rubin, the founder of a competing clinic? There's a lot of bad blood there that could be relevant."

The chief stared at Larson for what seemed like an eternity, then he spoke. "I'm not making my point, am I?" Larson started to speak but was immediately cut off. "I'm not interested in your theories and I'm not interested in your investigation—I'm only interested in unity in the department."

Larson sat quietly for longer than he needed to, then spoke as if he hadn't heard the chief. "I've turned up a lot so far. But obviously since I have to do all this without warrants and without the department's resources, it's taking me longer. In fact, it's making my job virtually impossible. But, Chief," Larson softened his tone, "I really think I'm starting to make progress. If you want, I'll put it all together for you in a report."

Bellamy clutched the sides of his desk and dramatically raised his voice. "I don't need a fucking report. I need you to stop. This is a department, a unified group of people who work together. You seem to have forgotten that. We don't just run around here half-cocked. What you do reflects on all of us, and right now your frustration is causing you to cross the line."

Larson shook his head and responded calmly. "No, Chief, it isn't. If anything, it's bringing me closer to the killer. I can feel it." Larson didn't know why that wasn't enough. "Why don't you sign off on a warrant and a wiretap? That'll help me bring this whole thing to a head."

Bellamy looked aghast. It was as if he were talking to his schnauzer and not a veteran detective. "And just whose phones do you intend to tap?"

"Let's start with the Oakwood's."

"Goddammit, Jack! Are you crazy? Do you know how that would look?"

Bellamy's sudden outburst caught Larson by surprise. "Why are you so caught up in how things look?"

"Because we arrested and charged someone for the murders!" Bellamy shouted.

"And in our courts, the accused is innocent until proven guilty," Larson replied, his jaw set hard. "Or have you forgotten?"

Bellamy's face turned red, and his collar looked as if it were choking the life out of him. "Don't give me that bullshit. You and I both know that's just some nice phrase people toss around so we seem more enlightened than some fucking third-world country. Most defendants are guilty, plain and simple, and this case is no exception. But it is different in that it is a highly sensitive case, one in which the very reputation of the department is on the line. Both this department and the D.A.'s office have all but said that Ms. Fielding is the killer. Can you imagine what would happen if word got out that we were still investigating other suspects while the trial was going on? Wouldn't make for a very strong case, now would it?" The chief was still feeling the sting from the last major murder trial in Los Angeles, when within days of the suspect's arrest, the D.A. proudly proclaimed that the killer had been captured—only to have to eat those words when the jury resoundingly said otherwise.

"But, Chief," Larson said, then paused. Arguing wasn't going to solve anything. Only time could prove that he was right. "Rebecca is not the killer. You're all dead wrong about her. And I'm going to prove it," he said with complete conviction. Larson could see in the chief's face that he was getting nowhere with this discussion. "Look, if you don't mind, I still have a lot of work to do on this case." Larson stood up to leave.

"Sit down. You're not going anywhere," Chief Bellamy said loudly and firmly. Larson sat back down and Bellamy seemed to soften with Jack's compliance. "Jack, I really like you. So I'm going to give you another chance. But listen to me carefully. You will drop your investigation. You will leave Hillerman, and whoever else you're bothering, alone. You will cooperate with the prosecution of Ms. Fielding. And finally, you will stop visiting the defendant in jail. This department has been good and loyal to you for nearly twenty years. It deserves the same from you. Here's what it boils down to. You can get in line or you can get out. Understood?"

"Understood," Larson said quietly. He stood slowly, turned and walked out, knowing what his answer ultimately would be.

"Valerie, may I see you in my office?" Hillerman's sugary voice did not seem to match his curt tone. She suddenly wished her office was not quite so close to his.

Hillerman ushered her in with a smile as wide as

it was fake. "Valerie, I think we need to have a little chat." He closed the door behind her. She sat on the edge of the chair, sensing there was no reason to get comfortable. Hillerman walked around and sat across from her, resting his head on his hands. "Is there something you want to say to me that you haven't for some reason? Anything, perhaps, you've been afraid to tell me?" he asked coyly.

Valerie quickly realized she was about to lose today's mind game. But then, since Hillerman always set the rules, he always won the games. "I don't know what you mean," she responded slowly, trying to read him.

"Well, how do you really feel about me? And you can put aside the warm fuzzies for now. I'd like to hear about the other feelings, the ones you haven't shared with me before."

Valerie cleared her throat. "You know how much I respect you. I don't know what I'd do without you. Where I'd be. You've helped me so much. I don't know how I could ever repay you for what you've done for me."

"Hmm," he murmured. Hillerman liked compliments but that's not what he was after today. "Given all that, isn't there a lingering negative feeling? Perhaps a small, niggling feeling?" He switched into his therapist mode. "Often we feel a tiny tinge of resentment toward the people we admire the most. Maybe you are suffering from a trace of that yourself." Hillerman played cat to Valerie's mouse, batting her around playfully before going in for the kill. He figured he owed himself that.

"Oh, no, Dr. Hillerman. Why would you say that?"

"You honestly do not know why I am asking?" he asked incredulously.

Valerie looked around helplessly and wished Hillerman's office came equipped with an escape route. "I'm sorry. It's just that I'm not sure what you're talking about."

Hillerman dropped the facade of a smile, sitting forward, glaring at her. "Don't play that game with me," he glowered. "Look who you're talking to. I know you better than anyone else and I know that you have been very curt with me the last few weeks."

"I didn't think I was." Her mind raced, trying to think of what had prompted this. She hadn't thought she'd been acting differently toward him.

Dr. Hillerman came over and sat down next to Valerie and took her hands. "Valerie, I've brought you too far to be treated like this. Now, perhaps you've felt a little stress recently. Perhaps you feel that I've put too much pressure on you?"

Valerie searched for the answer she thought he was looking for. "Oh, no. You've been absolutely wonderful to me, very patient, very understanding."

"So you don't feel the least bit, say, upset with me? There's nothing you'd like to share with me, no problem at all? No utter revulsion at the sight of me? No hatred of me? No thoughts of leaving me to go work for Dr. Rubin?" Hillerman added with deliberate emphasis as he dropped her hands. It was clear now that he already knew the answers.

Valerie flushed with fear. Omniscience was not a trait she had attributed to Hillerman before. So how could he know? How did he find out? She struggled to answer. "No, of course not. I'm very attracted to you—you're a very handsome man. It's just, well, you know—"

"Yes, I do know. Valerie, I know that it is in very poor taste to leave a Dear John letter on your computer. Especially a networked computer that anyone could access at any time. Don't you agree?"

Her heart began to pound. Oh shit, oh shit. Say something. A denial, an explanation, something.

"Oh, that." She tried to sound light, but her voice betrayed her. "No, no, that was just a writing exercise. It really had nothing to do with us."

Hillerman smiled devilishly. He enjoyed watching Valerie try to squirm out of trouble. "Not bad. Did you have that ready-made, or can you think on your feet that quickly?"

Valerie scrambled for the right words, and it showed. "Well, we had talked about, you know, maybe ending our relationship before. And I started to, I mean, back then I—uh, tried to get my thoughts together on paper, you know, get organized, and maybe I rambled on a bit."

"Oh. I wouldn't call them ramblings." Hillerman got up and walked over to his desk. He opened his drawer, pulled out a piece of paper, and pretended to read. "They seemed like sincere, pointed thoughts."

"No, no, you misunderstood. I think you're just wonderful, really. In fact, I worry that you really deserve someone better than me. Someone smarter, more accomplished, you know, a little more worldly." She studied his face as she spoke. Did she read him right? He always seemed overly susceptible to flattery. She thought she saw a sign it was working. She decided to continue. "If I really felt that way, I would have told you, I wouldn't have typed it up and never sent it to you, would I? I'm very happy with you, who wouldn't be?" She managed a seductive smile. "How can I prove it to you?"

Hillerman walked back over to where she was sitting. He stood in front of her and cupped her face in his hands. He smiled and flipped Valerie's flaxen hair over her shoulder and leaned down to whisper in her ear, "I suppose the way you always have."

33

The final days before trial brought with them a mixed emotional bag of hope, anger, and fear for Rebecca. As soon as she settled into one feeling, the others took hold. Preparing for trial was always nerve-racking and pressure-filled, but never before was it so achingly personal. Tom was luckier. He was so busy preparing for trial, he had little time to let any sensation other than exhaustion take hold. He had interviewed more witnesses than he could count, gone through the evidence with a fine-tooth comb, and searched for answers where none could be found. The biggest trial of his career and the best he could say after all this is, "Trust me. She didn't do it."

On the morning of the first day of trial, the media savvy political extremists were out in force to take advantage of the intense interest the case had generated. They crowded the courthouse, posters in tow, selling their brand of philosophical beliefs toward every red light that blinked their way. "Vengeance is ours, sayeth the children." "Six down, the rest to go!" "Child molesters have a constitutional right—To Die!"

"Don't give them freedom, give them death!" Virtually every car that passed honked their approval. Thumbs-up from passing motorists abounded. No one held any signs for the dead men.

Rebecca missed the throngs of people on the street. She was transported from the jail to the court-house away from the glare of the media spotlight. Inside, she was taken to a room where she could change into the conservative, tailored dark green business suit Tom had selected from her wardrobe at home. Tom had offered to bring her makeup as well, but she couldn't go along with the deceit. She spent twenty-three hours a day indoors, got at best two to three hours of fitful sleep a night, and spent both her waking and sleeping hours worrying. A little blush and lipstick wasn't going to fool anyone.

"All rise. Court is now in session. The Honorable Frederick H. Delacroix presiding." Rebecca had a pang of sadness. Delacroix. He'd been the presiding judge in her first felony case. Despite his reputation for dressing down rookies, he was surprisingly gentle and tolerant of her. She cherished the note he had sent her boss commending her performance. She had come before him a few times since then and always enjoyed the time spent in his chambers. When he was away from the bench he was charming, regaling attorneys with stories of his boyhood in his native Louisiana, arguing politics with the conservatively bent prosecutors, and proudly displaying pictures of his ever-growing brood of grandchildren. She felt as if she had somehow let him down, coming into his court as the accused and not as the accuser. It just wouldn't end, she feared. She was letting down everyone who mattered to her.

"Good morning," Judge Delacroix announced as he took the bench. A large man who dominated his courtroom both physically and mentally, he was all contrasts—with his shock of white hair atop deep mahogany skin and a booming, intimidating voice that gave way to ready laughter. "This is the matter of the People versus Fielding. Is Ms. Fielding present?" Delacroix inquired, knowing full well that she was. Sadly, Rebecca was the first defendant that Delacroix could pick out of a lineup.

"Yes, she is," Tom responded, confirming the obvious.

"Are the People ready to proceed?"

"Yes, Your Honor," Covington said, her voice strong as usual. She masked her excitement at trying the case of her professional life by maintaining her cool professional demeanor. She knew that the first words were always the hardest to get out, but once they were past, her nerves would give way to an adrenaline rush that would push her through to the end of the trial.

"Mr. Baldwin, are you ready?"

"Yes, Your Honor."

"Then let's proceed with picking a jury."

The words hit Rebecca hard. This was the day she had long hoped for, but now she was fearing it. Was it the beginning of the end or the beginning of the beginning? Rebecca wondered. She turned to the gallery of spectators, hoping to find some inspiration. It was there. Jack was in the last row, wearing a homemade button that said Be Strong. He winked, but instead of the usual twinkle, Rebecca could see the pain in his eyes.

After Delacroix advised each of the prospective jurors that there were no right or wrong answers, only honest ones, the process of selection began. The remainder of the first day and all of the next two were taken up with juror examination, each side trying to get not the proverbial impartial jury but one biased in their favor. Impartiality only got in the way of winning. Covington sought out for removal jurors who would be too sympathetic to Fielding, too emotional in their evaluation of the case, or those who seemed unable to send a pretty woman to the gas chamber. She wanted dispassionate bean counters who would vote with the facts, not with their feelings—those for whom two and two equaled four, and never anything else. The last thing Covington wanted was a juror who saw gray instead of black and white, or one who thought child molesters deserved a bullet or two in the head.

Tom used his shot at the jurors to tell Rebecca's side of the case. Eleven to one for conviction was still a victory for Rebecca, so Baldwin sought out the one person who believed that eyewitnesses can make mistakes, that innocent people are prosecuted, that child molesters receive sentences that are too light, or that it is not unusual for someone to care too deeply about her work. He knew, however, that picking a jury was only slightly more scientific than voodoo, although voodoo probably had a better record for accuracy. Tom had often joked that trying to choose twelve of your fellow citizens who you believed would see the case your way was like trying to pick a winner at the racetrack by talking to the horses.

The process yielded nine men and three women. Covington was satisfied. Even if the men were initially taken by Rebecca's beauty, she felt that a few crime scene photos of mutilated victims would quickly sober them up. As for the women, Covington was pleased that they were older retirees, very conservative, from the era when incest wasn't talked about or, for that matter, believed. Tom was too superstitious to admit to any contentment with the panel, but he felt pleased with two of the male jurors who kept smiling at Rebecca, and he hoped their ardor wouldn't fade.

With the jury seated and court adjourned for the day, Tom's attention turned to Rebecca. She had done a good job maintaining her composure, but it was clear that she was overdrawn at the emotional bank. As usual, Tom didn't have a clue what to do for her. At least he was consistent.

As Larson watched Rebecca being led away, his growing frustration consumed him. It was not helped any when he noticed an unfamiliar sight several rows in front of him get up to leave—Frank LaPaca in a conservative blue suit. Frank was just as surprised to see him and headed quickly out the door and down the hall to the escalator, but he was grabbed from behind. Jack spun him around and slammed him up against the wall. "So, Tinkerbell, you think I was harassing you before? You want to see some real harassment?"

"I—I don't know what you're talking about," Frank stammered, his eyes darting from side to side, looking in vain for help. "You better get your hands off of me, or I'll, I'll—"

Jack pulled Frank toward him then rammed him again into the wall. "Or you'll what, complain about me to the chief again?"

"You can't treat me like this." Frank tried to twist out of Larson's grasp.

"Oh yes I can. I'm getting real sick of you, Frankie. Or was it Barbie? You tell me what the hell you're doing here. What, you want to make sure Rebecca gets convicted so you're off the hook?"

"What are you talking about? I thought we were on the same side. I didn't mean to get you in trouble. I never complained about you to anyone. When Kingsley asked us if we had been contacted by the police, I just mentioned that you'd come by to ask me questions. She must have blown it out of proportion. I—I never meant to get you in trouble," Frank sputtered.

"I don't give a shit what you meant. Just tell me, Frankie"—he leaned in to whisper into Frank's ear—"how'd it feel to stick the knife up Knight's ass? Did you like it? Or did you wish it was your dick instead?"

Frank started crying. "I didn't kill anyone. I told you, it was Hillerman. He's the one you want."

Larson decided it was time to run a bluff. "Then why were hairs that match your wig found at the murder scenes? I know why, Frank. And pretty soon, everyone else will know, too."

Frank's eyes filled with panic as he shook uncontrollably. "Hillerman must be setting me up. I know he's got it in for me. He probably got Kingsley to get him some of my hair. It wouldn't be hard, you wouldn't believe how my wig sheds. I bet that's what it is. You've got it all wrong. It's not me. I swear it."

"You better come up with something better than that, Frank. I'm not about to let Rebecca take your fall. Now, are you ready to come clean?"

"I'm telling you the truth. Really, I am," Frank sobbed.

"I want you to listen to me and listen real close. When I come to arrest you, I'm gonna fuck you up so bad that they're going to have to unscrew your ass in order to find your head. You understand what I'm saying?" Frank nodded, eyes squeezed shut. Larson loosened his grip and Frank scampered down the hall.

"I thought we were friends. I was only trying to help you," he shouted back at Larson as soon as he was safely out of reach. "I guess I was wrong about you. You're just like everyone else."

34

Opening statements brought with them a packed courtroom. With a dearth of grieving family members, the seats were packed instead with journalists, trial groupies, and interested spectators. Covington knew that she would be all over the news tonight and had worked nearly as hard on her appearance as on her speech. She wore a peach-colored suit with a white silk scooped neck blouse and the requisite small strand of faux pearls. To complement her outfit, she pulled her hair back into a French braid and adorned it with an oversized orange bow. Unfortunately, rather than oozing femininity, Covington looked more like a pit bull in a tutu.

Covington stood slowly, walked over to the jury box, and began looking squarely at juror number one. By the time she finished, she would have made eye contact with each of them, holding their gaze firmly yet amiably, entreating them to accept what she was saying as the gospel and offering herself as the voice of truth. If she could have wrapped herself up in the flag, she probably would have.

"Good morning, ladies and gentlemen," Covington began.

The court reporter snapped into action as if a quarter had been dropped into her automatic fingers.

"As you know, my name is Diane Covington and I am the district attorney assigned to prosecute this case. What you are about to hear may sound shocking to you and, on some level, may even seem inconceivable. Indeed, it is unheard of for a respected prosecutor to commit murder. However, sometimes our expectations are shattered by the unthinkable. And the defendant in this case, Rebecca Fielding, has done the unthinkable." Covington allowed her voice to trail off for added effect. She let a few beats pass as her words penetrated the jury, then she roared back to life. "What started long ago as an honorable spark in the defendant to prosecute child molesters to the fullest extent of the law somewhere down the line exploded into a firestorm that flouted the law. That woman sitting over there," Covington angrily shouted while pointing at Rebecca, "is a cold-blooded, ruthless killer. Plain and simple." She watched with satisfaction as the entire jury reflexively turned to look at the accused defendant.

Rebecca was startled when she looked up to see Covington pointing directly at her. She wanted to scream, "No! Don't listen to her!" But her role as defendant required she just sit there quietly and take it while Covington engaged in cheap grandstanding tactics. Covington's reputation for theatrics apparently was not undeserved, she thought. Yet she knew she would do the same—and even more—to secure a conviction.

"The unmistakable truth is that the defendant abused her position as a district attorney to foster her own agenda, an agenda that included the brutal and savage slayings of six convicted child molesters.

Some may consider the defendant's agenda a noble one. However, it is important for you to remember that although these men may have committed offensive crimes many years ago, those crimes were not punishable by death. These men were serving their sentences as required by law. They simply did not deserve to die."

Covington paused and looked over at Rebecca, as if she were challenging Rebecca to stand up and tell the truth. Then she spoke. "You may ask yourself: what would possess this attractive young woman to toss aside her career as a successful prosecutor in order to become a self-appointed executioner?" Covington looked back over to the jury. "The answer to this question is simple," she said softly. "The defendant hated all child molesters, particularly those she perceived to have outmaneuvered her in a court of law. Rather than recognizing that her job was solely to prosecute these men, the defendant could not leave well enough alone. Her obsession grew out of control until she meted out her own brand of justice. An insidious and horrifying justice."

Covington noted with pleasure that the jury seemed to hang on her every word. "The contempt that initially motivated the defendant to make our streets safe for our children somehow mutated into a hatred that saw the law as weak and ineffective and in need of the assistance of a self-proclaimed vigilante. However, as a society we must"—she slammed her fist down on the podium—"demand that our prosecutors enforce the law in a court, and not with the barrel of a gun. Our prosecutors must strive for law and order, not reorder the law as they see fit. As a society, we must"—she slammed her fist down again—"send a strong message that not only must children be free from molestation, but the law must be free from molestation." From the looks on their faces, Covington half-expected the jurors to return her plea with a resounding "Hallelujah!"

It did not take long for Rebecca's inner strength to begin to falter. Although Covington's opening statement had only begun, Rebecca was already becoming demoralized, fearing that the jury would act simply as a twelve-member rubber stamp for the prosecution and bring home the verdict everyone expected. She had promised herself that whatever happened, she would maintain her composure and always look in control. She did not want the jury to smell fear. Unfortunately, she wore her emotions on her sleeve for all to see. Unsure what to do, Rebecca simply stared at the jury, hoping against all hope that they recognized her innocence as easily as they recognized her trepidation.

Covington had hit her stride and was alive with adrenaline. "The evidence developed in this case is largely circumstantial, but it is no less real and no less compelling. Taken as a whole, the evidence proves the defendant's guilt beyond a reasonable doubt. Starting on the third of September last year, the defendant embarked upon a vicious and brutal spree. Before it was over, Eric Penhall, William Matheson, Bradley Knight, Steven Jaffe, Harold Riddell, and James Hempstead were dead. The defendant admits to killing the last victim, Mr. Hempstead. Incredibly, even though the evidence will establish that all of the killings were related, the defendant contends that she had nothing to do with the other killings. The defendant's contention simply does not hold water, particularly since, as you will see, there is an abundance of facts that conclusively tie the defendant to each murder."

Covington paused, watching the jury scribble in their notebooks. She saw no reason to rush and certainly did not want anything she said to be missed. "Mr. Penhall was first. After lying in wait by hiding in the underground parking garage of Mr. Penhall's apartment the defendant shot him six times at close range. The fact that Mr. Penhall was killed at his apartment complex is itself noteworthy. Indeed, Mr. Penhall had only recently moved into that building. Except for his probation officer and therapist, Mr. Penhall had yet to advise anyone of his new address, including the post office. Why is this significant?" Covington looked over the jury box from end to end, almost as if she were waiting for one of them to raise their hand with the answer, then continued. "It is significant, because in the personal file that the defendant maintained on Mr. Penhall, she had his new address. Nobody else knew how to find Mr. Penhall, but the defendant did." Covington stopped and then innocently looked up. "Oh, and one more thing, immediately after the murder, an eyewitness spotted the defendant leaving the garage."

Tom flew to his feet. "Objection, Your Honor. This is outrageous. Ms. Covington knows better than to do that. May we approach the bench?" Tom knew that by objecting he may have just committed the cardinal mistake of highlighting for the jury a very bad fact, but he had to take that risk in order to find out about this supposed witness, a witness he knew nothing about.

Covington stayed at the podium. "Your Honor, with all due respect, Mr. Baldwin is completely out of line. If he has a specific objection, he should make it. 'Outrageous' is not a legally recognized objection. It is wholly inappropriate for Mr. Baldwin to interrupt my opening statement and prejudice the jury with his unnecessary acrimonious accusations." She looked over at the jury apologetically, as if sorry about her impudent colleague's performance.

"Counsel, please approach," Judge Delacroix signaled to the attorneys.

Tom was so infuriated he could not even look at

Covington. He hated being sandbagged. "Your Honor, at no point during any of the pretrial discovery did the government identify any witness in connection with the Penhall murder," he began.

Delacroix raised his eyebrows. "Is that true, Ms. Covington?"

"Yes, but—"

"Clearly, such a key witness should have been disclosed long ago," Tom interrupted.

"Let me explain," Covington began. "It was not until—"

Tom interrupted again, his voice raspy from the effort to shout quietly. "Your Honor, the only appropriate thing is for you to declare a mistrial. The first time that we learn of such a key witness should not be in opening statements. How can I prepare for my opening statement without knowing anything about this witness?"

Delacroix put his hand up. "Counsel, I can't and won't listen to both of you speak at once. Now Mr. Baldwin, you will have your opportunity. But I want to hear from Ms. Covington first. Ms. Covington, why was this eyewitness not disclosed earlier?"

"If I may explain, Your Honor." Covington cast a sideways glance at Tom. "Had the People known of this witness earlier, we, of course, would have disclosed his identity. But we did not learn of him until just last night. Apparently, he had seen reports of this case on TV and finally decided to come forward and tell what he saw."

"Ms. Covington, prior to yesterday, did you or the police have any inkling that there was an eyewitness to the Penhall murder?" Delacroix asked, his expression dubious at best.

"No," Covington said decisively. "Absolutely not. And I resent Mr. Baldwin's insinuations." She glared at Tom.

Delacroix knew Covington could swallow battery acid without changing her expression and his gut told him she'd push the discovery envelope as far as she could, but that wasn't enough to grant Tom the relief he sought. "All right, Counselor. At this time, I'm going to deny the motion for a mistrial. However, Ms. Covington, if I learn that your office or the police knew about this witness, I will throw this case out and dismiss all charges. I have no tolerance for prosecutorial misconduct. Now, I agree with Mr. Baldwin that he should not be penalized, so I assume, Ms. Covington, that you will turn over all the information you have about this new witness at the close of your opening statement so the defense can review it prior to their opening?"

Covington nodded. "Yes, Your Honor."

"Fine. Counsel, you may return to your seats."

"What was that all about?" Rebecca whispered, already knowing the answer.

Tom forced a smile on his face, feeling the jury's watchful eyes on him. "Evidently, they found someone last night who can place you at the scene of Penhall's murder."

Rebecca's fear was palpable. "Who?"

Tom patted her hand reassuringly, wanting to convey to her—and the jury—that this was not bad news. "I don't know yet. We'll find out when we break."

"If you are ready to proceed, Ms. Covington, you may continue," Delacroix instructed.

Covington was glad to have dodged that bullet. The last thing she wanted was to lose such a high-profile case during opening statements. She walked back to the podium, checked to find her place, then moved back toward the jury. "After Mr. Penhall, the defendant's next victim was Mr. Matheson. Mr. Matheson was shot four times—twice in the head and another two times in the knees as he tried to crawl away—with .22-caliber, hollow-nosed bullets. These were the same kind as those used to kill Mr. Penhall and later, three more of the victims. Remember that. Also, wool fibers from a jacket worn by the defendant were found on Mr. Matheson's door. In addition, long, blonde hairs were found next to Mr. Matheson's body. Those hairs are consistent with the defendant as well. And, most significantly, Rebecca Fielding's palm print was found on the door of Mr. Matheson's apartment.

"Third to die was Mr. Knight, another man the defendant had prosecuted to what the defendant considered an unsuccessful conclusion. This man was kidnapped in his own van, where he was stabbed repeatedly. Again, keep in mind the mechanism at work here—the kidnapping—as it will be relevant when we look at the murder of the final victim. Now, with respect to Mr. Knight, he was abducted after leaving a standing medical appointment, which the defendant had noted in her own date book. And, again, the defendant's hairs were left in his car, next to his bloodied body."

Covington looked down at her notes. She mulled over them for a minute and she then stepped back from the podium and continued, walking slowly over to the jury box. "The defendant then turned her evil attention to Mr. Jaffe, a man virtually unrecognizable by the time his rotting body was found. He was shot in the head at close range by the defendant. Again, .22-caliber, hollow-nosed bullets were used, the same as in the Penhall and Matheson murders. It is noteworthy that, in the months preceding his death, Mr. Jaffe had become something of a recluse, using a post office box as his official address and keeping a very low profile. And yet in her personal files, the defendant had up-to-the-minute information on his comings and goings, including quite accurate directions to his house in a remote area up in the hills.. Curious indeed." Covington knew that, other than the bullets matching those from the other gunshot victims, there was not a lot of evidence that tied Rebecca to the Jaffe killing. Yet she was not worried. The jurors all remained on the edge of their seats and seemed to be soaking in everything she said. Besides, five murder convictions were as good as six, she figured.

"The defendant's next victim was Mr. Riddell. The defendant surprised him in his apartment, shot his dog, then brutally and repeatedly stabbed Mr. Riddell. An eyewitness can place the defendant outside Mr. Riddell's apartment on the night of the murder." Almost in unison the jury turned to look at Rebecca. She knew she was supposed to meet their gaze, yet she couldn't bring herself to look at them. Diane observed this with supreme satisfaction. "And finally, the last victim in this horrible, but highly consistent, killing spree was Mr. Hempstead. The defendant admits to shooting and killing Mr. Hempstead while he was sitting, unarmed, in his car. The parallels between the Knight murder—where he was abducted from a strip center parking lot then killed in his vehicle—and the Hempstead murder are clear.

"One killer, six victims." Covington paused, not out of necessity, but simply for the drama. "It is important to remember that the defendant is not claiming insanity as a defense, nor could she. The defendant acted in a rational, clear-headed, and deliberate manner while she carried out these slaughters. Each victim had been carefully selected, stalked, and then ambushed and brutally murdered. The defendant's highly unusual, obsessive preoccupation with these men motivated her to mete out her own brand of punishment—death. The defendant mocked justice and her esteemed position as the defender of justice. She became what she detested, a shameless and unrepentant criminal, abusing her power as a tool for revenge." Covington stepped back toward the center of the jury box and leaned forward, putting her hands on the railing. She looked at juror number one, then moved her gaze slowly to each juror. "Yes, this is an unusual and difficult case. But the evidence demands only one result. Rebecca Fielding is guilty as charged of six counts of murder in the first degree. Thank you."

Covington bowed her head slightly then strode confidently back to her seat. She was still smiling when Delacroix spoke, surprising her with his bluntness. "Ladies and gentlemen," he said to the jury, "because of the failure of the People to notify the defense concerning one of their witnesses, we will have to delay the beginning of the defense's opening statement." Delacroix glared at Covington until she dropped the smile. "I apologize for this delay," he continued. "We will adjourn now and reconvene at one-thirty." He smacked his gavel down as he locked eyes with Covington.

Tom hoped the jury understood what had happened. He could use some good will before he began. He said a quick good-bye to Rebecca before she was taken out of court and then headed upstairs to the D.A.'s office to take a look at the file on the new witness, a file he prayed would not impress him.

Stan chose the privacy of a phone booth over the mobility of his cellular phone. Some conversations were open to varying interpretations. There was no need to make this one public.

"So?" was Hillerman's only greeting.

Stan let his usual reserve give way to a slight case of overconfidence. "Well, Bob, if it's true that most juries make up their minds after opening statements, you won't have to worry about Ms. Fielding anymore. She's as good as convicted," he crowed.

Hillerman exhaled loudly. "That's what I wanted to hear. But how can you be so sure?"

Stan looked at the throng gathered outside the phone booth, a jumble of cameras and microphones. He heard the muffled shouts as the reporters tried to get a quote from the lawyers heading down the hall. "Because there's enough for each murder—some hairs here, some fibers there, even a fingerprint or two. You should have been here. The D.A. wove the evidence together nicely. I don't see what the defense can do to overcome all that." The relief in his voice conveyed as much as his words.

Hillerman leaned back in his chair and put his feet up on his desk. "Stan, sometimes I think I don't pay you enough."

"Funny, I think that all the time."

"Where are you calling from? What's all that noise?"

"Don't worry, no one can hear me. I can barely hear myself." Stan watched with amusement as the show continued just outside.

"All right, as long as you're keeping a low profile."

"Not to worry."

Hillerman flipped on the television and found a live remote from the courthouse. He was pleased that Stan was nowhere in view. "So where do we go from here?"

"I'm not sure we need to go anywhere. I'll stick around for the defense opening, and after that I think we can just sit back and relax. I think we've done enough for now. I don't want to overplay our hand."

"Well, don't let up just yet. I want to make sure that we are well rid of her."

Stan smiled. "Look who you're talking to. I know

better than to let up now. But I think we should step back for a minute. After what I saw this morning, I don't think the D.A. will rest until she gets a conviction."

"Excellent. So you never told me, was that Covington woman at all suspicious about why we knew so much?"

"Hard to tell. I think she was just happy to have the information. I don't think she cared much about the whys or hows. But you certainly can take credit for giving her the little touches that make Fielding look like a scheming assassin."

"Excellent. Ms. Fielding should now understand the concept of what goes around, comes around."

Stan chuckled. "Bob, I gotta run. I've got a mob here lining up to use the phone. I'll be by later to talk with Valerie and Anita about their testimony."

"Thanks, Stan. I'm going to note this call for posterity. You so rarely call me with good news." Hillerman let out a hearty laugh, part amusement, part relief. "I still can't believe things are working out so well."

Covington looked across the salad bar to see Jack staring absentmindedly at the spread. She had just finished with Tom, enjoying the spectacle of his face turning pale as he learned the details about her new witness, and now here was Jack. A little verbal sparring would help keep her sharp for court this afternoon. "Well, if it isn't Detective Larson. You've been as elusive as ever. You wouldn't be trying to avoid me?" Jack didn't answer. "Don't you want to catch up on old times? Oh, I know, you must have lost my number. Or maybe your dog ate it."

In the light of day, Jack thought, Covington was quite the bitch. Too bad that bar had been so dark and he'd been so drunk. "Glad to see you don't hold any grudges, Counselor."

Covington smiled as she attended to her plate, speaking to Jack without looking up. "No, I don't have time for grudges. I've got this big death penalty case that takes up all my time. Maybe you've heard of it?" she said, quite amused with herself.

"Look, if you're pissed off that I never called you back, don't take it out on Rebecca."

Covington looked up from her salad. "You should give me more credit than that. I'm a big girl. I take responsibility for my own actions. Unlike others." The crocodile smiled, baring deadly teeth.

Jack found it interesting that someone who pretended she was so unaffected by their one-night stand couldn't pass up the chance to mention it every time she saw him. "This is ridiculous. This is someone's life we're talking about."

Covington's tone switched to deadly serious. "No, we are talking about six people who no longer have their lives. My job is to get a conviction, and that's what I intend to do. What are you trying to do? Protect your girlfriend, or maybe even your reputation? Let's see, you couldn't solve the murders even though the killer was right under your nose. Or was that right under your sheets?"

"You're very lucky we're in public," Jack said, seething.

Covington moved in closer, standing just under his chin, and looking up at him. "Or what would you do, seduce me to death?"

Jack had been looking for an outlet for his pent-up anger and frustration and this occasion fit the bill. "You know, I don't believe in hitting a woman, but that wouldn't stop me in your case. Fortunately for you, I'm not about to make a scene on your behalf. Just tell me, what are you going to do for a living after you lose the biggest case of your mediocre career? I suppose you could be a waitress in a truck stop. You sure know how to serve up shit."

She turned from him and continued piling food on her plate. "You know, Detective, I'm not the one who compromised the investigation because I decided to let my little head do all the thinking."

"What the fuck are you talking about? You're way off, sweetheart. Your killer's not downstairs. Try over at Oakwood."

Covington placed a couple of peppers on top and stopped to admire her well-stacked lunch. Then she turned back to face Larson, holding her plate between both hands. "Fine, Detective. Enjoy your little theories while you can. When it finally comes out how you had Henderson bumped off the case so he wouldn't find out about Rebecca, you're going to have plenty of explaining to do. Don't get too comfortable with that badge. You may not have it much longer."

Jack moved closer. "Are you threatening me?"

"Nope. It's a simple statement of fact. You've been uncooperative and stonewalling, and it's going to end. I can subpoena your ass and have you tell the world what you know. You either tell the truth or share your beloved's jail experience, it's up to you. But I know that you know plenty. It's going to be ugly." She smiled broadly. "But fun."

Jack's nostrils flared and his jaw thrust forward, but he kept himself from exploding, knowing nothing would be accomplished in the momentary release. And yet it was hard to ignore the overwhelming urge to push Covington's face into the potato salad. "The only fun is going to be watching Rebecca walk out of here a free woman and you trying to double-talk your way out of town. You're just going to be another in a long line of pathetic losing prosecutors."

Covington laughed. "Don't bet on it. More likely

that you're going to be another in line at the unemployment department. You'll look quite dapper in one of those security officer uniforms patrolling the mall, if you're lucky enough to get one of those jobs. Or you can become a walking stereotype and drink yourself to an early grave. I really don't care. You just think about this—it's your job or Rebecca. You choose."

He turned to walk away.

Covington called after him. "Oh, and by the way, Detective, if you ever get lonely, you know where to find me. I kind of enjoyed our time together."

As the afternoon session began, Tom rose, knowing that it was his job to explain away the unexplainable. A difficult job made more difficult by the fact the jury had a two-hour break to let the prosecution's opening sink in.

"Good afternoon, ladies and gentlemen." Tom looked at each juror for a moment, and smiled as he nodded in greeting. "My name is Thomas Xavier Baldwin and I am representing the defendant, Rebecca Ann Fielding." He gestured respectfully toward Rebecca, then spoke with measured emphasis. "Miss Fielding is not guilty of murdering anyone. She is not some vicious, cold-blooded, serial killer out to rid the world of child molesters. Instead, she is and has been for ten years a devoted and tireless fighter for the rights of the innocent, children whose lives have been irrever-sibly destroyed by adults who violated their trust. She has, it's true, tried to see that justice was done. But she has worked within the system, the system she believes in."

Tom walked slowly back and forth in front of the jury to keep their attention focused on what he was saying. "As the evidence will show, the prosecution's case is all smoke and mirrors. As one dead child molester after another turned up, the police were increasingly charged with dragging their feet in the investigation, putting out less than maximum effort because the victims were such vile, disgusting, criminal scum. To deflect the negative attention they were receiving, the police and the district attorney's office jumped at the chance to serve up Rebecca on a plate simply because she was forced to shoot Mr. Hempstead in self-defense after he abducted her.

"The evidence will show that Rebecca was the one who was stalked, followed by Mr. Hempstead as she left a television studio where she went on the air decrying the lack of tough sentences handed out to child molesters. Mr. Hempstead, himself a convicted child molester, had been drinking heavily as he watched Rebecca on television. He drove the short distance from his apartment to the studio, followed her, and then jumped her as she exited her car, dragged her to his car, and began to drive away with her as his hostage. Rebecca took the gun she carried in her purse for safety, and shot him. And thank God she did; otherwise, she undoubtedly would have been killed herself.

"Simply because Mr. Hempstead was a child molester, the police and district attorney thought, Wouldn't it be great if we could sew up all those unsolved killings by pinning them on Rebecca Fielding?" Tom leaned forward over the railing of the jury box as he looked from left to right at each juror. He was concerned. Already two of the jurors, a middle-aged man who worked in the insurance industry and an elderly woman, seemed disinterested in what he had to say.

Tom pressed on, with an eye to bringing them back to their sworn position of neutrality. "Since she had killed one child molester, why not just infer that she must have killed the other five?" Tom straight-ened back up. "But there is a problem with their the-ory. The killing of Mr. Hempstead is wholly different from the other five killings. He was killed in a public area, surrounded by witnesses, killed in a fit of panic and fear so great that Rebecca ran screaming from the car after she shot him, left her gun in the car, ran past those witnesses, entered her car, and drove home, where she collapsed in the same blood-soaked clothes after sobbing herself to sleep." Tom shook his head slowly, in disbelief at the prosecution's theory. "These were not the acts of a ruthless calculating killer trying to avoid detection so that she might kill again. These were the acts of a scared victim of vio-lence, frightened by her narrow escape from death, and desperate to get to the safety and security of her own bed." Tom's voice built to a crescendo of pas-sionate conviction.

"Rebecca has admitted to the self-defense shoot-ing of Mr. Hempstead. She was not trying to hide anything. There is no reason to. Anyone in her situa-tion would have felt the fear and panic she felt, would have felt their life was in danger, and would have acted to save their own life." Tom stared at the jury. "But, ladies and gentlemen, Rebecca Fielding was not involved in any way with the other killings.

"And just what is this evidence that the prosecu-tion is promising you?" Tom asked incredulously, looking around as if trying to find it. "What is this evidence that is supposed to convince you of Rebecca's guilt in the other killings? That too is noth-ing more than smoke and mirrors. Rebecca does not deny that she maintained files on these men, and on every other single defendant who she prosecuted— over a hundred different men and women. Did Rebecca leave her job at the office? No. She cared, maybe too much for Ms. Covington's tastes. But not

too much for the victims she wanted to help, who
were only too happy to find that someone in the system wanted to see justice done. Did she keep track
of the defendants she prosecuted? You bet she did."
Tom nodded, answering his own question. "No one
knows better than Rebecca how overworked the probation department is. And if she could act as a fail-
safe device, keeping tabs on the defendants, making
sure they were complying with their probation, then
she could sleep better at night. And so could we all."

Tom now reached the part of his prepared speech
about Mildred Walker, which he had hastily rewritten
over lunch to include the new witness. "Ms. Covington
is promising you eyewitness testimony. Now, from
watching television and the movies, you may believe
that eyewitness testimony is ironclad, put-'em-away
testimony. But listen carefully to the so-called eyewitnesses in this case. What you will hear is that they
each saw what looked like a blonde woman near the
scene of two of the murders. That's it. They don't know
if what they saw was really a man dressed as a
woman, or a black-haired woman wearing a wig, or
some woman who looks like Rebecca. And most significantly, they do not know if the person they saw was
the killer or just someone who happened to be in the
area. And they do not know if they identified Rebecca
as the person they saw simply because she looked
familiar from having been on television just before her
arrest. There is nothing magical about the prosecution's purported eyewitness testimony. It is of no use in
deciding this case."

Tom prepared to tread lightly. He and Rebecca
had still not decided whether she would take the
stand in her own defense, so he didn't want to
promise the jury they'd hear from her. Yet, he
wanted to impress upon them their responsibility to
withhold a final decision until the case was submit-

ted to them. "After you've heard all the evidence, and had an opportunity to get to know Rebecca, you will see that she is the victim here—the victim of overzealous prosecutors, frustrated police officers, and the natural desire that every mystery should have a solution. The killings of the five child molesters remain unsolved. The killer or killers are still free. The only mystery is why Rebecca Fielding, who has devoted her life to prosecuting criminals and defending the innocent, should herself be on trial for her very life. We may not be able to solve that mystery, but we can give Rebecca her life back. Thank you." Tom returned to his seat. Rebecca reached for his arm and gave it a gentle squeeze in thanks.

"Okay, this is a good place to stop," said Delacroix. "Let's reconvene at nine o'clock tomorrow."

35

Tom squeezed Rebecca's hand. "You ready?" he whispered.

She smiled and nodded convincingly, though her heart pounded in her chest as the fear of actually hearing the prosecution's witnesses swept over her. She watched the twelve sitting in judgment of her, looking for a sign of hope. Instead, they sat impassively, staring straight ahead, no one returning her beseeching gaze. Rebecca knew right then that Covington may have already succeeded in distancing the jury from her.

"Are the People ready to call their first witness?" Judge Delacroix asked.

"Yes, Your Honor. The People call Detective Jonas Henderson."

Henderson strode confidently up to the stand, leaving a wake of sickly sweet cologne in his path. He couldn't hide his enjoyment of what he viewed as a once-in-a-lifetime opportunity to even the score with a district attorney's office that always took credit for their victories while giving the police the blame for their losses. And what an added pleasure, getting to personally stuff Larson at the same time. That should teach him to keep his nose out of other people's cases, Henderson thought.

Covington stacked her notes on top of the podium. "Detective Henderson, by whom are you employed?" she began.

"The Los Angeles Police Department."

"Were you assigned to investigate the murders of the deceased?" Covington knew better than to refer to the dead men as dead child molesters. She left it up to Baldwin to remind the jury that the victims were no saints.

"Yes, I was."

"And as part of that investigation, did you have the opportunity to investigate the defendant, Rebecca Fielding?" Covington walked over to the jury, causing Henderson to turn and face them.

"Yes."

"And why was that?"

Henderson leaned forward. "When the third and fourth victims turned up dead, I decided that we should make a concerted effort to identify a common denominator among the four," he said, tossing an "aren't I smart" smile toward the jury. Henderson had no compunction about portraying himself as being in charge of the entire investigation and responsible for catching the killer. "The defendant's name came up in that context."

"And why was that?"

"Because she knew all the men and made no bones about the fact that she disliked them intensely," he said, nodding his head slightly in Rebecca's direction.

"Was she the only common denominator?" Covington wanted to dispel the rush-to-judgment notion.

Henderson shook his head. "Oh no, there were others. If she'd been the only one, we might have been able to save a few lives. No, she made it tough on us. She covered her tracks pretty well. But not well enough."

Baldwin sprang to his feet, incensed. "Objection, Your Honor, there is absolutely no foundation for any of this."

"Sustained. Detective Henderson, please save the embellishments for outside the courtroom." Judge Delacroix knew there was ample opportunity for both sides to put their spin on the evidence to anyone with a microphone or a camera, and both had already done more than their share.

"I'm sorry, Your Honor." Henderson looked at the jury apologetically, as if to say, "I'm only the messenger."

"Detective, please tell us what you did when you determined that the defendant was one of the common denominators."

"I directed one of the junior detectives, Jennifer Randazzo, to do a background check on the defendant—question the defendant's colleagues, review her personnel file, review her relationship with the deceased. That kind of thing."

"As a result of what you learned from Detective Randazzo, did you continue to include the defendant as a potential suspect in the killings, or was she excluded?"

Henderson nodded. "She was definitely included."

"But you didn't arrest her at that point?"

"Oh, no, we didn't have enough evidence yet."

"Okay. Now, at some time did you have the opportunity to meet the defendant?"

"Yes, I did."

"Can you point her out?"

"Yes, she's sitting right over there, next to Mr. Baldwin." Rebecca flinched automatically, feeling the accusatory nature of the identification. Unfortunately for her, it did not go unnoticed by the jury.

"And, how did you come to meet the defendant?"

Henderson opened his notebook and laid it out flat on the ledge in front of him. "On December second of last year, after she had been arrested for the murder of James Hempstead, she notified us that she wanted to talk to us. Myself, a court reporter, Ms. Fielding, and her attorney, Thomas Baldwin, convened for the interview."

Covington walked over to the counsel table, took some papers off the desk, and then approached Tom, handing him a five-page document with which he was all too familiar. He didn't bother to show it to Rebecca. Then Covington took another copy and handed it to Henderson.

"Detective Henderson—"

"Yes, this is it. This is the transcript of Ms. Fielding's confession."

"Objection, Your Honor, that document is not a confession. It's an explanation of the events surrounding Mr. Hempstead's death," Tom stated firmly.

"Wait a minute, Your Honor," Covington interjected. "When someone says 'I did it,' that is a confession. If Mr. Baldwin belatedly believes he was ill-advised to allow his client to talk to the police, I should not be penalized by having to call a horse a zebra."

A slight chuckle came from the jury box. Score one for the prosecution, Covington thought. She knew that no matter how the judge ruled on the objection, she had one-upped Baldwin in front of the jury.

"Ms. Covington," Judge Delacroix began, "why don't you refer to it as the statement and not a confession?"

Covington nodded her understanding, and continued. "Detective Henderson, you were saying that you met with the defendant concerning Mr. Hempstead's killing, is that correct?"

"Yes, that's correct."

"And the defendant had her attorney, Mr. Baldwin, present during this questioning?"

"Objection, leading."

"Your Honor, this is just foundational," Covington replied, surprised that Tom would object to such an innocuous question.

"Overruled, but watch your questions, Ms. Covington," the judge gently scolded.

"Detective Henderson, do you remember the question?"

"Yes I do and yes she did."

"And what did she tell you about the Hempstead killing?"

"She said, quote, 'I pulled out the gun and shot the man several times, until he slumped down and the car came to a stop,' end quote." Henderson stopped reading and looked up with a pleased smile.

Tom could feel Rebecca tense at hearing her own words used against her. He leaned over and whispered, "Don't worry, I'll get him on cross." Rebecca returned a weak smile.

Covington leaned back on the railing. "So the defendant admitted to you that she shot Mr. Hempstead?"

"Yes, ma'am. As sure as I'm sitting here, that's what she said. It's all in the transcript. She admitted to shooting Mr. Hempstead from behind with her own gun," Henderson said with a self-satisfied grin.

Covington couldn't help but smile. "From behind" was a nice ad-lib. Rebecca's face displayed a markedly different emotion. "Now, Detective, at the time of the Hempstead killing, was the defendant still considered one of the 'common denominators' linking the five other deceased?" she asked.

"She sure was."

"And did you have an opportunity to discuss her knowledge of the murders of the other men at that time?"

Henderson shook his head slowly. "No, ma'am. She and her attorney flat out refused to discuss anything other than the Hempstead killing. Clammed up rather tightly, I might add," Henderson said with a grin.

"So you're telling us she didn't even try to give you an alibi for the other murders? Is that what you're saying?"

Tom rose to his feet with an incredulous look on his face. "Your Honor, in all my years of practice, that is probably the most objectionable question I have ever heard!"

"What's your specific objection, Mr. Baldwin?" Judge Delacroix inquired, not considering "most objectionable" a sufficient ground.

Tom stood silent for a minute, not really sure why the question was objectionable—other than the fact that it was a lousy question that created a horrible inference. He blurted out, "Lack of foundation. It hasn't been established that she needed an alibi for the other killings."

"Overruled."

Tom sat back down, unsure whether any objection would have been sustained or whether he simply could not think of the right one fast enough.

Henderson turned toward the jury. "She just flat-out refused to discuss the other killings. That obviously made me suspicious."

"And why was that?"

"Well, Counselor, because innocent people have nothing to hide." Covington paused long enough for the jury to see the anger on Baldwin's face and the squirm in Rebecca's chair. "Detective, let's go back to the Hempstead murder for a moment. Did the defendant state to you that before she killed Mr. Hempstead, she saw a weapon on him?"

"No, she never mentioned him having any weapon.

She never even said she thought he had one, for that matter." A well-coached witness, Henderson knew what facts were good for the prosecution and would make sure they got out no matter how Covington phrased her questions.

"Was Mr. Hempstead armed with any weapon at the time he was killed?"

"No, ma'am," Henderson stated firmly. "When his body was found he was unarmed and there were no weapons anywhere near his body. We searched his entire car and the surrounding area, and no weapon of any kind was found. Other than the defendant's gun, of course."

"Mr. Hempstead didn't have a knife, a gun, an axe, a hammer, a baseball bat, anything like that?" Covington asked, feigning incredulity.

"No, he had no weapon of any kind in the car. He was completely unarmed." Rebecca looked over at the jury and saw their disapproving faces. She could read a jury with the best of them, and she knew these twelve were wondering why she shot an unarmed man. She instinctively sank into her chair, wondering why she ever thought that she could prove self-defense knowing that Hempstead was unarmed.

Covington walked back to the podium and flipped the page on her notes before circling back around to the side closest to the jury box. "Now, after you met with the defendant, what did you do next?"

"Well, like I said, I was real suspicious of her, so I started looking more closely at the evidence we had collected from the other murder scenes to see if any of it matched the defendant, which it did. So we got a warrant to search her house and her office."

"Were you present when the search warrant was served and executed at her home?"

"Yes, I was."

"And was anything found?"

"Yes, we recovered a knife from her kitchen, a half-empty box of hollow-nosed bullets, a blue jacket, and newspaper clippings concerning the murders of each of the dead men."

"A knife, bullets, and clothing?" Covington repeated for the benefit of the jury.

"Yes, ma'am."

"Did you oversee the forensic analysis of these items?"

"No, I instructed Detective Randazzo to do that." Henderson turned toward the jury. "She'll be testifying about what was learned," he offered, flashing a friendly "stay tuned" smile.

"Okay. Now you mentioned newspaper clippings. Could you tell the jury where they were found and what condition they were in?"

"Yes. Under the defendant's bed, there was a large, flat box, you know, the kind used for family photos, that sort of thing. Anyway, inside were articles concerning each of the first five killings. The articles for each murder placed in a separate folder with the deceased's name on it."

Covington looked at Rebecca and shook her head slightly. The jury picked up on the nonverbal rebuke. "All right, now, Detective, were you also present when the search warrant was executed at the defendant's office?"

"Yes, ma'am."

"Was anything recovered?"

"Quite a bit, as a matter of fact. We found a file cabinet that contained what we later determined to be her personal files on the men she had prosecuted. The files for each of the dead men had a large red X across the front, as if to say 'closed.' These files contained not only the victims' court files, their arrest warrants, indictments, and all the paperwork up through the disposition of their cases, but they also contained information about the victims after their court cases were concluded."

Covington interrupted to slow Henderson down and allow the jury to digest what they were being told. "What else was found in the defendant's office?"

"The defendant had detailed notes about the lives of the victims. There were reports from a private investigator apparently retained by her at her own expense. The PI supplied her with information about what the dead men were up to while they were on probation."

"You mean, after their trials were over?" Covington asked incredulously.

"Yeah. If you can believe it."

Rebecca looked over at Tom, wondering why he wasn't objecting. Someone had to stop this. Her every movement was being twisted around to something evil and sinister, and Tom was doing nothing about it. It was as if he had become paralyzed, she thought. Paralyzed by doubts, she feared. Covington was doing more than just swaying the jury.

"As part of your job as a homicide investigator, have you had an opportunity to work with the district attorney's office?"

"Yes, of course."

"On how many different cases would you say you have worked with the district attorney's office?"

"I'd say hundreds, maybe more."

"Have you ever known any district attorney to keep such personal files?" Covington asked deliberately, forecasting the answer for the jury.

Rebecca looked at Tom for help. He looked back at her sheepishly. Finally, he stood up. "Objection. This witness can't possibly know what each district attorney does." He knew that even if his objection was sustained, the damage had already been done.

Some questions never need to be answered in order to have a devastating impact. This was one of them.

"Withdrawn," Covington said with a wave of her hand. She headed over to the blackboard and nonchalantly posted six color photographs of a bloodied figure only vaguely resembling a human. Audible gasps came from the direction of the jury, and she had to stifle a smile. "Do these photographs accurately depict the nature and extent of Mr. Hempstead's fatal wounds?"

"Yes. As you can see, Mr. Hempstead was shot at point-blank range with hollow-nosed .22-caliber bullets—that's why there's so little left of him. And this was done to him by the defendant, who shot him from behind."

"From your analysis of those photos, and from your analysis of the crime scene, does it look to you like the defendant was in danger when she shot Mr. Hempstead?"

"Objection, calls for speculation."

"Your Honor," Covington responded, "the witness can testify as to his observations and the conclusions he reasonably draws from those observations. Obviously, we don't have to take the defendant's word for what happened."

Tom stared at Covington. "Better that, Counselor, than the word of someone who was not even there," he shot back.

Judge Delacroix was not amused with the extraneous comments. "Detective Henderson, please limit your answer to what you personally know."

"I know Mr. Hempstead was shot from behind. And I know he was unarmed. I find it impossible to believe an unarmed man would attempt to kidnap someone—a young, able-bodied, grown woman—without knocking them unconscious or tying them up in some way, then walk around to the driver's side door, which had its window down, and then start to drive away. If the defendant was in the car against her will, why didn't she run out when he went around to the driver's seat? I never got an answer to that question."

Covington knew that there was no better time to stop than now, with the simple facts left hanging in the air. "I have nothing further, Your Honor. Your witness, Mr. Baldwin."

As Tom headed to the lectern, Rebecca grabbed his arm and motioned for him to lean over. "Tom, we can't win this unless you have faith in me. Don't just go through the motions."

Tom figured it best to say nothing and just start strong, even if he didn't feel particularly strong. Luckily Henderson had left him a big enough opening, one he was surprised Covington hadn't closed. "Detective Henderson, when you conduct an investigation, do you normally just do half of the investigation?"

"No, of course not."

"And when you read a prisoner his rights, do you only read him a portion of those rights?"

Covington stood up with a puzzled look on her face. "Your Honor, I'm not sure what the relevance is of this line of questioning."

"Your Honor, the relevance of this line of questioning will become obvious in a moment," Tom promised.

"Well, Mr. Baldwin, don't take too long getting there," Delacroix drawled.

"Please answer the question, Detective Henderson," Tom said.

"Of course, I read the whole thing."

"Why?" he asked, leaning on the podium.

"I think that's obvious, Mr. Baldwin."

"Why don't you tell us then, Detective?" Tom

asked, gesturing to the jury with a sweeping motion of his hand.

"Because if I didn't read the whole thing I might miss something," Henderson answered, stating the obvious a bit snidely.

"And one more thing, when you read a book, do you read only the odd-numbered pages?"

"Your Honor!" Covington said with exasperation.

"Mr. Baldwin, why don't you get to the point?" Delacroix instructed.

"Gladly, Your Honor. Now Detective Henderson, can you please tell the jury why, just now, when you quoted from Rebecca's statement, you only read part of the statement?"

"I don't know what you mean." Henderson looked over at Covington.

"Sure you do. In fact, Detective Henderson, you intentionally left out the most important part, didn't you?"

"I most certainly did not," he said indignantly. "I read the important part, the part that explains what happened. Not the defendant's self-serving additional comments, if that's what you're after."

"Detective Henderson, why don't you read for the jury the whole statement regarding the shooting and permit them to form an opinion about what the statement means?"

Henderson shifted in his seat and looked down at Rebecca's statement. "Let me look. Uh, here it is. 'Believing my life was in danger, I pulled out the gun and shot the man several times, until he slumped down and the car came to a stop. At that point I ran out of the car and into my own car. I drove home.'" Henderson stopped and looked up.

"Please keep reading," Tom said, pointing to the paper.

Henderson continued reading in a flat monotonous

tone, depriving Rebecca's words of any intensity or passion. "'I didn't know what else to do. I wasn't even sure the guy was dead. He still could have been following me for all I knew. I was running on adrenaline I guess, because when I got home, I just collapsed on the bed in my clothes.' Is that enough?" Henderson asked, looking up.

"Yes, thank you. Now, Detective, that part of her statement which began 'believing my life was in danger,' you just decided not to read that to the jury?"

"Well, I don't believe her life was in danger."

"Sir, with all due respect, that's for the jury to decide." Tom glanced at his notes. "Let me ask you a question. Did Rebecca Fielding in any way try to hide the fact that she had to kill James Hempstead?"

"Objection to the use of the phrase 'had to kill,'" Covington stated.

"Rephrase your question, Mr. Baldwin," suggested Judge Delacroix.

"Did she in any way hide the fact that she killed James Hempstead?"

"Well, no. But it would have been useless for her to try to deny it—"

"You've answered the question. Didn't she volunteer to make a statement?"

"Yes."

"And didn't she explain in that statement"—Tom placed both hands on either side of the podium, leaned forward, and raised his voice until it filled the courtroom—"that she was kidnapped by James Hempstead and dragged into his car against her will, that she was threatened by him, and that she was in fear for her life when she shot him?"

"Well, of course. What else could she say? Everyone knew she killed him. She left her wallet in his car, after all. She couldn't pretend it didn't happen."

"Motion to strike. Nonresponsive and calls for speculation," Covington shouted.

"Sustained." But Tom didn't care. The jury had already heard Henderson's answer.

"Detective, isn't it true that Ms. Fielding had bruises on her body consistent with her version of what happened, that she was grabbed by a much larger . . . how big was Mr. Hempstead?"

"Oh, I'd say, about six feet, one eighty."

"How 'bout six foot two, two hundred pounds—does that sound about right to you?" Tom asked, looking at the coroner's report.

"If that's what it says."

"Ms. Fielding, could you stand up please?" Tom asked. She rose slowly, unsure what he was doing. "Detective, what would you say—about five foot seven, one hundred and fifteen?"

Henderson looked at Rebecca. "Well, she was heavier when I arrested her."

"Yes, jail can do that to you."

"Counselor," Judge Delacroix scolded. Rebecca sat back down.

"Well, her driver's license indicates five foot seven, one hundred twenty-five pounds—does that sound about right?"

"Yes."

"Good, now let's discuss the bruises. You saw bruises on her arms the morning of her arrest." Tom walked over, pulled down the photos of the deceased and replaced them with pictures of a frightened, dazed Rebecca and her bruises. He grabbed a pointer and smacked it against the photos. "These bruises, Detective Henderson, did you see these bruises when you arrested Ms. Fielding?" Baldwin asked, his voice filled with indignation. "Weren't these bruises consistent with her statement that she had been grabbed in the parking lot, dragged against her will into his car, and thrown in the back of his car?"

"They could have come from many things. She could have done it herself to make it look like she was in a fight. I don't know."

Tom concentrated on not losing his temper, but the answers he was getting from Henderson were not helping. He thought of the notion of quitting while you're ahead and wondered if he'd ever get to such a place. He tried again. "The question is: are these bruises consistent with her statement?"

"I guess you could say that."

"Would you say that?" Tom asked, pointing the stick at Henderson.

"I don't know how the bruises got there and neither do you. Is it consistent with her statement? Sure, but that doesn't mean that the bruises happened the way she said. She could have made the whole thing up. Anyway, since she had the gun, why didn't she just tell him to pull over and get out of the car? Why did she shoot him?"

Tom thought it best to ignore Henderson's gratuitous questions. "All right," he began, "now, Detective Henderson, you conducted interviews with witnesses to the crash of Hempstead's car, isn't that correct?"

"Yes, I did."

"And were their statements consistent with Ms. Fielding's claim that the car was moving when she shot Hempstead and that after he slumped over, the car continued until it crashed into a light pole?"

"The witnesses stated that they heard some shots, looked in their direction, and saw a car come to a stop at a light pole. You know, come to think of it, maybe that's how the defendant got her bruises."

Tom quickly had the last part of Henderson's answer stricken, but it was a hollow victory. He wasn't having any success making his points with this witness. He had failed to calculate how Henderson's desire to incriminate Rebecca would make him a difficult witness to manipulate. Tom looked over at Rebecca and saw in her face his failings reflected back at him. He went back to the counsel table for a sip of water and to refill his confidence, then started walking back to the podium. "Is it your position that Ms. Fielding planned to kill James Hempstead in such a way as to endanger her own life and draw attention to herself? Shooting a man in a moving car in a parking lot filled with witnesses?" His voice filled with disbelief.

"The witnesses say the car wasn't moving that fast, so I doubt she was imperiling her life. She got out of it okay."

"You want this jury to believe that Ms. Fielding planned to shoot Mr. Hempstead in the parking lot, in front of the store, while the car was running and while she couldn't control the car." Tom knew this was the best set of facts for his case and moved in closer to the witness. "That's what you want us to believe?"

Henderson looked over Tom's shoulder at the jury. "It's not my responsibility to tell you what to believe," he said, grinning slightly.

"Oh, really? Did you also feel that way a couple of minutes ago when you told the jury that you didn't believe that her life was in danger?"

Henderson locked eyes with Tom. "I don't need to tell you what to believe or what not to believe. The facts prove that Ms. Fielding's life was not in danger."

Tom winced inside. He knew that he had asked one question too many and was not going to get any further with Henderson. "Nothing further, Your Honor." Tom sat down. Never before had he felt such intense pressure. He couldn't face Rebecca, so

he fumbled with his notes to avoid the contact.
Rebecca weakly muttered, "You did fine," but Tom
didn't believe it, and neither did she. It wasn't a good
start.

It was just after eleven when Covington climbed into
her warm bed with a small tub of chocolate Healthy
Choice Frozen Yogurt and watched one news anchor
after another recount what unanimously was considered a very good day for the prosecution. The trial
analysts in particular gave Covington high marks for
the swiftness with which she debunked Rebecca's
self-defense theory on the Hempstead murder.

Tom, on the other hand, was not having as good a
night. He knew enough to keep the television off, not
wanting to have his fumbling endlessly replayed. He
sat at Rebecca's kitchen table poring over the evidence Covington had provided, hoping to find some
little hole in it. It didn't have to be a large one. Any
hole would do at this point. The loneliness of Tom's
search was interrupted by a loud pounding on the
door.

"Who is it?" he yelled. With the crime scene photos of Matheson still very much on his mind, Tom
did not use the peephole.

"Open the door, asshole," a familiar voice shot
back.

Tom did as he was told. "Jack, what the hell are
you doing here? Are you crazy?" he asked, still holding the doorknob.

"Tom, I gotta talk to you." He looked hard into his
friend's eyes. His self-imposed exile—separated from
his partner and from the case they were working
on—left Jack desperately needing to connect with
someone who was on the same side as him. "Come
on, let me in."

"All right." Tom opened the door and let Jack in. After he closed the door, he motioned Jack over to the living room couch, away from the mess of notes on the kitchen table. "You still haven't answered my question. Why are you here?"

"I'm not," Jack said, sitting down. It felt strange, being here without Rebecca. And yet all he could focus on was a way to help get her out and bring her back here, where she belonged.

"You're what?"

"I said, I'm not here."

Tom got the message and sat down across from him. "So then, why are you not here?"

Jack looked around the room, lost and uncomfortable. "Well, I just wanted you to give a message to Rebecca for me. Tell her that I'm getting more heat than ever now from the chief and that I'm not intentionally staying away from her. It's just that if I go down there to visit her, I might as well hand them my badge."

"Jack, I've got my own problems without getting in the middle of yours. Why don't you just tell her yourself? Why do I have to be your messenger?"

"Because, moron, there are no sign-in sheets here."

"Oh. Right." Tom realized he was so punchy from late nights on the case that he apparently did need a ton of bricks to fall on him.

Jack leaned forward, looking at Tom squarely. "And by the way, I hope you're working on someone else's cross-examination. I told the D.A. I wasn't going to testify."

Tom was puzzled. "I thought they subpoenaed you for tomorrow."

"They did. But I just got off the phone with Covington before I came here and I explained to her why she should withdraw the subpoena."

"What did you say?"

"I told her that if she called me, I'd tell the jury that Rebecca was completely innocent and totally incapable of committing these murders. I added that I'd also tell them that Henderson jumped on Rebecca as a suspect to wrestle back control of the case and to get the 'big bust.' And for good measure I'd throw in that Rebecca is being used by the D.A.'s office to get a conviction after a string of high-profile losses and by Covington as a political stepping stone to further her career. I think I made my point because she didn't have a response. She just hung up on me."

Tom erupted with a long, resounding laugh. "Good for you!" He could picture Covington's face, and thinking of her stunned reaction gave him a moment's pleasure. "I'm sorry I missed it. Covington stunned into silence. That's great!" Jack smiled. It felt good sharing a laugh, especially at Covington's expense. "So what exactly did the chief say to you?"

"It's not important. Just tell Rebecca that I love her. And also tell her that the plane won't leave without her."

"That sounds kinda cryptic. You planning a jail break?"

Jack got up to leave. He looked at Tom, seeing in him all his hopes for Rebecca's acquittal. "Just get her off, buddy."

"Easier said than done," Tom said grimly.

Jack's eyes narrowed. "Are you not up to the challenge?"

"It's not that. It's just that there're too many coincidences here. Rebecca's tied in some way to each of the murder scenes. No amount of fancy footwork will ultimately hide that fact."

Jack's face dropped, and a cold feeling passed through him. "What are you saying? Rebecca didn't do it, it should be easy for you to prove that."

"I'd like to agree with you. I mean, I don't think Rebecca's capable of murder. It's just there are a lot of things that are hard to explain away, even for me. When I look at some of the evidence they have, it makes me stop and wonder." Tom shrugged his shoulders as if to say, "You know."

"Wonder what?" Jack snapped.

"You know about Rebecca's past, don't you? With her father and all?"

"Yeah, so?"

Tom looked away and sighed, afraid to utter his doubts, as if keeping them silenced prevented them from being true. "I keep wondering, you know, when someone goes through a trauma like that, it's possible that they may not be aware of what they're doing. I've spoken with a psychologist who specializes in treatment of sexual abuse victims, and she said some people do tend to split off, where they might not be aware that they have another side to themselves. They may have black-outs—periods when some other part of their psyche is working."

"That's not Rebecca. You're talking like you think she did it." Jack registered the look in Tom's eyes. Tom wasn't sure.

"Why are her prints at Matheson's? Why did two people see her at the victims' apartments? Why did she have a gun? Why did she keep the clippings on the killings? Why couldn't she just stay away from these guys?" Tom looked to Jack for the answer.

Jack took a couple steps toward Tom. "You're supposed to be her attorney. You can't have doubts like that. You have to believe in her," he implored.

"I'm only human. I can't just tune everything out because you want me to get Rebecca off. The more I learn, the worse I feel. There's a lot here, a lot more than I expected." Tom looked at the floor and was

silent for a long time. "I don't think—I don't think I
can get Rebecca an acquittal," he said finally.

Tom expected to see a flash of anger in Jack's
eyes. Instead, he saw a calmness that scared him
more than anger. "Listen to me carefully, because
I'm only going to say this once. You're overtired and
you're frustrated. I'm going to forget what you said
and you are never going to repeat what you just told
me, and you are never going to entertain those
thoughts again. You are going to do everything in
your power to get her off. I don't want to hear anything else, ever. Too much is at stake, way too
much."

36

Over the next several days, Covington continued placing the pieces of her puzzle together. Item by item, fact by fact, the jury was being led to only one conclusion—that Rebecca was a methodical, cold-blooded killer who stalked and butchered each victim. Covington skillfully—and, to some extent surprisingly—was able to humanize the deceased with the help of the coroner, who detailed the last few minutes of the victims' lives with graphic testimony and equally graphic autopsy pictures. Those reporters covering the case found particularly effective the drawn-out accounts of the injuries suffered by each man and what pain and terror each must have suffered before his death. To Covington, the gasps from the jury, and their quick, furtive glances from the autopsy pictures to Rebecca, were proof that she was making headway.

Tom was relegated to hairsplitting and obfuscation, since he couldn't explain away the evidence. He asked unanswerable questions of the criminalists to distract the jury—why wasn't any of the victims'

blood found in Rebecca's car, why didn't they take
tire or foot impressions around some of the murder
scenes, why weren't there more fingerprints? He tried
to imbue these questions with importance by his
tone and manner, asking the jury to believe that the
real answer lay in those questions. After years as a
prosecutor, judging a good day by whether he had
proved what needed to be proved, it was difficult for
Tom to get used to his new role where his entire
approach centered on merely planting a seed of
doubt. But his efforts at least comforted Rebecca,
assuring her that her attorney was not just going to
roll over for the prosecution—that he was going to
fight for her after all. Tom never mentioned the
details of his meeting with Jack, but its impact was
evident. Less tentative and bumbling, Tom did his
best to resemble his old confident self.

Covington hoped Randazzo's testimony would be
strong enough to keep Larson as far from the jury as
possible. While he would have been the preferred
choice in ordinary circumstances, this trial was by no
means ordinary—and he was by no means an ordinary witness. She did not want the trial sidetracked
by jousting with what promised to be the witness
from hell.

Randazzo had eased her jitters answering the
foundational questions about her training and experience and the initial investigation of the case, and
now was ready to plunge ahead into the heart of her
testimony. She took a deep, relaxing breath, and sat
back in her seat.

"Detective Randazzo, as one of the detectives
investigating these murders, what evidence did you
discover which caused you to believe that the murders were the work of one person?"

"We looked at various factors in reaching that
conclusion, but primarily the fact that the victims

were all convicted child molesters, the same weapon was used in the first three murders, each of the first five were near the end of their probationary term, and the fourth and fifth murders were each marked with similar mutilation of the victims." Randazzo ticked off each fact robotically.

"Were there any other factors?"

"Yes. The victims were all prosecuted for their crimes by the same prosecutor, the defendant." Randazzo paused and looked out at the spectators, uncomfortably noting Larson's looming presence. She hadn't seen him when she arrived and had naively hoped he would skip today. She quickly decided to clarify her answer, convincing herself that Jack's being there had nothing to do with her decision. "Those weren't the only similarities. They were also each in therapy, each having gone to the same treatment center at one time, and they were each under the supervision of the same probation office." Covington's scowl told Randazzo that the extra information was more than she wanted.

"Detective, what other evidence pointed to these murders being related?"

"Similar evidence was found at the scenes of the different killings. And the same person's hair was found at three of the scenes—long and blonde. And the same type of bullets were used in each of the killings except for the stabbing of Mr. Knight. And a woman was spotted at the sight of the Riddell killing and was described as tall, with long blonde hair, which matched what we found at the crime scenes. The whole thing was just much too coincidental to realistically suggest more than one killer," Randazzo said, her voice more relaxed and conversational. She looked over at the jury occasionally as she spoke.

"Now, Detective, was any physical evidence discovered at the scene of any of the murders which later tied the defendant specifically to the crime?" Covington asked, her voice strong, telegraphing confidence. She wanted to make sure the jury took notice of the question and answer.

"Yes. A palm print was located at the apartment of the second victim, Mr. Matheson. Initially, we were unable to get a match on the print because our database does not include palm prints. But, once the defendant was arrested in connection with the Hempstead mur"—Jack's eyes, fixed on her— "uh, matter, we were able to compare her prints with those at Mr. Matheson's and found them to be similar."

"Her prints were similar to those found at Mr. Matheson's apartment or they were the same?" Covington asked in mock confusion.

Randazzo hated the falseness of Covington's question, but she understood that the courtroom was often a theater for the dramatic. "No, not 'similar to.' They were her prints," she said firmly, establishing her part in the drama.

"No doubt?" Covington asked, emphasizing the point beyond necessity.

"No doubt." Randazzo's mouth went dry and she reached for a drink of water.

"Now, Detective Randazzo, in addition to the evidence found at the actual murder scenes, are you aware of evidence recovered pursuant to two search warrants served at the home of the defendant?"

"Yes, I am."

"And did you cause any of that evidence to be subjected to examination and comparison analysis?"

"Yes, I did."

"Please tell the jury about the examination of evidence seized at the defendant's home." Covington walked over to the jury box, arms resting at her side, to direct Randazzo's answers in the jury's direction.

She nodded supportively as Randazzo spoke, drawing her out.

"Okay. A blue wool jacket was recovered at the defendant's house. It was taken to the FBI for forensic examination to determine whether the fibers from the jacket matched blue fibers found on the door jamb of Mr. Matheson's apartment."

"And are you aware of the FBI's results?" Covington asked, fully knowing the answer.

"Yes, I am."

"And what were they?"

"They matched."

Rebecca's face flushed red with anger. She knew the rules of evidence as well as she knew her own name and couldn't understand Tom permitting a witness to testify as to something someone else had told her. "Why aren't you doing something? This is hearsay," she whispered fiercely. Tom patted Rebecca on the hand, but kept his eyes fixed on Randazzo. "Don't worry," he said.

"Was any other evidence submitted to the FBI for analysis?"

"Yes, the bullets found at the defendant's home were taken to the FBI and compared with the bullets found in the bodies of Mr. Penhall, Mr. Matheson, Mr. Jaffe, Mr. Riddell, and Mr. Hempstead. And the bullets were found to match each other, caliber and type."

"Did the ballistics also match?"

"Since the bullets used in the murders were hollow-nosed, they distorted greatly upon impact, particularly if they hit bone. So, we were unable to make a ballistics comparison."

Covington nodded. "Were forensic analyses conducted in connection with this case?"

"Yes. We compared the hairs found at the scene of the Matheson, Knight, and Riddell murders with hairs from the defendant." Randazzo paused, looking uncomfortable as she waited for her cue.

"And what was the result of that comparison?"

"The hairs matched."

Covington looked at the court clock. She could try to stretch out the testimony so that it could end at a break, giving it time to make its impact with the jury. She decided against a stall. It was time to put it all together for the jury. "Now, sometime after the defendant's arrest, did anyone come forward to identify the defendant as having been seen at any of the murder sites?"

"Yes." Randazzo shifted uncomfortably in her seat as she again looked out at Jack. How could just telling the truth feel so much like a betrayal? "Two different people identified the defendant."

Covington walked back over to the podium and pretended to shuffle through papers as she let the information sink in with the jury. Long pauses were the better part of reinforcement, she reasoned.

Rebecca noticed where Randazzo was looking and turned back toward Jack. She tried to send him support, which she herself needed now more than ever. Jack suppressed his anger and frustration and smiled warmly at Rebecca. She smiled back, then closed her eyes, taking emotional sustenance from his presence.

Covington paused, looking back at Tom. "Your witness." Try to tap-dance your way out of this one, Baldwin, she thought smugly.

Tom took the opening Randazzo gave him.

"You said that there were other people besides Miss Fielding who knew and had interactions with each of the first five victims. I think you mentioned that each was seen at the same probation office and each had received therapy at the same treatment facility, is that correct?"

"Yes."

"So were these people also added to the list of possible suspects—the people who work at the probation department, the people who work at or receive treatment from the treatment center?"

"Yes."

"But since none of them were abducted by James Hempstead and had to shoot him in self-defense, none of them is sitting here in court today, isn't that correct?"

Covington popped up like a jack-in-the-box. "Objection, Your Honor."

"Sustained. The jury will disregard the question."

"But so that there's no misunderstanding, there were any number of other people with whom the dead child molesters had interacted who were on your list of possible suspects?"

Randazzo thought for a moment. "I wouldn't say 'any number,' but yes, there were other people on the list besides the defendant."

"How many more?"

"Less than a dozen."

That sounded like a big enough number for Tom to offer the jury, and not knowing the answer, he didn't want Randazzo to bring the estimate downward. He moved on. "All right. Now, Detective, the bullets found at Ms. Fielding's apartment, those were hollow-nosed .22-caliber bullets?"

"Yes, they were."

"And that's a very rare type of bullet, isn't it?"

Randazzo seemed perplexed. "No, not really."

"Actually, it's very common, isn't it?"

Randazzo nodded slightly. "I believe so."

"And, in fact, the FBI was unable to match the gun used in the other child molester killings with the gun fired by Ms. Fielding in self-defense, isn't that correct?"

"Well, they couldn't include or exclude it."

Tom stared at Randazzo, cocking his head slightly. "Is that a yes?" he asked finally.

"Yes, they couldn't match the gun."

"Okay," Tom continued, after flipping a page in his notebook, "now, with respect to the hair samples, the ones that were recovered at the crime scenes, DNA tests were conducted on them, right? In fact, that's how they were determined to have matched Rebecca's hair, right?"

Randazzo shook her head. Either Tom was an idiot or he was playing her for one. "No, we could not conduct DNA tests, since the hairs did not have the follicles attached to them."

"Oh, I'm confused then. What was done?" Tom asked, his eyes wide with bewilderment.

"Microscopic examinations."

"And precisely what does that entail?"

"The crime lab compares the recovered hairs to the defendant's hair by placing the two under a microscope side by side. In this case, all the hairs had very similar characteristics."

"And from these examinations, it can be said with one hundred percent certainty that the hairs found at the crime scenes came from Ms. Fielding, right?" he asked innocently enough as he looked around the courtroom.

"Well, no. You can't be one hundred percent certain."

"You can't?" Tom pretended to be shocked.

Randazzo knew she was being patronized and didn't like it much. "DNA testing can get you close to one hundred percent. It's very reliable."

"Well, how close does microscopic testing get you?"

"It can give you a high degree of certainty."

"But nothing like DNA, right?"

"That's true."

"In fact, microscopic testing leaves plenty of room for doubt, doesn't it?"

Randazzo hedged. "I wouldn't say plenty."

"What would you say?"

Randazzo thought for a moment. "That microscopic examination is a good indicator of whether the sample hair and suspect's hair are similar. If they are, then the suspect can be included in the group of the possible contributors of the hair."

"In other words, all the microscopic examination can tell you is that Rebecca is among the thousands of women in Los Angeles County whose hair matches those found at the crime scene?"

"I don't know if it's thousands."

Tom leaned in. "In fact, you don't know if it's more or less than thousands, do you? There's no data on how many women share the same hair characteristics, is there?"

Randazzo shrugged. "Not that I'm aware of."

"So, would it be fair to say that all the microscopic examination can tell us is that Ms. Fielding is among an unknown number of women in the Los Angeles area who could have contributed those hairs?"

"Yes, that's a fair statement."

"But it does not mean that she is the one who left the hairs."

"Right."

Tom walked over to the witness stand and leaned an arm on it, looking first at Randazzo and then back at Larson. "And if your partner, the lead detective on the case, discovered that the hairs also matched a wig worn by a cross-dressing fellow patient of each of the murdered victims, himself a convicted sex offender, then that would mean he could be included in that group as well, doesn't it?" Tom threw the sucker punch so fast, Randazzo didn't have time to flinch. But it propelled Covington to her feet.

"Objection, assumes facts not in evidence, violates reciprocal discovery—"

"Calm down, Ms. Covington. Sustained." Delacroix sent a disapproving scowl toward Tom.

Tom knew that Delacroix's rebuke could have been much harsher. However, he still couldn't stop himself. "Your Honor, my apologies. I thought the district attorney had done a complete investigation and was well aware of this other suspect," Tom said as he walked back to the podium, past the jury, a slight smile on his face. He was relishing Jack's clandestine help.

Delacroix was not amused by Baldwin's tactics. "That's quite enough, Mr. Baldwin. Proceed."

"So, Detective Randazzo, the hair samples alone establish nothing, isn't that correct?"

"I don't know what you want me to say." Randazzo remained calm, her voice steady. "I look at all the evidence taken together, not just one piece."

"Even if each piece establishes nothing by itself?"

"But each piece is significant."

Tom ignored the comment, not wanting to highlight it for the jury. "Let's move on to the wool fibers recovered off of Matheson's door. Those could have only come from one piece of clothing, right?"

Randazzo knew where this was going. "The fibers that were recovered matched a jacket seized from the defendant's closet."

"And you discovered that to be a unique jacket containing some unique fibers that would point to Ms. Fielding as the only source for those fibers?"

"No, Mr. Baldwin. The jacket we discovered at the defendant's home was a navy blue one hundred percent wool jacket. And no, it's not unique."

"I see. So any number of women may have similar jackets in their closets right now. Transvestites as well?"

"I suppose so. Although I didn't know trans-vestites went for business suits," Randazzo added, clearly annoyed with Tom's attack.

"Then the wool fibers alone establish nothing con-clusively, isn't that correct?"

"The wool fibers in conjunction with everything else establish a lot," Randazzo said, exasperated.

"That wasn't my question. Please answer my question."

"Your question only focuses on one piece of the puzzle."

Tom turned toward the judge. "Your Honor, please admonish the witness to answer the ques-tion."

Delacroix leaned over to the witness. "Detective Randazzo, please answer Mr. Baldwin's questions as phrased." He turned toward the court reporter. "Please read back Mr. Baldwin's last question."

Randazzo took another sip of water as the ques-tion was read, then replied, "Alone, the wool fibers indicated that the defendant is included in the group of people who may have left the fibers at the scene of the Matheson murder."

"Now the palm print—that we can be sure is Rebecca Fielding's. Right?"

"Right."

"And we can be sure that it was left at the time of Mr. Matheson's murder, right?" Tom asked offhand-edly.

Randazzo let out a long breath. "No, we can't tell when it was left."

"You can't?" Tom seemed shocked. He looked off in the distance, as if considering her answer for the first time. "So the print could have been left weeks before Mr. Matheson's murder?" he asked finally.

"Possibly."

"Or even years?" he asked hesitantly, still asking

the jury to believe he had no idea what the answer might be.

"Well, that's unlikely. You'd have to assume that no one cleans the area, or paints over it, and that it's not covered up by dirt or other prints."

"But it's possible that it could be years old, right?"

"Sure."

"Hmmm." Tom nodded his head slowly, as if contemplating her answer. The delay gave the jury enough time to soak up the inference. "Oh. Where was this print found?" he asked, his eyes narrowing quizzically.

"On Mr. Matheson's door."

"On the inside?"

"No, on the outside," Randazzo sighed, tiring of Tom's trapdoor questions.

"Where inside his apartment were Rebecca's prints found?" Tom asked with more than a hint of irritation, his voice filling the courtroom.

"Nowhere."

"*Nowhere?*" Tom was getting adept at looking aghast at Randazzo's answers. "What about at the scene of the other killings—leaving out Mr. Hempstead of course—Rebecca's prints were found there as well, right?"

Randazzo sighed heavily, weary from her ill treatment and weary from being the sacrificial lamb for the defense. "No, Mr. Baldwin. We were only able to identify the print she left at Mr. Matheson's."

"Would you consider having her print on the outside of the door to be proof that Rebecca was ever inside his apartment?"

"No, but why would—"

Tom was quick to cut her off. "Detective, please do not speculate. Let's stick with what we know. Now, Detective Randazzo, had Ms. Fielding not killed Mr. Hempstead, would you have attempted to have an arrest warrant issued on the other five killings?"

"Objection, calls for speculation," Covington called out.

"Your Honor, Detective Randazzo was one of the detectives investigating these killings. She certainly has knowledge whether the police intended to arrest Rebecca for the other killings. She knows what evidence she had."

"I agree, Mr. Baldwin. Overruled," said Judge Delacroix.

Randazzo thought for a moment. She hated lawyers, how they ask the precise question that they know you'll have to answer their way. While she had suspected Fielding, she hadn't had sufficient evidence to get an arrest warrant until after the Hempstead killing. "I can't answer that. Our investigation was heading in many directions. We may very well have sought a warrant somewhere down the line."

"Did you investigate the circumstances surrounding the killing of Mr. Hempstead?"

"No, not originally. That investigation was conducted by another detective in the department, Detective Henderson."

"Do you know the circumstances of the killing?"

"Yes, I've spoken with the other detectives investigating that killing and I've read their reports."

"From your experience investigating the other five homicides and based on the differences among the killings and the victims, do you believe it possible that the killer of the other five men was someone other than the person involved in the Hempstead homicide?"

"Do I believe that the real killer is still out there? Is that what you are asking me?" Randazzo challenged Tom.

Tom grabbed both sides of the podium and leaned forward. "Yes, Detective. Do you believe that it is possible that the real killer is still on the loose?"

Randazzo was now sorry that she had rephrased Tom's question. Anything is possible, she thought. He's not gonna back me into this one. Her irritation caused her to momentarily forget Jack and what her answer might do to him. "No, Mr. Baldwin, I don't believe that. The evidence is much too strong to think that."

"But you do see the differences between the Hempstead homicide and the other five killings, don't you?"

"There are some, but there are more similarities."

"Isn't it true that whoever killed the others attempted to cover up their involvement in those killings, whereas in the Hempstead case, Ms. Fielding did nothing to hide her involvement in the homicide?"

"Objection, calls for speculation," stated Covington.

"Your Honor," Tom started, "if this question calls for speculation, then the entire prosecution case calls for speculation."

"Please rephrase your question, Counselor."

"Fine." Tom breathed deep, trying not to let his frustration show. "In the other killings, the killer did not leave their identification—credit cards, driver's license—did not leave their gun with fingerprints, did not leave screaming from the scene attracting attention, driving past witnesses in a car with traceable license plates displayed, isn't that correct?"

"That's correct."

"Wouldn't you say that's a difference?"

"Maybe."

"Thank you, Detective. I have no more questions."

Covington was on her feet before Tom returned to his chair. She knew that she needed to show the jury that his questions were meant to confuse them rather than help them search for the truth. She could easily expose his game by reemphasizing the notion that the individual pieces of testimony could not be viewed in the abstract, so she had Randazzo reiterate that it was not just the hairs or the fibers or the bullets alone but these three factors combined that pointed to the defendant. And when you added the palm print and the eyewitnesses, this was not a case about coincidences or happenstance. Statistically, the totality of the evidence still only incriminated one person, and Tom Baldwin could not change that fact.

Randazzo was dismissed and left the courtroom. As she headed down the corridor, finally released from the ordeal of testifying, she walked silently past Larson. Neither spoke, both unsure what to say to the other. Larson could not understand how she could show such a lack of faith in his instincts. How could she ignore his beliefs? And she didn't understand how he could expect her to do anything but honor her profession by testifying as truthfully as she could.

Randazzo paced her cramped living room, still tense and irritable from her day on the stand, feeling torn between her job as a cop and her duty as a partner. She had no one to talk to, now that Ben was camping out all night at the law library, at least no one who would understand what she was feeling. She couldn't believe Ben was going to turn into one of those asshole lawyers, twisting people's words around, backing them into corners, doing and saying anything to try and get their clients off. Would it change him? Could he—could anybody—do that for a living and have it not? She had to hope that Ben was different and would resist the lawyers' sickness of believing that even if they were not God almighty, they would certainly be the first person He would call if He were ever in trouble.

It was all Jack's fault. If he hadn't fallen in love with Rebecca, it would have been him up on the stand and she could have been out in the audience supporting him. But then, she figured, if he hadn't fallen in love with her, this wouldn't be a problem. As it was, she took the heat while Jack stayed in the background, lost and adrift in a sea of loneliness. Randazzo wanted to reach out to him today but didn't know how. Or perhaps she was afraid of what he'd say.

Randazzo stared at the phone, irritated with its silent reminder that her partner was but a phone call away. What are you, a coward? the phone taunted her. "No, I'm not," she shot back. "All right, I'll call," she said to her Touch-Tone heckler.

"Hello?"

"Jack. Hi." There was no response. "It's Jennifer."

"Yeah, I know. I still recognize your voice. What do you want?" As she'd feared, he was cool and aloof.

"Jack, c'mon. Don't talk to me like that."

"Like what?" he asked, keeping his emotional distance while leading with safe sarcasm. She could hear his television blaring in the background and noticed he wasn't lowering the sound.

"Like that. Like you don't know me. I don't want us to be like that. This case shouldn't come between us."

"Then maybe you shouldn't have put it between us by lining up on the other side. You should have trusted me. I'm right on this one. But you, like everybody else, are going to see to it that Rebecca gets convicted anyway."

"Jack, it's not a matter of trusting you. You and I just see things differently. I look at all the evidence and it seems so clear to me. I don't know if you're blinded by your feelings for Rebecca or why it is you think she didn't do it."

She could hear Jack click off the TV. "I can put my feelings for Rebecca aside. It's my feelings about the evidence that I'm talking about. When you've done this as long as I have you get a feel for things."

"God, you're just like my father. 'When you're my age, you'll understand.' I'm sorry I'm young, but that shouldn't invalidate my opinions. Can't we just agree to disagree and still stay partners? Why does this have to put a wedge between us?" Randazzo looked over to the framed picture sitting on her TV—the entire Randazzo clan smiling and beaming with pride at her police academy graduation. She acutely felt the loss caused by the three-thousand-mile separation, and she needed to recapture that feeling of connection with Jack. "When I was a kid and I'd listen to my dad talk about his partner, it was so special. It was like he was talking about his right arm. I thought they were closer than he was to my mom, and they have a great relationship. It was just that 'partner' meant something special. That's part of what I wanted when I joined the force."

"Well, you have a partner—Ben."

Jennifer sighed. "You know what I mean. I want us to get past this. I'm not the bad guy here. All I did today was tell the truth as I know it. That's all I could do."

"But you're wrong, Jennifer. You're dead wrong about Rebecca. And you know it. I saw the way you reacted to Tom's questions. You're not so sure anymore."

"I don't know. What about the witnesses who say they saw Rebecca? Why'd she go to Matheson's? Why was she carrying a gun?" Randazzo stopped, realizing she was going down a path that led further away from Jack. "Look, forget it. I did my job today, let the jury do theirs. Maybe you're right and the system'll prove me wrong. That's what it's all about. But don't get mad at me for doing what I had to do."

There was a long pause, then she heard Jack's voice, softer now. "I'm not mad at you, Jennifer. I'm mad that Rebecca has to go through this. I'm mad that the killer is sitting out there laughing at us while this farce is going on, and I'm mad that I'm not allowed to do anything to help Rebecca."

"You're sticking by her. That's more than most people would do."

"Oh, a lot of good that's going to do. Do you know how much the department has hamstrung me? I was getting someplace and then, bam, the fucking chief slams the door on me. I can't even go to the bathroom now without being followed by Internal Affairs."

"I'm sorry," was all Jennifer could offer. "I guess all I wanted you to know is that if you still want me as your partner, I'll be there. For whatever that's worth."

Randazzo heard nothing and wondered if Jack was still there, if he'd heard her. If her words meant anything to him anymore. Then she heard what sounded like a tearful break in his voice. "It's worth more than you know."

37

Larson leaned against the wall, soaking in the coldness of the marble, waiting for the courtroom doors to open, his eyes closed, thinking about the case, about Rebecca, and about how fucked up everything was. The tap on the shoulder nearly sent him airborne. "You're not still mad at me, are you?" The fake lashes fluttered and the ruby red lips parted in a smile. The new wig threw him for a moment, but the voice was unmistakable. "I know you were just feeling frustrated, so I didn't take it personally."

"Great. God knows, I wouldn't want to upset you." Larson was too emotionally exhausted to gird himself for battle with Frank.

Frank sidled up next to him. "Well, what do you think?"

Larson cast a quick glance before turning back to stare at the opposing wall. "I think Rita Hayworth's probably spinning in her grave right now. That's what I think."

"You don't like? Your loss. Oh well, believe it or

not, I wasn't talking about me. I was talking about the Oakwood."

Larson turned toward Frank, a blank look on his face. "What about the Oakwood?"

"Don't tell me you haven't heard!" Frank's face radiated with excitement.

"Heard what?" Larson demanded, not much in the mood for Frank's games.

Frank took no notice, too thrilled with his role as bearer of good tidings. "Someone tried to burn it down."

Jack had thought he was beyond being shocked by anything that happened anymore, but Frank's news stunned him. "You're shitting me!"

"No, it's true. On my honor." Frank gave a Boy Scout salute. "Gutted the rear conference room, smoke all through the place. Hillerman got real lucky—the boys from the station caught it before it spread. Unless Hillerman was banking on the insurance money, then he's probably real pissed. Anyway, can you believe someone tried to torch it?"

"What makes you think it was arson?"

"Well, what else?" Frank asked flippantly. "It's not like they've got a kitchen in there, you know. It ain't no restaurant."

Larson looked at his watch. Court was about to start. "Frank, I gotta make a phone call. Don't go anywhere." He headed for the pay phones and rang up Randazzo. "Jen, did you hear?" He could barely contain his elation.

"I assume you're talking about the Oakwood?"

"You bet I am. What do you know about it?"

Randazzo leaned back in her chair, across from Larson's empty one, keeping her voice low. "Not much yet. It looks like your basic gasoline and a match. It started in one of the conference rooms around midnight, consumed the room pretty bad, but didn't spread. The guard who walks the parking lot noticed the smoke and it was put out right away."

"Any windows broken? How'd they get in and out?"

"Don't know yet."

"You know what it means, don't you?"

"I'm not sure." But Randazzo knew what he thought it meant.

"It means I was right. Our killer is still out there," Jack said, euphorically.

Randazzo looked around the station to make sure there were no prying ears. "Now just slow down. Aren't you jumping to conclusions?"

"Come on, don't start with me. This is big stuff. You're the one who doesn't believe in coincidences, remember?"

Randazzo winced. "All right, you got me on that one. But I don't see how you get there. What does someone torching the Oakwood have to do with the killings? It could be like when people bomb abortion clinics—somebody may not like what they do there and decided to let them know."

Larson shook his head. "Nah, I don't think so. Think back to all the info you got from the FBI about serial killers—how they need to keep killing? Look, if the killer can't kill anymore 'cause he or she wants us to think we've caught the real killer, then he or she's likely to burst. Right? Since the killer can't go after them one at a time, maybe the killer decides just to burn the whole place down. Makes sense to me. And hey—guess who told me about the fire?" He didn't wait for an answer. "Frank LaPaca." Larson looked down the hall. "Damn! He's gone."

"Huh?"

"He came down to the courthouse to tell me about the fire and I told him to wait. But I guess he split while I was on the phone. This guy, I can't figure him out. He always seems to know too much."

Randazzo had never given much weight to Larson's theory about Frank, but something had to explain the fire, and Frank was as good an explanation as any. Yet she knew how desperate Larson was to hang the murders on someone else. "You used to think he might be the killer. Rebecca's attorney sure wants the jury to think that."

"Well, he's connected somehow. I just haven't been able to check into him the way I'd like to. Maybe now you can get the chief to let me investigate him, and the Oakwood as well." Larson paced as far as the telephone cord would allow. "He can't say no after this."

"I don't know. The chief's gone out on a limb on this one and he's not about to go back." As she spoke, Randazzo realized she was cupping her hand around the phone and whispering, like a mole in a spy novel.

Larson heard the secretiveness in her voice and felt that what she might lack in enthusiasm for his theory, she more than made up for in personal allegiance, so he went for it. "Then you gotta do me a big favor. You gotta check out the Oakwood yourself and you gotta do it fast."

Randazzo hesitated. "I don't know, Jack. I could get fired."

Good, he thought, she didn't say no. "Look, sometimes you just gotta do what's right. Can I count on you? Are you gonna be there for me—partner?" Jack added, harkening back to last night's phone call.

There was a long pause on her end of the phone. "Boy, you play dirty, don't you?" she said at last.

Jack smiled. "Thanks, you won't regret this. Unless, of course, you get canned, in which case it was a really bad career move. Okay, look, you go out to the

Oakwood and snoop around. Call me at this number at one o'clock. I need to go talk to Tom and then I need to find Frank."

"Who's Tom?"

How could she have forgotten? "You know—the guy who tried to give you a second asshole while you were on the witness stand."

"That would have been my third one. You were my second."

By now, Rebecca's routine for the trial was pretty much set. Up at five, pick at her breakfast, get showered and dressed, and be transported to the courthouse for an early morning meeting with Tom. He'd bring her clothes for the day and they'd talk for a while. Ostensibly strategy sessions, they also gave Rebecca the illusion of her old life, where she could simply sit and have a private chat in a place where there were no glass partitions, no metal dividers. This morning was no different as they sat drinking bitter courthouse coffee and exchanging ideas about the cross-examination of the upcoming witnesses. As it neared nine o'clock, Tom quickly stuffed his papers back in his briefcase and stood up to leave. He'd see Rebecca in a few minutes back in the court after she changed out of her jail clothes and into the smart, conservative—but never navy blue—suit of the day.

Rebecca got up slowly, stretching her body as she rose. "So, Tom, do me a favor. You'll have done your job today if you keep me from leaping out of my seat to strangle Ralph," she said.

"You'll do fine. You've been amazing, so far. I really don't know how you do it."

She shrugged. "You do what you have to do. What should I do, sit in court each day sobbing or mumbling incoherently to myself? Although I guess that'd be good for an insanity defense," Rebecca said with a weak laugh. "I just have to hold it all together. I've got to be strong or I'm no use to you and I'm no use to the case."

"Speaking about being strong, we've got to make a decision soon about whether you're going to testify," he reminded her.

"Of course I'm going to," she stated firmly. "I have to."

"Well, you remember what happened the last time you talked to anyone about this case."

"Yeah, I know." Rebecca bowed her head slightly. "But if I don't testify, the jury will think I have something to hide."

"At least we don't have to make the decision today. So any message du jour for Jack?"

"No, just hug him for me."

When Jack caught him before the court day started, Tom was afraid he'd have to carry out his client's instruction. Instead, he was stopped dead by the news about the Oakwood.

He fell back against the wall in the hallway just outside of the courtroom. He saw Covington hurry down the hall, then stop when she saw him talking to Jack. He turned his back away from her to keep his talk with Jack private. "So what does it mean?" Tom asked.

"Could be that someone heard about Oakwood from the trial and just wanted to torch it as an antipervert political statement. But I've got this feeling it's the work of the killer."

"So, then, the killer really is still out there?" Tom joked.

Jack grinned. "You're such an asshole."

Tom put his hand up to his head, a little dazed by the news. He looked back at the door and saw that everyone was going in. "So is anybody looking into this?"

"Randazzo is doing a little snooping. You may end up owing her an apology."

"Hey, if she can dig up something to help Rebecca, you name it."

Jack clapped his arm around Tom's shoulder. "In the meantime, keep plugging. I know it's looking bad, but you can't let up. You're doing great. Just keep it going."

Tom started for the courtroom, then turned back. "Thanks for the vote of confidence, even if you don't mean it."

"The People call Ralph Simpson." Covington cringed slightly as she saw her next witness saunter up to the stand, grinning broadly as he passed Rebecca. She knew that cockiness doesn't play well to a jury and was sorry that her efforts to convey that message had been lost on him. She grabbed the reins as she began her direct examination, intending to hold on tight. "Mr. Simpson, you've had the opportunity to work with the defendant in the prosecution of several cases involving child molestation, isn't that correct?"

"Yes, we were co-counsel on many cases."

"And did you ever become aware of the defendant's feelings toward the child molesters she prosecuted?"

Ralph puffed up, enjoying his role as the insider who was going to let the jury in on the real Rebecca Fielding. "I certainly did. She loathed each and every one of them. With a passion, I might add. It was as if each case was personal, like she had a score to settle or something." Ralph liked his perch on the witness stand from where he could look out and watch Rebecca react to his testimony. Seeing her seethe caused his eyes to gleam devilishly.

Covington, though still irritated with his arrogant posture, was pleased with his volunteered statement and eased up a bit, giving him a little more rope. "And what specifically did you observe, Mr. Simpson?"

Ralph beamed. "She would become absolutely livid when things didn't go her way in court, shouting at the judges, yelling at opposing counsel—we're talking way out of control. She'd carry on about how child molesters didn't deserve to breathe the same air as the rest of us, what lowlife scum they were. Unlike everyone else in the office, she seemed to really despise the guys she was prosecuting. It wasn't just a job. She seemed to take it very personally."

"Did you ever observe any unusual behavior on the part of the defendant with respect to how she conducted her job?"

Ralph nodded enthusiastically. "Oh, yeah. She kept tabs on all the guys she prosecuted. She even hired outside private eyes to follow these guys to try to dig up dirt about them. She tried to get the department to okay an expenditure for this kind of investigation. But when they nixed it, she used her own money to spy on them. I don't know any other D.A. who would do something like that. She kept files, records, had people checking up on them. She was obsessed," he added as a conspiratorial aside.

"Motion to strike." Tom raised his voice, letting his irritation show.

"Sustained as to the last part. Mr. Simpson, please keep your answers responsive and relevant," Delacroix said with some annoyance. This witness should know better.

Covington looked down at her notes, then back up at the witness in an offhanded gesture meant to make her next question seem foundational. "Do you know of any facts that you believe may account for the defendant's extreme feelings of hatred for the child molesters she prosecuted?" she asked, looking at the jurors.

Tom was caught off guard for a moment, but was back on his feet before Ralph could begin his answer. "Objection, calls for speculation."

"May I make an offer of proof, Your Honor?" Covington asked.

"Fine, at sidebar."

Covington leaned in, her arms resting on the judge's desk. "Your Honor, this witness has information about the defendant which I believe establishes a motive for the killings beyond her anger at having lost the cases against the victims," she said.

"And this information would be what, Ms. Covington?" asked Delacroix.

"This witness will testify that the defendant was herself an incest victim and became personally involved in her cases to avenge her own abuse." Covington was gesturing with her right hand, pointing her finger between Ralph and Rebecca. The confused jurors looked back and forth between the two, trying to figure out what was going on. Covington continued, her arms back at rest, crossed in front of her. "Later, we will bring in a psychologist who is an expert on incest survivors who will discuss that latent, unresolved anger at the perpetrator may be acted out against replacements."

"And just how does the witness know that Ms. Fielding was an incest victim?" Tom asked accusingly.

Covington raised her eyebrows. "I believe he learned it from Ms. Fielding's secretary, Joan. She felt sorry for your client, and when Ralph was teasing her one afternoon, Joan took him aside and scolded him for his insensitivity. She explained all about your client's history. We can call Joan, if you would prefer it coming from her."

Tom could keep the testimony out of Simpson's mouth on hearsay grounds, but then again, he didn't want the testimony coming from Joan. First, she was unimpeachable, so he couldn't attack her in cross. But more importantly, Rebecca needed all the support she could find, and having Joan testify against her, even unwillingly, was an insult Rebecca didn't need. "Withdraw the objection. But remember, Counselor, you picked this fight. My client's going to be the most sympathetic accused killer you've ever seen."

"Go for it, Mr. Baldwin," said Covington deridingly.

Tom returned to the defense table, leaned over, and whispered to Rebecca. "Ralph's going to testify about your history. It was either him or let them drag Joan in to testify. I think it works out better for us to have Mr. Sour Grapes tell the jury about it. Should build sympathy for you."

"I don't want sympathy," Rebecca hissed.

"Well, you also don't want to be convicted. So take whatever you can get."

Rebecca shook her head. "I don't like it."

Covington took her time walking back to the lectern, a slight smile moving across her face. "Now, Mr. Simpson, you were about to tell the jury about what may have accounted for the defendant's excessive hostility toward the victims in this case, beyond having lost each of the cases she tried against these men."

Ralph straightened up. He had wanted to sell this tidbit to the tabloids when Rebecca was first arrested, but then he figured the prosecution wouldn't call him as a witness. Now he finally had the opportunity to spread his gossip and help the prosecution at the same time. "Rebecca claimed she was herself a victim of child molestation, and that she took an extra interest in the cases she prosecuted because of her history."

His tone let it be known he wasn't convinced Rebecca had been molested, but he thought her claim explained her intense interest. "The cases weren't just cases to her—they were personal."

"And how did you come to understand this?"

"Well, I noticed that her crusade always seemed to go too far. She just couldn't put the cases behind her. It's like she never forgot a case she lost. She'd continue to talk about the defendants in the office, she'd follow their progress through probation, and, like I said before, she'd go absolutely ballistic when she'd lose a case. You know, not lose per se, but when she couldn't get jail time. She considered that a loss. She'd come back to her office and rip it apart."

"And you came to understand that her anger and frustration stemmed from her personal history?"

"Yeah. One day I was asking her secretary, you know, what the heck's wrong with Rebecca? Why is she such a nutcase about—"

"Your Honor?" Tom couldn't believe Simpson was this incapable of tailoring his testimony to the rules of evidence.

"Mr. Simpson, you are not qualified to render opinions on anyone's state of mind. Objection sustained."

"I'm sorry, Your Honor," said Covington, trying to convince the jury, if not the judge, that she was not responsible for her witness's irresponsibility. "Mr. Simpson, exactly how did you learn that the defendant was herself an incest victim?"

"As I was saying, her secretary told me that it was hard on Rebecca prosecuting these guys because she herself had been molested."

"Thank you, Mr. Simpson. I have one more question. Did the defendant make any statements to you about any of the five deceased in this case, concerning their murders?"

"Yes, ma'am. She said—I remember it to this day cause it sent a shiver down my spine when I heard it—she said Matheson died too quickly. I always wondered how she knew that. She said these guys should really suffer a slow, painful death. And then when I heard that some of the later guys were really carved up, well it just got me thinking . . ."

"You bastard! You lying bastard! I never said that!" Rebecca was on her feet, screaming at Ralph, moving toward the stand. Tom jumped up and grabbed her around the waist, struggling to hold her back. "How dare you lie like that!"

Delacroix pounded his gavel, shouting above Rebecca's screams, "Order! Order! Counselor, if you do not control your client I will have the bailiffs remove her from court this instant. I said order!" Rebecca, oblivious to the banging of the gavel and the judge's harsh warning, kept pulling toward Ralph, screaming at him, his placid, smug grin provoking her even more.

All around her, the courtroom exploded in a sea of noise and confusion. The spectators were stunned by the outburst, the media frantically scribbling notes, the jury abuzz, confused and a little frightened, the bailiffs propelled into action, one escorting the jury out of court, the other surrounding Rebecca, Tom whispering to her, trying to calm her down. All the while, Covington stood by impassively, stifling a broad smile at Ralph's big payoff. Rebecca had showed the jury that hair-trigger, explosive side of her personality Covington could only allude to. Perhaps that rage was what the victims saw just before they died. She hoped the jury made that connection.

Tom pulled Rebecca back down to her seat, repeating into her ear an urgent "calm down, calm down."

"I'm okay. I'm fine." Rebecca's breathing slowed

as she started to get a hold of herself, suddenly aware of all the attention focused on her. "Oh, shit, Tom, I'm sorry. I can't believe I did that."

"Just don't do anything. Let me talk to the judge." Tom turned toward the judge, dismayed to find him glaring down over his glasses, his face hard and angry. "I'm sorry, Your Honor. Everything's fine. My client apologizes deeply and would like to tell you herself if that is possible. There won't be any more outbursts, I can assure you of that."

His jaw set firmly, Judge Delacroix's words resonated with barely tempered fury. "No, I think it is I who can assure you of that. If I hear so much as a peep from your client while she is at the counsel table, she will be physically removed in front of the jury, tied up and gagged, and then returned to the counsel table in that condition. This is a court of law, not a wrestling match. Consider yourself warned." Judge Delacroix turned to the bailiff. "All right, you may bring the jury back." After admonishing the jury to ignore what they just witnessed, Delacroix instructed Covington to resume.

"Actually, I have no more questions, Your Honor." Covington smiled broadly. "Thank you, Mr. Simpson."

Tom didn't wait for Covington to sit down before starting in on Simpson. Damage control was of utmost urgency. "Now, Mr. Simpson, what was your position in the hierarchy at the Van Nuys branch of the district attorney's office prior to Ms. Fielding's arrest? Who was your immediate superior?"

"I don't have a superior," Ralph answered blandly, looking away.

"Isn't it true that Ms. Fielding was appointed to head the sex crimes unit of the department, and you were not?"

"Rebecca was technically above me in the department, if that's what you're asking." Ralph shifted in his seat and looked over at the jury, shrugging his shoulders as if to say, "Big deal."

Tom crossed his arms. "And did you convey your displeasure with that fact to any other members of the District Attorney's office?"

"Sure, I thought I was more deserving of being the head of the unit than Rebecca. I've apparently been proven right," he added smugly, tossing his head back.

Tom walked back and forth behind the podium, prowling like a caged tiger. He turned to face the witness. "Mr. Simpson, wouldn't it be fair to characterize your feeling toward Rebecca as one of intense jealousy?"

"I am not jealous of Rebecca. I just happen to think she was promoted for reasons other than competence."

Tom continued to pace slowly, nodding his head, as if fully understanding Ralph's intense jealousy. "You believed you should have had her position at the sex crimes unit, correct?"

"Yes." Ralph leaned forward. "But that doesn't mean that I would mischaracterize my conversations with her. She said the child molesters got what they deserved. That's the gospel truth."

Tom looked up at the seal behind the judge, as if pondering some troublesome fact. "While Ms. Fielding is on administrative leave pending the outcome of this trial, who is in charge of her unit?"

"Well, I am."

Tom opened his eyes wide, then nodded and grinned slightly. That seemed to make everything perfectly clear to him. He looked over to the jury and exchanged knowing smiles. "Thank you. I have nothing more for this witness."

"Any redirect?"

Covington realized that for all the juicy tidbits he

had to offer, Ralph was the kind of witness whose obnoxious personality might impact the jury more than the substance of his testimony. And she worried that Tom had done an effective job of pushing the jealousy button. "No, Your Honor. No more questions."

Covington looked over at Tom and Rebecca, sitting fairly pleased with themselves after the cross on Simpson. That would have to change. As she called the first of her two eyewitnesses, a wiry young man with a nervous laugh, she thought she saw a shudder pass through them.

The man's testimony was as direct as it was short. "It was her, plain as day," he drawled convincingly, unshaken by Tom's repeated attempt to question both his memory and motive. "No, sir, I'm one hundred percent sure that's the lady I saw at Eric's place the day he was killed." And then he pointed at Rebecca for good measure. Covington tied Rebecca to the Penhall murder that simply. The next witness, Mildred Walker, was a sweet, plump, gray-haired grandmother so endearing that Covington half expected the jurors would give her a hug as she left the stand. She seemed sorry with her role and yet equally certain that she had seen Rebecca on the street outside Harold Riddell's apartment.

By the end of the day, Covington had admirably steered her two disparate eyewitnesses safely through their testimony, which she knew juries put an undue amount of faith in. Tom and Rebecca knew that as well. After their testimony, Covington began to give in to the conceit that a win was now inevitable.

Covington's office was surprisingly neat, especially for someone in a death penalty case—the floors devoid of boxes, the desktop bare, no oversized exhibits or blowups on the walls. The war room for the Fielding case was set up down the hall where two other attorneys and a law clerk were crowded among all the trial materials. The receptionist rang her to say her witness had arrived, and Covington turned to the clock and smiled. Six o'clock on the nose, punctuality was a good sign of a cooperative witness.

"Come in, sit down." Covington motioned to Valerie Kingsley. Kingsley seemed to hesitate and Covington recognized the signs of pretestimony jitters. She rose to shake Valerie's hand and start the process of relaxing her about tomorrow. Covington was about to walk the fine line between witness preparation and witness coaching as she discussed Valerie's testimony. "Can I get you some coffee or something to drink?"

Valerie sat down, smoothing her skirt under her and pulling it straight. "No, that's okay, I'm fine." She let out a sigh, then seemed a little embarrassed by her show of nerves.

"I hope you don't mind if I eat my dinner while we talk. I'm a little pressed for time, as you might imagine," Covington said, laughing. "So are you ready for tomorrow?" she asked, about to take a mouthful of chow mein, straight out of the take-out container. "You seemed a little upset on the phone." And you're sitting here like you're about to jump out of that chair, she added silently.

"Well . . . I guess I'm just a little . . . I guess you would say . . . nervous about testifying. You know, I've never had to do that before. Personally, I think you'd be better off with Dr. Hillerman."

Covington did not share Valerie's belief. She had interviewed Hillerman and feared that he wouldn't fare much better in front of the jury than one of his patients. But Valerie was young, female, and attractive, perfect to convey the prosecution's message—so long as she took Covington's advice to come to court a little less buttoned down. "Valerie, you'll be fine. We've gone over all of this before. Just remember to stay calm, listen to the questions, and give truthful responses."

"But what if I don't know all the answers? I'm not as experienced as Dr. Hillerman." Valerie was showing more nervousness than when they had spoken originally, and it made Covington uncomfortable. She put her food down.

"There are only two rather distinct areas that I'm going to question you about. First, what you observed about the defendant's obsession with the deceased men. Second, how the deceased had made genuine progress in therapy and were cut down after you and your fellow therapists had successfully cured them of their problems."

"Well," Valerie offered, "you know, we don't really cure them. That word just doesn't really fit with what we do."

Covington was about to lose her appetite. Valerie wasn't quite getting it and she needed to before tomorrow. "We want to convey the right message to the jury. Keep in mind at all times that what you say and how you say it are critical. So use words they can understand. Okay? Cure is a word everyone knows and can relate to. To the lay person it means 'get better.' And really, that's what you try to do—help these men get better. So I think there's no problem with us using that word." Covington thought she had pushed the right button. Doesn't every therapist try to help their patients, after all?

Valerie thought about it for a moment, seeming to grapple with the suggestion. She finally nodded, accepting Covington's terminology. "Well, yeah, I think I get what you're saying. It's just a term of art—it's not meant literally. I can go along with that. I just hope I don't forget tomorrow. There's so much to remember, I wish we could just write out what I'm supposed to say." Valerie fingered her necklace. "I've watched trials on television before and I have to tell you, the idea of testifying scares me a little. Especially answering questions from her attorney."

Although it took some effort, Covington smiled in reassurance. "Just relax. We've already been over all the questions and the answers. It should go very smoothly." She said the words as cheerfully and confidently as she could, but Valerie's cold feet were causing her concern. "Watch. 'Ms. Kingsley, can you tell the jury about your observations of the defendant?' Then you say, 'She used to call me to check up on the victims, trying to dig up dirt on them to get their probations revoked. When I told her they were doing well, she'd get very angry and hang up the phone on me.' See? Simple."

Valerie looked a little embarrassed. "I know, you're right. It's just that Dr. Hillerman is very upset right now, you know, with the fire and the trial and everything, and if I say something . . . I know he's sending the center's attorney to watch me. He's worried that the Oakwood doesn't look bad in all this."

Great, all I need. More pressure on the witness. "Don't worry. Ignore all that and just focus on me. I'll help you along. Just follow my lead and you'll do fine." It seemed that Valerie had relaxed, that whatever pressure she felt had been lifted. "Why don't you go home, take a nice long bath, get a good night's sleep, and I'll see you in the morning. Okay?"

Valerie nodded then stood up and gave Covington a firm handshake. "Okay."

38

Covington wore her hair down today. She was feeling relaxed, particularly since it promised to be another day of strong testimony for the prosecution. Another string of witnesses telling the jury what swell guys the deceased were and what an obsessed, hate-filled, explosive woman the defendant was. But then, the jury was now well aware of the side of Rebecca that could fly into an uncontrollable rage.

Jack showed up this morning with a rose and a note for Rebecca, which the bailiff grudgingly passed along to Tom. The note read: "Roses are red, Violets are blue, Last night I beat up Ralph for you." Watching her laugh meant the world to Jack. He knew she'd need the good feelings to carry her through another difficult day.

Covington called Valerie to the stand, pleased to note that she had taken her suggestions for modifying her appearance for trial. Valerie looked softer, more attractive, with her hair tumbling off her shoulders and glasses forgone for contacts. Stripped of her usual matronly outfit, Covington thought she looked as if she

could be Rebecca's kid sister, which would make her
testimony all the more damning. Covington began by
having Kingsley provide sympathetic depictions of
each of the deceased, portraying them as confused,
troubled men who were benefiting greatly from their
treatment and who had turned their lives around, just
as those very lives were brutally cut short. That accomplished, she then turned her attack toward Rebecca.

"Now, Ms. Kingsley, as the treating therapist for
William Matheson and Harold Riddell—"

"And also for Mr. Knight and Mr. Jaffe."

Covington hated being interrupted. "Yes, yes, of
course. Those two, also. Well, can you tell the jury
whether any of these men voiced concerns about
their safety, specifically fear of retribution by the
defendant?"

"Objection, hearsay."

"May we approach?" Covington asked. She and
Tom gathered in a corner behind the clerk's table.
"Your Honor, the witness had heard these men discuss their fear that the defendant might come after
them. They told this witness that the defendant
threatened them after their trials and continued to
harass them while they were on probation. The victims told her that the defendant said 'I'm not done
with you' and 'Look over your shoulder'—those
types of threatening remarks."

Tom responded quickly. "That's double hearsay,
Your Honor. There is no exception for conversations
the witness may have had with the deceased that
would make the statement reliable."

While the sidebar was continuing, Randazzo quietly entered the court and sat down next to Larson in
the back of the courtroom.

Larson turned his head toward her. "I tried to call
you last night. Have you learned anything yet?" He
tried to keep his voice down.

"No, nothing yet. Nobody's saying much," she whispered as she looked at the witness box. "What's Rebecca doing testifying today?" she asked, loud enough to get shushed.

"That's not Rebecca, that's Kingsley. Remember? Matheson's therapist."

"Oh." Randazzo looked again, squinting slightly. "Geez, you're right."

Larson reached into his pocket and pulled out his glasses. "You want to borrow these?" he kidded. "You're too young to be going blind."

She smiled, then nodded up at the sidebar. "So what are they talking about with the judge?"

He shrugged. "Who knows? We all think they're discussing some fine point of law and they're probably ordering lunch." He kept his voice down to avoid a scolding from the judge.

"Well, I snooped around all I could, I think your buddy Frank was right. The fire looks like an inside job," Randazzo said, drawing disapproving stares from audience members rows ahead. She flipped them her badge and they quickly turned back around.

"The jury is to disregard the last question," Delacroix boomed. "Next question, Counselor. And please, I'll have quiet in the court, or I'll clear it."

Covington returned to her post, hoping to get the examination back on track and establish a rhythm. "Ms. Kingsley, were you contacted on more than one occasion by the defendant with respect to the progress of any of the deceased?"

"Yes. She called me many times, sometimes more than once a day," Valerie added.

"Please tell the court about these discussions." Covington took two steps over to the edge of the jury box, and Valerie turned toward them.

"Ms. Fielding would call as soon as someone was sent to us for treatment and give me this speech about how we were the only punishment they were getting so it shouldn't be a walk in the park. She wanted me to know that she didn't care what we thought about these guys, but that she thought they were dangerous, vile criminals who shouldn't be allowed to go free and that we should treat them as such."

"Were those the only calls you would get from the defendant?"

Valerie looked annoyed. "Oh, no. I wish. She'd call every week, sometimes more than once a day, about certain of her old defendants. She'd ask what they were doing, were they attending their meetings, that sort of thing. And there was always a call when one of them would reach the start of his last year on probation. Like clockwork. Always checking up on them, trying to get some evidence that they were violating probation so she could get them sent to jail. And she was always reminding me that I had a duty to report any such violations, that I didn't have to look the other way if I learned anything." Valerie sighed deeply, conveying her exasperation with Fielding's calls.

Covington smiled to herself. Valerie was right on track. "Would she ask you any personal questions about the men who were in treatment?"

"Oh yes, she wanted to know everything she could. She said that once they were off probation, they'd be unsupervised and could return to their old habits, so this was her best chance to keep them off the streets. She'd ask if I thought they would reoffend once they were off probation—were they living with or working around children, did they have any unsupervised access to children, that sort of thing. Also, were they drinking or using. She'd call repeatedly, right up to the day they were released from probation, always trying to dig up dirt."

"And what would you tell her?"

Valerie shrugged helplessly, conveying, What could I do? "I always told her to contact the probation officer, that I didn't want to compromise my relationship with my men by reporting to her on such an informal basis."

"Did that stop her calls?"

Valerie shook her head firmly. "No. She continued to call. But I told her that if there was a problem, I'd inform their probation officer."

Covington walked back over to the podium. "But there was a problem with Mr. Penhall, wasn't there?"

"Yes," she said offhandedly, apparently trying to downplay any problems. "We were a little troubled because we had some evidence that he had fallen off the wagon, as it were. He was supposed to refrain from drugs or alcohol while on probation, but he started coming to group obviously on something. Of course, we reported it to the probation department immediately," Valerie said, looking directly at Rebecca.

"And when the defendant called you about Mr. Penhall, did you tell her about this?"

"Yes," Kingsley answered wearily. "I told her that we knew the law and we were dealing with the probation department about it, and that she should contact them. But that didn't seem to satisfy her."

"Objection," Baldwin declared, "lack of foundation."

"Sustained."

Covington didn't miss a beat. "And how long before his death did that conversation with the defendant take place?"

"Oh, I'd have to say a week or two." Valerie took a sip of water.

"A week or two," Covington stressed. She took the four steps back toward the jury as if they were four miles. "Okay. Did you ever receive a call from the defendant about William Matheson?"

Valerie sat up and straightened her jacket. "Yes, she called to tell me that she thought it was a mistake for me to set up a meeting between Mr. Matheson and his family, that it could be very damaging for the family. I told her that I thought he was ready for the meeting and that it would go just fine."

"And did it?"

"Well, no, actually. It was very surprising, considering all the progress he had made up to then. I told her afterward that the meeting hadn't gone well. That he hadn't behaved well. She was very upset."

"And this was . . . ?"

Valerie looked at the jury. "A few days before he was killed."

That was a nice touch, Covington thought, making eye contact with the jury. "Did you have a similar telephone call prior to Mr. Knight's murder?"

"Yes." She turned back toward the jury, as if talking with friends. "She was supposedly on vacation, and yet the defendant called me three times one day to ask about my guys, and one of the guys she was particularly worried about was Brad Knight. She thought he was manipulating us into letting him switch treatment centers, that he was getting the upper hand and that he couldn't be adequately monitored," Valerie said flatly, as if mimicking Rebecca's chastising tone.

Covington leaned back on the railing and crossed her arms in front of her. "Did you find Ms. Fielding's frequent calls to you to be normal?"

"Oh no, not at all. It was highly unusual. No other district attorney ever called to check up on some guy after he was sent to us. It was a little scary, to tell you the truth," Valerie said apologetically.

Covington couldn't end on a better note. "I have nothing further." She knew she had done all the damage that she could. The jury now knew that a therapist found Rebecca's obsessive behavior to be far from the norm.

Tom approached the podium slowly, not quite sure what to do with Kingsley's testimony. In a fit of anger, he simply chose to lash out at her. "Ms. Kingsley, please tell the jury what occurred at the meeting between Matheson and his ex-wife and step-daughter just before he was killed."

"Well, briefly, I arranged a meeting for Matheson and his ex-wife and her daughter, what was to be an apology session where he would discuss what he had learned in therapy and take responsibility for the hurt he caused. It was his final step in therapy—accepting accountability for his actions."

Come on, he thought, let's remind the jury what a stand-up guy Mr. Matheson was. "His actions?"

"Molesting his stepdaughter."

Tom walked away from her, nodding to himself, then stopped and turned around. "When you say 'molesting,' what exactly does that mean?"

Valerie tilted her head to one side and crossed her arms. "He had intercourse with his stepdaughter without her consent." She kept the "Are you satis-fied?" to herself.

Tom smiled a sarcastic smile. "So Mr. Matheson raped his twelve-year-old stepdaughter and you"—he filled his voice with rage and disbelief—"you thought he should have a session with her to show what a great guy he was?"

Valerie looked at the audience, worried as she saw Stan scribbling notes. She took a long drink of water and asked the bailiff for a refill, her mouth still dry.

"No," she said when she was ready. "It was for him to hear what she had to say and apologize for what he did. It's not like he could take back what he did. I was helping him learn to take responsibility, that's all."

"Did he do that in the session? Take the blame for raping his stepdaughter?"

Valerie looked down nervously. She played with the bottom button of her jacket, avoiding Tom's eyes. "No," she said finally.

"In fact, he was anything but apologetic, isn't that true?" Tom's voice filled with contempt. Tell them what he did, he thought. Let's hear about your guys.

"That's correct. He dumped all of the blame onto them, saying it was all their fault that he had a record and had to go to therapy and be on probation. Everything. The session went quite badly," Valerie said, keeping her eyes downcast.

"Evidently," said Tom as he faced the jury, his back toward Valerie. "How did the ex-wife react?"

"She was devastated . . ."

"Objection, relevance?" Covington sounded exhausted. She thought this line of questioning had already gone on too long and too far afield.

"May we approach, Your Honor?" asked Tom.

"Yes." After the two attorneys and the court reporter had settled into a semicircle around the front of the judge's bench, Delacroix leaned forward, directing his comments to Covington. "You have a problem with Mr. Baldwin's questions, Counselor?"

"I certainly do, Your Honor. Mr. Baldwin is making a rather transparent attempt to put the character of Mr. Matheson on trial here, and I am not going to allow that to happen. If Mr. Baldwin is not stopped and directed to ask only questions that pertain to his client's guilt or innocence, then we will have witness after witness describing the crimes these men committed many years ago solely for the purpose of having the jury not care that these men were murdered."

"Your Honor," Tom began, "I can see that my colleague is uncomfortable with testimony concerning just who these men were. She clearly does not want the jury to know that these men were manipulative, child-abusing, rapist bullies, but I believe it is crucial to the defense for the jury to understand that many more people than my client may have had a motive to kill the deceased."

"I'm sorry, Counselor," Judge Delacroix said to Covington, "but I tend to agree with the defense on this issue. I think that this line of questioning falls under the category of sauce for the goose being sauce for the gander. Your Mr. Simpson was quite eager to discuss the defendant's feelings of hatred toward the deceased as motive for murder. I'll allow the defense some leeway in exploring other possible suspects. You may return."

"Thank you, Your Honor," both attorneys said in unison, albeit only one of them sincerely.

As the attorneys retreated to their respective tables, the judge spoke for the record. "The objection is overruled. The witness may complete her answer if she recalls the question."

"I don't remember, Your Honor," Valerie said, a little confused. She put her hand to her forehead, massaging it gently. She could feel her head tightening, the blood vessels constricting. As she looked at Tom, his features began to blur. She tried to focus on what he was saying, but the throbbing in her head was distracting.

"Ms. Kingsley, you were telling the jury the reaction of Mr. Matheson's ex-wife to his performance at the last meeting, a week before he was killed."

"Oh, yes." She closed her eyes. Testifying was more grueling than she had imagined, and Stan's constant stare wasn't helping matters. She struggled to stay focused, to concentrate. "Mrs. Matheson, I mean Jenkins, Ms. Jenkins was extremely upset, very agitated. She was angry at me, angry at him, angry at the center. She was yelling at me how I had hurt her and hurt her daughter. I think she threatened to sue me. I tried to calm her down. I wanted to help her." She stopped, then looked up. For a moment, she forgot where she was. She felt herself back in the session, looking helplessly at the distraught mother and her devastated daughter. Her own anger at Matheson began to stir.

"Ms. Kingsley, did you tell Ms. Fielding about the ex-wife's reaction?"

"Yes, I believe we discussed it."

"And what did you tell her?"

"That the ex-wife was"—Valerie looked at the judge, waiting for instructions. With none forthcoming, she continued—"devastated. That she was enraged and the daughter was very hurt. It was a fiasco. He was shouting at them, they were shouting back, the daughter in tears. The wife was so mad, I thought—"

"You thought what?"

"I thought Ms. Jenkins was going to kill him."

"Motion to strike," Covington shouted.

Tom ignored her, focusing solely on the witness. "And this occurred how long before he was killed?"

"Sustained," said Delacroix, in unison with Kingsley's answer: "Less than a week before he was killed."

"The jury will disregard that last question and answer. Counselor," he said, looking at Tom, "when there is an objection, please wait for the ruling before asking any more questions. Ms. Kingsley, please try to do the same. Thank you. Proceed."

"Yes, Your Honor." Tom walked back over to the podium, looked down, then started his next line of questioning. "Now, Ms. Kingsley, were you familiar with the first victim?"

"Henry MacDonald, yes. I was his therapist for about—"

Tom looked down at his notes. "No, the first victim. Mr. Penhall."

Valerie swallowed hard. "Oh yes, Mr. Penhall."

"Right," Baldwin said, staring at the witness. The last thing he needed was more confusion. "Okay, isn't it true—"

"Jack," Randazzo said, louder than was acceptable for the courtroom observers. Larson was met by a strange look in Randazzo's eyes. "Did you hear what she just said?"

"No, what?"

"Kingsley said the first victim was MacDonald."

"Yeah?"

"He was the suicide." Randazzo paused, thinking, but only one thought popped in her head. "Why would she say that MacDonald was the first victim unless . . . ?"

Jack's eyes widened. "Are you sure she said MacDonald?" he asked, holding his breath as time stood still.

"Positive. And the only person who would consider MacDonald the first victim . . ."

Larson exhaled. "Is whoever killed him," he said, finishing Randazzo's sentence. Larson's mind raced as he looked back and forth between Kingsley and Fielding, feeling alive again for the first time in months. "She looks a little like Rebecca at least from a distance. You were fooled yourself a few minutes ago when you walked in. It all makes sense. Oh, shit. I've got to talk to Tom. He doesn't have a clue. He missed it completely. Hell, *I* missed it completely."

Jack slinked from his back of the courtroom seat to the railing behind the defense counsel table. "Tom," he whispered to him in midsentence. Tom turned around, not quite sure why anyone was calling him. "Tom, get a recess." A stage whisper that caught everyone's attention.

"What?" Tom turned back toward the judge, "Excuse me, Your Honor. May I have a moment?"

Judge Delacroix nodded and Tom turned around to Jack. "What's going on? Why do you want me to—"

"Don't ask me why, just get a recess. I think I may have something to blow open the case." Jack looked over and winked at a dazed Rebecca.

"What is it?"

"Just get a fucking recess. I'll tell you later."

"What'll I tell the court? I've got to tell the judge something. He won't grant a recess simply because I ask for one."

"Tell him anything. Tell him Chicken Little was wrong, just get the recess. And, by the way, tell Rebecca to start packing. They just started boarding our plane."

Judge Delacroix had seen enough. "Counselor, this interruption is uncalled for."

Tom looked back up and started walking toward the counsel table. "Your Honor, I apologize. I need to request a brief recess."

"And why is that, Mr. Baldwin?"

"May I request a sidebar, Your Honor?" Tom asked, not knowing what he'd do if his request were granted.

Valerie looked at the goings-on with a quiet fear. She instinctively realized something was wrong. A small trickle of sweat rolled down her back.

"Mr. Baldwin. I certainly hope there is a splendid explanation for what's going on."

So do I, Tom thought. "Your Honor, one of the homicide detectives in this case has requested that I obtain a short continuance. While I am not sure of the reason, I have no doubt that there is a very good excuse. Thus, if we could recess until tomorrow, I would greatly appreciate it."

"Mr. Baldwin, although your candor is commendable, I'm hesitant to recess this case without an adequate reason. Ms. Covington, do you have any objection?"

"Absolutely, Your Honor. This detective has been linked romantically with Ms. Fielding. This stunt is nothing more than an excuse to disrupt this trial and delay the inevitable. I find this whole thing highly questionable."

Delacroix rubbed his chin, then glanced over at the clock. "I tend to agree, Counselor. However, being as we are nearing the lunch break, why don't we just call it a day and reconvene tomorrow morning? I expect that this should all be sorted out by then, Mr. Baldwin."

"I think that's right, Your—" Tom began.

Delacroix put his hand up to silence him. "Mr. Baldwin, that was an order, not a question," he clarified.

Tom bowed his head slightly. "Yes, Your Honor. And thank you. I apologize. And I can assure you this was not planned."

As the jury filed out, Valerie looked confused. Covington walked over to her to apologize for the interruption. She tried to explain what was going on, but that was difficult, since Covington herself did not know. Valerie pretended to listen, though her attention was focused on the conversation that Larson and Randazzo were having in the back of the court. After agreeing to return tomorrow for the continuation of her testimony, Valerie stepped down off the stand and headed briskly out of the courtroom. Stan tried to intercept her to find out what Covington had said, but Valerie brushed right past him.

"Excuse me, Ms. Kingsley, may we speak with you for a moment?" Larson called out as Valerie burst out of the courtroom and into the corridor. He knew he couldn't detain her on a hunch, but he hoped she wouldn't know that. He followed her down the corridor.

Valerie didn't turn around, continuing toward the exit to the street. "Sorry, Detective. I'm late for an appointment," she muttered as she maintained her quick pace out of the courthouse, with an over-the-shoulder wave to Larson.

Larson called after her again, trying to get her to stop. "It'll just take a minute." This time, Valerie didn't even turn around. Larson ran back into the courtroom and found Randazzo standing in the back with a still-startled Tom.

"Jennifer, let's go, now!"

"What is it?"

"She left the building." Larson grabbed Randazzo by the arm. "Tom, this will all make sense later, I promise. But we gotta go." Larson led Randazzo out the courtroom and they raced back down the corridor to try to find Valerie.

"She said she had some appointment, but she didn't say where she was going," Larson said.

Randazzo looked at the time. "That's bullshit. How can she have an appointment? Court ended earlier than expected."

"Good question. I hope we can find her to ask."

They moved quickly, out the door, through the parking lot, and climbed into their car. Randazzo picked up the radio and called the D.A.'s office. "Hi. Who's at the search warrant desk?" she asked, hoping not to hear the name Ralph Simpson. She relaxed upon hearing the name of Rachel Myer, a D.A. she had worked with on a gang shooting last summer, and someone to whom she'd given a nice baby shower present. "Good, put me through. Thanks. Hi, Rachel. This is Jennifer Randazzo. How're things going?" Randazzo didn't wait for the answer. "Look. I need a favor. I need a warrant to search the house of Valerie Kingsley. Now don't ask any questions, just take this down. You gotta trust me on this." Randazzo hoped Rachel hadn't heard this line from a desperate cop too often to fall for it. "I don't know the address."

Larson pulled a small notepad out of his breast pocket and handed it to Randazzo. "It's 14323 Sycamore Road, Sherman Oaks," she said, reading his notes of Valerie's testimony. Randazzo looked at him, surprised, then turned her attention back to the phone.

"Did you get that? Great." She handed the notes back to Larson. "Okay, get it and meet us there. Grounds? Put down reasonable cause to believe occupant is guilty of the child molester murders." Randazzo was not surprised by the stunned "What?!" on the other end of the phone. "I know it sounds crazy, but we've got something on her. Let's just say that the suspect knows more than she should know unless she's the killer. But put it in language that'll get us past a judge."

Randazzo listened as the D.A. formulated the request for the warrant in perfect legalese and offered her as much additional information as she could, hoping it was enough to get a judge to sign off on the warrant. Rachel then asked Randazzo the expected cover-her-ass question. Randazzo replied: "No, Covington doesn't know. Yet." She looked over at Larson and smiled. "I think I'll let my partner explain it to her later."

39

Valerie gripped the steering wheel so tightly her knuckles were white, and she could feel her heart pounding in her chest. Still, she forced herself to maintain her speed, not wanting to attract attention by darting around the traffic. They knew, they had to know now. What was the old saying? A slip of the tongue can sink a ship. Stupid!! She had stayed in the background so long, quiet, letting Rebecca get all the credit—wanting to continue the work she'd started, yet knowing she had to stop till the trial was over. The fire had been a smoldering monument to nothing—incomplete and misconstrued—not the statement she had wanted it to be. Now time was running out.

She instinctively turned toward the Oakwood. She had to go there first, before he could be warned. She knew what she had to do. She had to stop them.

Valerie nearly rear-ended the car in front of her, which had stopped when the light turned yellow. Nobody stops at yellows, she seethed. She slammed her hand on the steering wheel in anger and frustration.

"Go, go, go!" she yelled both at the car and the light, commanding it to turn green. She continued through traffic, driving almost automatically until she reached the Oakwood. She parked on the street, about half a block away and sprinted to the office, passing the office staff heading down the stairs for lunch. Anita stopped in front of her. "You're back so soon. How'd it go?" she asked.

Valerie continued up the stairs, not interested in small talk. "Fine. Nothing exciting."

Anita called up to her. "Want to join us at BJ's?"

"No. I've got some work to catch up on. But thanks anyway." Her voice was bright.

Valerie hurried through the doors—thankful no one was there—and straight into Hillerman's office. He was surprised to see her, happily so when she closed the door and walked seductively up to him. Moments later Valerie emerged from his office and switched on Hillerman's do not disturb light, closing his office door behind her. She rushed back toward the parking lot, opened the door to Hillerman's Mercedes, and drove off.

Larson and Randazzo waited for what seemed to be an eternity for the search warrant to arrive. They kept their eyes on Kingsley's apartment but noticed no activity. Finally, with the warrant in hand, Larson knocked on the door. In a scene out of the worst cop movie, when he was not met with a response, Larson reflexively announced that if the door wasn't opened, he'd break it down.

"Break it down? Who's going to break it down?" Randazzo asked him with some amusement.

"I will," he said, pumping himself up for the challenge.

After two unsuccessful runs at the door, Randazzo

offered a sarcastic, "You want me to get that?" His glare told her no.

Fanned as much by his irritation as the hope that beyond the door lay the truth, or more accurately, the lies Kingsley had kept hidden, Larson found success on his third attempt. The rush of adrenaline kept him from feeling the aching in his shoulder.

Larson and Randazzo split up once inside the apartment. Moving around inside with their guns drawn, Larson took the dining room and kitchen, while Randazzo went to the rear of the apartment. The apartment was immaculate though devoid of much in the way of decoration, the kitchen lemon fresh, the living room orderly, precise. But not so the bedroom.

"Jack!" Randazzo yelled from the bedroom. "Get in here."

Jack ran in, then stopped abruptly, his eyes scanning the room in shocked disbelief. Covering one wall, the bed, and most of the floor were press clippings on each killing. The haphazard display of the newspaper and magazine articles was out of sync with the room, its bed made, its furniture freshly dusted. Situated in the center of the bed was a large photo album in which some of the articles and photos had been neatly placed. Randazzo pulled out a pen and used it to flip to the first page. Henry MacDonald. His probation report on one page, his one-inch funeral notice, and a postmortem Polaroid on the next. The unfinished scrapbook of her killing spree. "Oh, man, will you look at this?" said Randazzo, pleased with her find, but now shuddering, suddenly aware of her role in almost sending an innocent woman to her death.

"No, look at this," Larson called from the head of the bed. Polaroids, close-ups of the victims' death masks, were arranged neatly in a semicircle on the nightstand next to her bed. The photographs faced her pillow—so she could grab a final glance before slipping off to sleep? "This woman is one sick puppy," Larson thought out loud.

Randazzo turned toward the tall bureau across from the foot of the bed. She was drawn to an eight-by-ten photograph prominently displayed. Fuzzy with faded colors, it appeared to be a family picture—a father, a mother, and a daughter. Randazzo guessed from their clothing it was taken in the post-polyester early eighties. The father was handsome, rakish, with his jaw thrust forward and head tilted upward, his arm around the girl like a fisherman displaying a prized catch; the mother on the other side, less attractive, distant, awkward, and uncomfortable. The daughter appeared to be around ten. She bore some resemblance to Kingsley, though the frozen smile made it difficult to notice at first. She was posed uncomfortably with her waist pulled tight against the father, yet her upper body bent away from him. The father looked strangely familiar as well. It took Randazzo but a moment to realize where she'd seen that look before. "Jack, whaddya think?" she asked, gesturing toward the picture. "That pompous grin. He kinda reminds me of Hillerman."

Larson looked and nodded slowly. "Yeah, I see it." He went back to the other mementos on the dresser, searching for clues behind the woman with the secret. Next to an ornately framed photo of Valerie's mother was a small, pink envelope containing a yellowed newspaper obituary attesting to the woman's death, from a long bout with cancer, at the age of thirty-nine. She was described only as the wife of famed child psychiatrist Dr. Herman Kingsley, and mother of their thirteen-year-old daughter, Valerie. Also inside the envelope was a handwritten note on stationery framed in pink roses. The note was addressed to "My darling daughter." Larson started reading aloud. "I'm so sorry I let you down when you needed me most. I want you to know that I do believe you now. And your father has sworn to me that it will never happen again." He looked up. "Do you want to guess what it was that Dad won't do again?"

Randazzo looked back at the picture of the three of them. "I think we know now." Randazzo shook her head, angry with herself. "Shit! I can't believe I missed it! I mean, there she was—blonde hair, nice-looking, slender. Just like Rebecca. She had access to all the victims. Listening to them day after day, knowing what they did. I just never thought . . ." Randazzo looked at Larson apologetically.

"It's okay," he reassured her. "Neither of us did. But it was right there. If you think back to the profile we had of the killer—she was likely a victim of incest herself, acting out a revenge fantasy of sorts on sur-rogate dads. Someone fed up with the fact that none of these guys were punished for what they did. You thought it pointed to Rebecca. But Rebecca didn't have to kill them, she got to prosecute them. She got to help the victims. Kingsley, on the other hand, just sat in group with them day after day, being sympa-thetic and understanding. So if she had been molested herself, I mean, can you imagine her sitting there, listening to their BS? It must have eaten her alive. I guess after a while, she just snapped." Larson stopped, suddenly struck with an overwhelming sense of relief. He wasn't sure his legs could hold him as he felt the months of tension leave his body. He was free to feel again, and the first feeling was euphoria. "I knew Rebecca didn't do it. Jennifer, she didn't kill them. I told you she couldn't do that. I told you!"

Randazzo's face lit up as she watched her partner come back to life. "Enough with the I-told-you-so's. We've gotta get moving. There'll be plenty of time to celebrate with Rebecca afterward." She smiled. "Years and years to celebrate." Randazzo recognized the old glint in Jack's eyes.

Jack fought to stay in the present. He wanted to run to the jail, to carry Rebecca out of there to their life together. He let his heart drift to Rebecca and called on his head to stay focused on the work still to be done. "Okay, where the hell would she go now? She's got to know we're looking for her. Where's she running to?"

"I don't know. But she's got a little head start on us." Randazzo instinctively reached for her radio and called in an APB for Valerie Kingsley. "We don't even know if she's still in town. If she knows it's over, that we're on to her, she's gotta try to get away. But where?" Randazzo scanned the room, looking for clues into Valerie's mind. "Maybe Hillerman'll know. He's got to have some idea where she'll run to."

Valerie wound her way up and down the well-tended streets in Woodland Hills, one of the few remaining affluent pockets of the West Valley, before pulling up to her father's estate-sized, Tudor-style house. The house had always appeared to Valerie as a rather imposing structure, seemingly thrust up from the ground to lord over the neighborhood. She pulled her car through the opened gate, past the lush garden and neatly manicured lawn, up the long, circular driveway, and parked it next to another car belonging, she surmised, to the mother of one of his patients. She sat quietly for a moment staring at the house. The windows were shrouded in dark paisley drapes, pulled closed, as usual.

Valerie grabbed her purse and climbed out of her car. Something propelled her to the house first, not for any reason, but out of some irrational need to see it one last time—to be reminded of it, as if its dark memories weren't with her always. She walked quickly, her thoughts spinning wildly as the last few steps of her journey neared, yet not knowing what she would find at the end.

She took out her key and quietly placed it in the lock, pushed the door open, and stepped silently into the house. She would have known she was home even blindfolded as the scent of her father's favorite Davidoff cigars lingered, despite the maid's greatest efforts to remove their scent. Valerie stood in the expansive marble entryway and took a look around. Everything was the same—the large dining room, fully set as if a dinner party for twelve were scheduled for that night, the living room, still decorated in her mother's favorite English style with patterns of floral chintz and jacquard weaves, in hues of dark rose and blue. She walked along the back of the couch, running her hand across the smooth damask upholstery, trying to remember way back to when her mother's laughter had filled the room. She looked up the spiral staircase, toward her bedroom upstairs. As she started up the stairs, the floor beneath her feet creaked a too-familiar sound, the sound of her father heading up to her room. Valerie froze as a lifetime of memories overwhelmed her, coming back as they always did, like an incurable cancer. She turned around and headed back down to the foyer and out the door, around to the rear of the house to her father's office.

Larson and Randazzo arrived at the Oakwood just as the staff slowly filtered back in from lunch. They stopped Anita, remembering her as one of the few people there they could count on for a straight answer, and began questioning her about Valerie. "Yeah, I saw her when we went downstairs for lunch," she offered. "She seemed to be in a big hurry. Passed on lunch. It looked like she had something on her mind."

"Do you know where she went?" asked Randazzo.

"No, I'm sorry, I don't know." Anita sensed the urgency in her voice. Her eyes shifted back and forth between the detectives. "What's going on? Did something happen at trial?"

Randazzo maintained a hint of a smile. "You might say that. We're very eager to find Ms. Kingsley. Do you know where Dr. Hillerman is?"

"He was in his office." Anita looked down the hall and noted his do not disturb light was on. "I hope he's not taking a nap, he really hates being interrupted."

Randazzo and Larson looked back at his office and Randazzo put her hand on Anita's shoulder. "Don't worry about it. It's an emergency. I'll take the heat." She and Larson hurried to the door and knocked hard. Anita cringed at the pounding, waiting for Hillerman's bombastic explosion. Instead, there was an eerie silence. "Dr. Hillerman?" Larson called. Again, no reply. Larson jiggled the handle, then turned to Anita. "Anyone have the key?"

"Yeah, there's a spare one in the drawer over here." Anita quickly retrieved the key and handed it to him. Larson opened the door and saw Hillerman seated, facing away from them, his head slumped down in his chair. "Dr. Hillerman?" Larson said as he walked over tentatively toward him. He turned the chair around and saw two bloody holes where Hillerman's eyes used to be, streaks of red running down the still-surprised face. He heard Anita's stunned gasp from behind him as he leaned in for a closer look. Larson checked for a pulse, a useless gesture. Hillerman was still warm, but lifeless. "Well, at least she's consistent. She always did tend to pick pretty unsympathetic victims."

"Jack, please . . ." Randazzo motioned over to Anita.

Anita stood staring at Hillerman's bloody corpse, her body shaking uncontrollably. "I—I can't believe it. How could she do that? She just walked right in . . . like it was nothing. Just going to work." She looked at the detectives confused, searching for answers, then stared at the floor as if remembering something. "When I saw her, she was smiling."

"I don't doubt it," said Randazzo.

Anita looked at her oddly, then gazed off into the distance and began chewing on her thumbnail. "I just don't understand this. She really admired him— she always said he was like a second father to her. What's going on . . . ?" Her voice trailed off as she started to hyperventilate.

Anita's offhand comment struck a chord in Randazzo. She spun Anita around and away from Hillerman's body and looked her square in the eyes. She had a hunch. "Anita, we need your help. Do you have any idea where he works? Valerie's father."

"No, I, uh, I'm sorry. I—I can't help you. I just don't know." Anita started sobbing, her head in her hands. "Oh, my God. How can you just stand here? He's dead. Do something."

Randazzo grabbed her by the shoulders. "Anita, we're trying to do something. We're trying to prevent another killing, but unless you can help us find her . . ."

Anita bit her bottom lip and tried to think. "I—I'm sorry. I know he's a psychiatrist, so his office's got to be listed." She wrapped her arms around herself but still couldn't control the shaking. "I'm sorry, I just can't think."

Directory information proved more helpful than Anita. The office of Dr. Herman Kingsley was less than a half hour away. Randazzo called ahead for a backup unit to meet them there. She added that Valerie might be armed and dangerous, although she thought that she might only be half right. Randazzo then called Dr. Kingsley's office to warn him but reached only an unhelpful answering service, which kept repeating that emergency or not, Dr. Kingsley could not be contacted directly while he was in session—that he would check his messages between sessions. The service failed to mention that Dr. Kingsley was at his home office on Wednesdays.

Valerie entered her father's office slowly. Inside she found an attractive, thirtyish woman sitting in the waiting room, nervously flipping through the pages of a magazine. Valerie remained standing, pretending to examine the artwork adorning the outer office. In a corner, a small clock ticked off the time. At precisely fifteen before the hour, the door opened and Valerie watched as a small, blonde-haired girl started out of the office. She looked to be about eight or nine, with long, braided pigtails and wearing a red corduroy dress and white tights. Just behind her was Herman Kingsley, his hand patting the little girl gently on her back. He followed the child over to her mother, a sweet, yet insidious look on his face. One that Valerie recognized.

Dr. Kingsley looked up and was startled to see his daughter standing in the office. He stared right at her, but said nothing. Instead, he turned to speak with Mrs. Sorenson, not acknowledging Valerie's presence.

Valerie cleared her throat, not wanting to be rude to the woman, but desperately wanting her to leave before the next patient arrived. Her father noticed her efforts to get his attention and said, "I'll be with you," as if she were another patient, and continued the conversation. "Mrs. Sorenson, we had a wonderful session today." Valerie watched as the little girl shifted uncomfortably, her head downcast. "Our Courtney is making tremendous progress. Aren't you, dear?" Dr. Kingsley said, looking down at the little girl, his voice dripping with honey.

Valerie was growing increasingly impatient. Her stomach churned as she watched her father's hands rubbing the little girl's shoulders. She glanced back at the door and could feel her breathing quicken. Just say good-bye, she thought. It's time to say good-bye.

The mother spoke. "Well, we'd better get going. C'mon, Courtney." Valerie exhaled deeply at the mother's words. "Thank you again, Dr. Kingsley."

"My pleasure, Mrs. Sorenson." He turned Courtney around and kneeled down to her eye level. "You remember what we talked about, okay?" Dr. Kingsley flipped one of the little girl's pigtails over her shoulder, a simple move that might have gone unnoticed by someone else, but Valerie noticed. A sick feeling came over her, a mix of repulsion and fear. She didn't hear what Mrs. Sorenson said to Courtney. She was flashing back to the little gesture, so innocent, so familiar. She said nothing as she stood watching them walk out to their car, the silence lingering in the air.

"Valerie." Her father's booming voice snapped her back. "What are you doing here?" He crossed his arms in front of himself and cocked his head. "It's not time for another tuition payment, is it?" He bent down to straighten the magazines on the table, then stood back up to his full height. Even at his age, he still struck an impressive figure. Tall, handsome, with a wicked smile and stunningly blue eyes, Dr. Kingsley had the bearing of a man who had moved effortlessly through life attaining whatever he wanted and assumed it was ordained to be that way.

"It's not Father's Day." He paced the small outer office while rubbing his hand along his chin, imitating a pose of contemplation. He stopped suddenly and pulled his hand away, as if he'd found his answer. "I know. It must be take-your-daughter-to-work day and I forgot." He added a grin that was meant to diminish the sarcasm in the comment.

Valerie returned her father's smile. "No, Dad. I don't need any money. In fact, just the opposite, I'd like to think I'm here to pay you back . . . for all that you've done." Valerie paused. "So, do you have a few minutes?"

Her father looked put upon by the inquiry. He sighed heavily and checked his watch. "Well." Another sigh. "All right. You have a little time before my next session. What precisely do you want?"

Valerie paced the office, looking at the walls, avoiding her father's eyes. "That's an interesting question to answer right now. One I probably haven't given enough thought to." She stopped herself and frowned. "Sorry. I just ended a sentence with a preposition, didn't I? That should have been to which I haven't given much thought." She nodded. "Yes. That would sound much better."

Dr. Kingsley dropped the amused look. "Look, Valerie, are you going to tell me why you're here? Or are you simply going to continue babbling on incoherently?"

Valerie tilted her head up. "Aren't you happy to see me?"

He looked down at her sternly. "Let's not start that again." He looked around for something to do and grabbed the back of a chair and repositioned it a few millimeters closer to the table. "I'm just surprised to see you here today. Besides, wasn't today the day that you were supposed to testify in the Fielding murder case?"

"Oh, I didn't know you were following the case that closely. Although I shouldn't be surprised"— Valerie paused, and her eyes turned cold—"considering who all the victims were."

Her father avoided her gaze as he moved to dodge the innuendo. "I was just surprised they were calling you to testify. You are only an intern, after all. Why didn't Hillerman or one of the therapists testify?"

"I don't know. Maybe they thought I had more to offer. You'd be very surprised by what I can do." She walked over and stared at a reproduction of a Dali, her back to her father. "In fact, I can honestly say that I have been far more successful with my patients than any other therapist at my office. Their recidivism rate is way down." Valerie barely stifled a laugh at her private joke.

Her father mumbled a disbelieving "Really?" as he headed back to his office, deciding he'd stood long enough. Valerie walked first to the front door and quietly turned the sign on the door around so that the do not disturb side was facing out. Then she shut and locked the door. She walked back to her father's office and found him seated behind his desk. He turned on his answering machine, listened to the first breathless message from an anxious parent and jotted notes. Valerie sat down in the chair across from him, her purse on her lap. She looked around the office, his sanctuary. The tools of his particular trade were all there, the dolls used for play therapy, the paper and crayons for art therapy, and the requisite couch. The walls attested to his exalted expertise and his esteemed position as the one in whom countless parents innocently entrusted their children. Valerie knew him differently. She looked back toward the waiting room and thought about little Courtney and all the other little patients who had filed through that door. She looked back at her father, the monster in an expensive Italian suit and hundred-dollar haircut, and shuddered. And knew she was right to be there. Right not to look away anymore, but to face the truth.

"So, Dad, tell me something." Valerie settled back in the chair, ignoring the pounding in her chest while trying to maintain the appearance of calm. "What do you think about the Fielding case?"

Her father observed her struggle to appear relaxed but was so accustomed to the pose he gave it no importance, thinking her question was no more than natural curiosity. He punched the button turning off the machine, exasperated with the interruption. "What is it you want to know?"

"Well, why don't we start with this. Do you think it's okay to kill incest offenders for what they've done?"

Dr. Kingsley laughed. "Only you would ask such a ridiculous question."

Valerie tried not to let her reaction show, wanting for once to stay strong in the face of his evil. "Oh, yes. How could I forget. You don't think child molesters should be punished at all, do you?"

He picked up the half-burned cigar resting in his prized pewter ashtray and lit it, sucking hard and blowing thick clouds of smoke in her direction. "I think this whole topic has been overblown by everyone concerned." He looked at her playing with the strap of her purse, wrapping it around her fingers as she moved to the edge of the chair, and noted the familiar signs of her nervousness.

Valerie recrossed her legs and considered her father. "Oh, really. Is that how you see it? Child molestation is all some big media invention? It never really happens?"

"I really don't think we need to get into this now," he stated forcefully. Dr. Kingsley had kept this topic at bay for years and wasn't about to let that change.

"Well, I disagree. I think it's time we deal with this. We should discuss it sometime before you die." Valerie's mouth went dry. "And, there's no time like the present."

Dr. Kingsley revealed nothing, his face impassive. "Just what are you talking about?" he asked evenly.

Valerie stared into his eyes and steeled herself to go on. "I'm talking about you. And about all the other men like you. I may only be an intern, but I think I've come up with a terrific approach to deal with people like you. I'd like to show it to you. I think you'll be impressed." She cast a look down at her purse and tingled in anticipation, barely aware of her father's reaction.

He sat back, adopting his aloof posture. "I really don't have time for this. If you have something to say, then say it. Otherwise, please go. This is starting to get boring." Dr. Kingsley had no intention of dealing with her accusations, veiled or otherwise. He kept his eyes fixed on her, watching the anxious mannerisms—tapping her fingers on her purse, her leg bouncing in the air—and enjoyed the signs of her discomfort. Then the movements stopped and she leaned forward.

"How do you do that? Pretend you don't know what I'm talking about?" She considered him with genuine mystification, almost in awe of his brazen defiance. "But I guess that's all part of it. Being able to act as if you know nothing about it. As if you couldn't write the book about incest."

Dr. Kingsley dodged her words once again. "Don't embarrass yourself like this, dear. You are speaking to the leading expert in this area." His eyes narrowed disapprovingly. "Tell me, how many awards have you won? How many books have you published? How often are you sought after as an expert in this field? Isn't your only claim to fame—besides being my daughter, of course—is that you have spent more time on an incomplete dissertation than anyone else at your school?"

"I am well aware that you're the expert, Dad. But perhaps I just have trouble accepting that anyone listens to you."

"You had no trouble accepting my name and all that it can do for you. You had no difficulty accepting the money I've sent you. You had no problem accepting my letter of recommendation to get you into that graduate school you didn't even finish. And now you want to question me and my opinions? It may be understandable that your jealousy issues would manifest in this way, but it's not at all pleasant to listen to."

Valerie lowered her eyes. "I can't help it. I have trouble accepting your opinions when I know about all your extracurricular activities. You're a dangerous man and I let you get away with this far too long. I was afraid of you. I was embarrassed." Valerie's voice quavered in defiance of her words, but she forced herself to look back up at her father. "But not anymore."

Dr. Kingsley leaned back and crossed his arms on his chest, somewhat amused that she was making the game a little harder to win this time. "So what's your point, exactly? I have patients to see."

"That's not going to work. Don't pretend you don't know what I'm talking about. You know what you are and what you did." His eyes remained blank. "You had a little girl and you destroyed her. You took away the Valerie who ever trusted, who ever felt safe, who ever felt happy. You killed her. You betrayed an innocent little girl who looked up to you, who loved you, who believed in you. You stole her childhood. Can you understand that?" Valerie stopped, seeking the strength to speak in her own voice and not behind distant pronouns. She looked him dead in the eyes. "I was humiliated by what you did to me. I felt guilty because I thought for the longest time it was my fault. I wanted you to stop, I wanted you to go away. I begged you, but you wouldn't." Valerie fought back tears. "Now you're going to beg me and we'll see if I stop."

Dr. Kingsley huffed deeply with every breath, but he had to maintain his composure, not knowing when his next appointment might show up. "I'm not going to listen to this. You've created some fantasy in your mind about what I supposedly did to you, but that's all it is. Your fantasy. You come in here and want to talk about you, how you feel, what happened to you. But it's all filtered through your distorted little mind. You try to blame me, but I didn't do anything wrong." He read her face and saw the same old weaknesses. He took the opening. "But you did. Telling your mother about us. You didn't care about hurting her, when she was suffering so. That's what ultimately killed her, not the cancer—your telling her about us. She wasn't equipped to handle it. Tell me, Valerie, you want to start pointing fingers? Well, how does it feel to know you killed your own mother?"

Tears rolled off Valerie's cheeks and she quickly reached into her purse and pulled the gun out, shaking as she pointed it at her father. "How dare you say that!"

Her father's eyes moved to the gun. "What are you doing with that?" he demanded. His eyes went wide, and Valerie thought she saw a flicker of fear. That small crack in the facade of his superiority filled Valerie with an uncommon feeling of power. "Put that thing down before you hurt somebody."

"I'm your daughter and you taught me well. If you want to get someone's attention, subtlety doesn't work. But people do respond to fear." Valerie waved the gun at his face. He recoiled and tried to move away from its direction. "See? Isn't it amazing how well it works?"

Her father's nose was flaring and he was breathing so heavily he seemed like a bull restrained in a stall, waiting for someone to open the door so he could bolt. But she hoped that while she held the gun he would stay seated and listen to her. She took a deep breath.

"You know what I learned at the Oakwood about child molesters? I learned that they were all like you. They were a bunch of manipulating, self-serving scum who cared about nothing but their own pleasure. And those were their good qualities. They didn't care that they had ruined their child's life." Valerie's voice broke and she clutched the gun for strength. She swallowed hard and went on. "No. They were only sorry about getting caught, not about what they had done."

She looked at her father and flashed on Hillerman's face. It was there, that same disdainful look, that same obvious indifference. The hint of fear she had seen in him was gone, and he was once again poised to dismiss what she had to say as the rantings of a hysterical girl. She had to find that fear again, to convince him she was deadly serious.

"What they needed was a taste of what they had done." She moved the gun slowly, aiming it up and down his body. "Tell me. How many of your so-called patients have you molested?" She glanced around the office, holding the gun level. "Where do you do it, on the couch? On your chair? What do you tell them to keep the secret—that they're your best patient? Do you tell them how special having a secret is? What a big girl they are?"

Her father's face showed no sign of the rage building within. He knew better. So he forced a placid expression and an overly relaxed, patronizing tone. "Valerie, why don't you take a deep breath and let it out. You've been under a lot of strain lately. . . ." He smiled, the phony, toothy smile that offered such sincerity. "I understand how people can sometimes fall apart under stress. Maybe testifying was too much for you. Why don't you go upstairs, get some sleep. When you are feeling better we can sort out all these confused feelings you're having." He didn't add the pat on the head, but Valerie still felt it pushing her into the ground.

Valerie could barely catch her breath, his dismissive tone more than she could take. Her eyes filled with tears and when she could speak her voice came out desperate and plaintive. "Why? Why do you do it? How can you live with yourself?" The unanswerable questions hung in the air. Her father looked away, as if exasperated by the emotional display. Valerie pulled the hammer back and her father's head snapped back toward her. "Now," she said, seething. "Let me hear you beg me for forgiveness. Me and every other child you ever took advantage of." She leveled the gun at his head. "Beg."

Her father's jaw set firm, but his voice remained calm, even indifferent. "No, Valerie. I will not beg for forgiveness because I did nothing wrong. Don't you see how you're projecting your own guilt feelings onto me?" He crossed his arms and shook his head disapprovingly. "I'm very disappointed that after all this time, you continue to refuse to accept that. I understand the need to blame me, so that you don't have to reconcile your own feelings of responsibility over what happened, but you should be beyond that by now." He tilted his head up, nose in the air as if offended by the fetid smell of false accusation. Only he knew it wasn't false.

Valerie moved the gun closer, aiming in between her father's eyes. "Say it. Say 'I'm sorry. I did a terrible thing. I don't deserve to live. I should get a bullet in the head.'" He stayed still, saying nothing. "Say it!" she yelled.

Her father pushed himself forward, leaning on his desk and looking up at his daughter with an eerie calmness. "You want me to say 'I'm sorry.' Well, I won't!" Dr. Kingsley could see the hurt flash in her eyes and knew she could not pull the trigger. "Valerie, this isn't about me, it's about us. It's about a relationship that's apparently too complex for you to understand. I loved you, just like you loved me. It's a natural thing for a little girl to want to please her daddy."

Valerie's eyes went wide and felt his words like a slap in the face. "I was eight years old! I was just a terrified little girl who didn't want to make you mad. I just wanted you to love me." The words caught Valerie by surprise, yet they seemed to hold the secret to her pain. She felt her heart grow heavy as a sick feeling came over her. Then the tears came and she could barely speak. "How can you sit there and say what you're saying?" Valerie stood there trembling, sobbing, her whole body aching from the hurt in her heart.

He watched the tears stream down her face as the clock chimed for the top of the hour. "You have it all wrong. Don't you see how you've distorted the memory in your own mind? It wasn't like that at all. I never threatened you. I never hurt you in the least! You want to make me out to be some terrible monster, but it's just not true."

Valerie stood quaking, her finger frozen around the trigger, her body aching. He rose slowly from behind his desk, his arm stretched forward, his voice syrupy. "Valerie, neither of us did anything wrong. You couldn't help yourself. I don't blame you. It was natural and beautiful. It's nothing for you to be ashamed of. It's okay. I know you wanted me as much as I wanted you."

"No!" Valerie screamed as she emptied the gun into him, squeezing the trigger again and again until she heard the impotent clicks of the trigger. She slowly lowered the gun, looked down, and watched the blood pour out of her father's chest. Feeling nothing, she was aware only of the man she had feared and loved and hated, dying on the floor. She watched as he took his last breaths.

Valerie did not know how long she had been standing there when she heard the buzzer ring. But she wasn't frightened by what was on the other side of the door. Her fear was gone.

The police photographer moved around Dr. Kingsley's office quietly, efficiently, snapping pictures from every angle. He stepped carefully over the pool of blood surrounding the body as he moved in for closeups of the fatal wounds then moved back for overall shots to give perspective to the murder scene. Larson stood off to the side and watched the photographer's work with respect yet certain it was a colossal waste of time. There would be no trial. Something told him that Valerie would never be found. She could blend in almost anywhere and start a new life. Who would ever suspect her? And even if someone suspected her, who would ever turn her in?

Larson walked over to the outer office, where Randazzo stood taking notes as she talked to the mother of Dr. Kingsley's next patient. "So you only saw a dark-colored car parked in the driveway? Not a white Civic?" Randazzo asked the shaken woman as Larson joined them.

The woman twisted a tissue between her hands.

"No. I mean, yes. I wasn't paying a lot of attention. I didn't know it would be important." She looked over at her daughter, who was being entertained outside by one of the female officers.

"That's okay. Did you see the woman drive off? Do you know which way she went?" Jack stood listening as Randazzo rattled off a dozen more questions that all went unanswered. What he was able to gather was that the woman had knocked on the door of the waiting room and had been escorted in by an attractive young lady who told her to wait on the couch and that Dr. Kingsley would be with her in a minute. She had no reason to suspect the woman of anything and hadn't taken particular notice of her. Now she was being told that the woman was the notorious child molester killer who had just killed again. It was far too much for her to take in, especially the nagging question of why Dr. Kingsley would be one of the killer's targets.

Randazzo handed the woman her card and thanked her for her help, then watched as the woman and her daughter left hurriedly. When they were out of sight, she turned back to Larson. "Damn. I can't believe we were so close." Her hand went instinctively to her silent radio to make sure it was on the right channel. "Why haven't they found her yet? She can't be very far."

"They're not going to find her." Larson said it matter-of-factly. "Some young, nice-looking white girl is just not gonna attract that much attention." He shook his head. "Nope. There are too many ways out of this town for anyone who wants out. I'll bet we've seen the last of Valerie Kingsley."

Randazzo took it all in without reaction, taking a few laconic steps out the door and squinting up at the afternoon sun.

Larson was surprised by her lack of emotion. "You

don't look all that torn up about it. I thought Randazzos always catch their man."

"Well, there's a first time for everything, I guess." Randazzo ran her hands through her hair. "This isn't exactly the typical homicide, anyway. Maybe it's better if there isn't a second trial. The first one was confusing enough. We should just let it rest."

Larson walked up behind her, looking out the door. He shoved his hands into his jacket pockets and took in a deep breath of Valley smog, wrinkling his nose at the lingering acrid smell. "I thought you liked being a witness for the prosecution."

"Yeah, right. I almost lost my partner, I almost helped convict an innocent woman, and I had to defend the honor of child molesters in the process." Randazzo sighed deeply, her shoulders rising and falling with the release of the memory. "No, I'm not gonna do that again. From now on I stick to nice, simple homicides where I can tell the good guys from the bad."

Larson nodded slowly. "I tried to tell you this wasn't an easy case."

Randazzo looked down at her shoes. "That you did." She shielded her eyes as she looked back up at Larson. "So what do you think Valerie will do now?"

Larson thought for a moment. "Well, she's killed her father, so the source of all that pain is gone. Maybe that'll be enough—maybe she'll be free now to go on with her life. What do you think?"

Randazzo shrugged. "I think this case is too complicated for simple answers."

Jack smiled. "You've made quite some progress, Detective. I think our training is over." He extended his hand. "Congratulations, partner."

EPILOGUE

When she had allowed herself to dream about freedom, which wasn't often, Rebecca had imagined walking along a sandy beach, warmed by the sun, her hair blowing in a gentle breeze. But then the blare of the morning siren would startle her awake, hurtling her back toward the grim reality of her imprisonment. This morning, when Rebecca awoke, there was no siren, only the comforting realization that this was the day she and Jack would be boarding a plane heading for Kauai, making her most impossible dream a reality.

Rebecca had walked out of court a free woman, the D.A.'s office quickly dismissing all charges. Covington was selected as the one to be taken out and publicly shot, the whole of the blame for the wrongful prosecution rested squarely on her sagging shoulders. She was not at all surprised by her demotion to hard-core gang. Baldwin was a surprise beneficiary of the win—knowing how little he actually had to do with it—and got enough calls to his new office from potential clients to hire both a secretary and his own receptionist. When his new receptionist informed him that a representative from the Council on Judicial Appointments was calling about his request for a seat on the bench, Tom took the call and respectfully withdrew his request. He was far too busy with his new practice to even think about leaving.

Randazzo was credited with cracking the case, homing in on the misspoken words of the killer. Her moment in the sun was dimmed only slightly by the fact that Valerie had eluded capture and was still out there, somewhere. But in a matter of weeks, Valerie's escape was no longer of concern, and there was no public clamor to find her. For many, she was a hero whose legacy would forever be embedded in the continued debate over the problem of how to adequately punish child molesters.

Much hand-wringing ensued from the apologists in the psychological community, following disclosure of Dr. Herman Kingsley's history of incest and his daughter's murderous revenge. It was agreed that no one was immune to human failings and that Dr. Kingsley was, sadly, no exception. As for the Oakwood Center, its patients spread out among a number of other therapy centers, with Elmhurst inheriting enough to hire three new therapists. None from the Oakwood.

The buzzer rang just as Rebecca placed her suitcase near the front door. Apparently Jack was as excited about the trip as she was, because he was uncustomarily punctual, she thought. She buzzed him in and left open the door while she dashed around the condo, checking to make sure she hadn't forgotten anything. When she returned, she was startled to find Randazzo standing in the doorway, with a bottle of Dom Perignon. "I wanted to send you guys off in style. Where's Jack?" she asked, peeking her head in.

Rebecca looked confused. "I thought you were him. He was supposed to be here by now." Randazzo stood a little awkwardly in the doorway, waiting for an invitation from Rebecca, who seemed momentarily flustered by the unexpected visit. "C'mon in," she said, suddenly remembering the protocol. She took a step back and waved Randazzo in. "You know, knowing Jack, he probably turned off his alarm and went back to sleep. We'll end up needing a police escort to get to the airport on time."

"He'll be here, he'll be here." Randazzo walked in and handed the bottle to Rebecca. "I wanted to talk to you before you guys flew off." She paused in the entryway and looked down at her feet. "I just wanted you to know how sorry I am, you know, about everything."

Rebecca nodded. "I know, Jack's told me." She turned away and walked into the kitchen to put the bottle on the counter, then took a long moment before returning to the entryway. She appreciated how hard this was for Randazzo, and yet she wasn't ready to give her total absolution. She looked at Randazzo squarely. "Listen, what's done is done. We can't go back and change things. And I have no interest in dwelling on the past anymore. I just want to get on with the rest of my life." Rebecca thought how for the first time this statement resonated with truth. "We all make mistakes and the important thing is to learn from them. I've learned a lot myself. Although I'm not yet to the point where I can say any of this was for the best," she added with a smile, then turned solemn. "But I want you to know that I realize that I wouldn't be out now if it weren't for you."

Randazzo nodded slowly. "I just wish I had listened to Jack. And I should have looked more closely at the people at the Oakwood. I just couldn't believe that the killer came from inside."

"Why not? Who better to appreciate how messed up the system is?"

"Yeah, I guess you're right." Randazzo paused and looked back at the door. "The only thing that still bothers me is, sure we figured out who the real killer was, but the system's still screwed up. That hasn't changed. I'm afraid nothing's going to change that."

Rebecca was gratified to have Randazzo come over to her way of thinking. "Unfortunately, it's easy to point out what's wrong, but it's a lot harder to decide what to do about it. Well, not for me. I say, lock 'em up and throw away the key. First offense—we cancel your membership card to society. I've said that for a long time, but no one listened. Maybe now they will." Rebecca looked a little wistful, then sighed. She did not want all the unanswered questions to weigh on her today. "I hope so. I hope things will change now, because one thing I do know is that the answer is not to go back to the way it was. Kids deserve better."

The two women nodded in unison, finding agreement at last, yet still feeling a little uncomfortable together. Suddenly, the buzzer sounded again and Rebecca's heart skipped a beat. This time she was sure it had to be Jack, and she was happy to discover she was right. He strode into the condo eagerly, ready to start their new life together, the two tickets to Kauai sticking out of his shirt pocket, bearing today's date, but was caught by surprise seeing Randazzo there with her. He stopped suddenly and pretended to gasp, as if remembering what had happened the last time Rebecca and Randazzo were together. Randazzo picked up on Jack's attempt at humor and turned to Rebecca. With a straight face, she said, "So, Rebecca, you're sure you don't know anything about that judge who committed suicide last night?"

Jack looked at Rebecca. "Don't say anything without your lawyer present!" He grabbed Rebecca's suitcase and her hand and bolted out the door. Halfway down the corridor, they stopped and looked back to find Randazzo laughing hysterically.

For further information regarding the treatment and prevention of child sexual abuse, contact the following organizations:

Mothers Against Sexual Abuse (MASA)

A national nonprofit organization based in Monrovia, California, MASA provides psychological, emotional, and legal services to adult survivors of sexual abuse, and to nonoffending parents and families of children who have been sexually abused. MASA also provides educational programs about child sexual abuse to schools, colleges, social service agencies, and law enforcement agencies. For their network of resources across the United States as well as some Canadian provinces, call MASA at (818) 305-1986 or write to 503-1/2 S. Myrtle Avenue, #9, Monrovia, CA 91016.

Childhelp USA

Childhelp USA is the largest child abuse treatment and prevention organization in the U.S. It operates the Childhelp National Child Abuse Hotline and Child Advocacy Centers and assists victims with residential/outreach treatment facilities, foster and group homes, and parent education programs. Childhelp USA also contributes to child abuse and neglect research and actively supports legislation benefiting children. To reach the Childhelp National Child Abuse Hotline, call 1-800-4-A-CHILD or 1-800-2-A-CHILD (TDD).

The Rape, Abuse, & Incest National Network (RAINN)

RAINN operates America's only national toll-free hotline for survivors of sexual assault. The hotline (1-800-656-HOPE) provides callers free, confidential counseling and support 24 hours a day, from anywhere in the country.

RAVES FOR
FATAL CONVICTIONS

"Move over, John Grisham. Shari Geller's courtroom scenes crackle with tension as they careen toward a surprising revelation. Randazzo is the other surprise here—this female cop is sharp, witty, and practically screaming out for a sequel of her own."

—Tess Gerritsen
Author of *Harvest*

"Remarkable . . . an enthralling novel."

—*The Toronto Star*

"*Presumed Innocent* meets *Death Wish*."

—Andrew Vachss
Author of *False Allegations*

"Fast-paced and riveting, *Fatal Convictions* takes the thriller genre to new heights. Every now and then, you read a first-time novelist, and you just know in your soul that she's destined for great things. Add Shari P. Geller to your list!"

—John Gilstrap
Author of *Nathan's Run*

"A promising debut in the tradition of Nancy Taylor Rosenberg."

—*Library Journal*

"A brilliant, thought-provoking, and conscience-prodding indictment of the justice system. This novel is well executed and plotted, a thoroughly entertaining legal and police procedural."

—*Bookpage*

"Welcome to a fresh and exciting new talent. *Fatal Convictions* is a glittering, literate mystery and legal thriller, better than Grisham's first. Shari Geller tells a powerful story, the tension building toward the climax as if a hand were tightening around your throat."

—Jameson Cole
Author of *A Killing in Quail County*

"Shari Geller makes an auspicious debut in this nerve-jangling roller coaster ride of a thriller. *Fatal Convictions* is a compassionate and compelling page turner; it packs an emotional wallop and lingers long after you've put it down."

—Harlan Coben
Author of *Fade Away, Deal Breaker,* and *Dropshot*

"An engrossing thriller [that] plunges into the searing world of vengeance."

—*Greensboro News & Record* (NC)

"If you are tired of the traditional chiller thriller, in which psychopaths terrorize and brutalize female victims, you will find *Fatal Convictions* refreshing. This novel turns literary convention on its head; the suspects are primarily female, and their victims are dangerous men. Each character in this novel is distinct and unforgettable. . . . Shari P. Geller shows promise as a new writer of crime fiction."

—Paula Sharp
Author of *Crows Over a Wheatfield*

"*Fatal Convictions* is a suspense thriller with heart, and also with a brain. . . . The fact that this is Shari Geller's first novel is astounding. . . . My hat is off to her. . . . one last, tantalizing word: whodunnit? If you can figure this out before the last few pages, my hat will be off to you, too."

—Dianne Day
Author of *The Strange Files of Freemont Jones*

"An engrossing read . . . we can all look forward to the second [book.]"

—*The Mystery Review*

"Shari Geller is a terrific author. . . . She never falters in presenting this complex and engrossing story. . . . I felt I was in the hands of a master."

—*Deadly Pleasures*